T0205390

Biological Magnetic Resonance

Volume 31

More information about this series at http://www.springer.com/series/5693

Takeji Takui • Lawrence Berliner
Graeme Hanson
Editors

Electron Spin Resonance (ESR) Based Quantum Computing

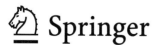 Springer

Editors
Takeji Takui
Department of Chemistry
Osaka City University Grad
  School Science
Osaka, Japan

Lawrence Berliner
Department of Chemistry and Biochemistry
University of Denver
Denver, CO, USA

Graeme Hanson (deceased)
Centre for Advanced Imaging
The University of Queensland
St. Lucia, QLD, Australia

ISSN 0192-6020
Biological Magnetic Resonance
ISBN 978-1-4939-8108-3   ISBN 978-1-4939-3658-8   (eBook)
DOI 10.1007/978-1-4939-3658-8

Printed on acid-free paper

This Springer imprint is published by Springer Nature
The registered company is Springer Science+Business Media LLC New York

Preface

The intimate connection between information and quantum physics has received considerable emphasis in the past two decades, in large part due to the successes of quantum information science (QIS). The field of quantum computing/quantum information processing is revolutionary in physical science for the future of information technology. There are a wide variety of platforms that may be adapted for useful information-processing protocols. This book specifically addresses the areas of electron spin-qubit-based quantum computing and quantum information processing with a strong focus on background and applications based on EPR/ESR technique/spectroscopy, and organization of the book places emphasis on relevant molecular qubit spectroscopy. The issues have never been included in a comprehensive volume that covers the theory, physical basis, technological basis, and a selection of various applications and new advances in this emerging field. QIS links the advanced electron magnetic resonance technology and sophisticated chemistry/materials science for preparing realistic molecular spin qubits and their physical models as matter qubits. An idea of quantum entanglement overlooked so far in applied and natural sciences has attracted much attention in many a branch, recently. The authors are well-known experts in the field who draw together aspects of pulse-based magnetic resonance and computational science in the world. The philosophy and approach to this volume stem from the fact that the field of quantum computing/quantum information processing is not only a revolutionary approach for the future of information technology but also underlies disruptive methodological advances in magnetic resonance and molecular spectroscopy. "Quantum control of spin qubits" is a current and important technological issue in manipulating many addressable qubits to realize quantum computing, providing feedback on the advanced spectroscopy. EPR/ESR spectroscopy can afford suitable platforms for this issue, in spite of the fact that electron spin qubits have been the latest arrival in the emerging field of quantum computing and quantum information processing.

The volume begins with a comprehensive introduction to quantum computing or quantum information processing from the viewpoint of electron magnetic resonance superbly done by Sushil Misra. The next chapter, one of two involving nuclear spins as well, relates to quantum effects in electron-nuclear-coupled molecular spin systems by an expert team spearheaded by Robabeh Rahimi Darabad and one of our coeditors, Takeji Takui. Next, Hideto Matsuoka and Olav Schiemann address molecular spins in biological systems. Biological spin systems relevant to the target issue have their own right. Then, emphasizing the electron spin-based computing aspect more heavily, Takui's group addresses adiabatic quantum computing, different from quantum circuit approaches, on molecular electron spin quantum computers, followed by a chapter on free-time and fixed end-point multi-target optimal control theory applied to quantum computing by Mishima and Yamashita, followed by a chapter by Koji Maruyama and Daniel Burgarth on gateway theoretical schemes of quantum control for spin networks. Both chapters above are important in terms of future development of control technology for matter spin qubits. Coming back to nuclear spins and related topics, the group of Raymond Laflamme from the Waterloo Institute for Quantum Computing provides two chapters, one covering NMR quantum information processing and the other on heat bath algorithmic cooling with spins. We note that NMR quantum computing and quantum information processing have their own disadvantages, but there have been many pioneering achievements in this particular field on the basis of the inherent advantages.

As the reader can garner, we have a world-class team of contributors addressing a relatively new, perhaps a paradigm shift in our use of this emerging technology. It is also important to avail the reader of our ongoing plans to compile a second comprehensive volume on this technology that addresses yet some of the topic areas that we were unable to include in this book.

Lastly, it is with deep regret that our coeditor Graeme Hanson left us early in 2015 as a result of a devastating cancer. Graeme worked at his endeavors up to the day he passed away and serves as an excellent role model for the rest of us. And, of course, Graeme remains as a coeditor of this book.

Osaka, Japan   Takeji Takui
Denver, CO   Lawrence Berliner
St. Lucia, QLD, Australia   Graeme Hanson (16th July 1955–25th February 2015)

Contents

Quantum Computing/Quantum Information Processing in View of Electron Magnetic/Electron Paramagnetic Resonance Technique/Spectroscopy

Sushil K. Misra

Abstract This chapter discusses spin-based quantum computation and information processing using Electron Magnetic Resonance (also known as Electron Paramagnetic Resonance—EPR, Electron Spin Resonance—ESR; the term EPR will be used hereafter). The technique of pulsed EPR can be exploited to design quantum computers. New quantum information applications can be established by the development of EPR-based spin manipulation methodology on self-assembling, interacting nanoscale structures, e.g. fullerenes. The details and implications of these in the context of quantum computing are covered. As well, the various relevant jargons used in quantum computing are briefly described.

Keywords Quantum computing (QC) • Quantum information processing • Electron paramagnetic/spin resonance (EPR/ESR) • Pulse EPR/ESR Fourier transform (FT) spectroscopy • Spin manipulation technology • Electron-nuclear spin qubit systems • Quantum entanglement • Pulsed electron-nuclear double resonance (ENDOR) • Time-proportional phase increment (TPPI) technique in pulsed ENDOR • Electron-nuclear hybrid spin qubits • Molecular magnets • Endothermal fullerenes • Quantum gates • Di Vincenzo's criteria • Bell states

1 Introduction

A quantum computer can outperform any classical computer in factoring numbers [1], and in searching a database [2] by exploiting the parallelism of quantum mechanics. Whereas, Shor's algorithm requires both superposition and entanglement of a many-particle system [3], the superposition of single-particle quantum states is sufficient for Grover's algorithm [4], and has been successfully implemented [5] using Rydberg atoms.

S.K. Misra (✉)
Department of Physics, Concordia University, 1455 de Maisonneuve Boulevard West, Montreal, QC, Canada H3G 1M8
e-mail: skmisra@alcor.concordia.ca

© Springer New York 2016
T. Takui et al. (eds.), *Electron Spin Resonance (ESR) Based Quantum Computing*, Biological Magnetic Resonance 31, DOI 10.1007/978-1-4939-3658-8_1

In quantum computing, one brings together ideas from classical information theory, computer science, and quantum physics. Information, propagating from a cause to an effect, plays a fundamental important role in it. The mathematical treatment of information, especially information processing, is quite new so that the full significance of information as a basic concept in physics is only being discovered in quantum mechanics recently. The theory of quantum information and computing leads to some profound and exciting new insights into the use of quantum states to permit (i) the secure transmission of classical information, known as *quantum cryptography*, (ii) the use of quantum entanglement for reliable transmission of quantum states, known as *teleportation*, (iii) the possibility of preserving quantum coherence in the presence of irreversible noise processes, referred to as *quantum error correction*, and (iv) the use of controlled quantum evolution for efficient computation, known as *quantum computation*. In all these, the use of *quantum entanglement* is the common theme as a computational resource.

A qubit (quantum bit) is a two-state system quantum mechanically; see Appendix 1 for more details. It is capable of providing an arbitrary superposition of quantum states, and it is much more complicated than a classical bit. An electron spin with spin-1/2 is an example of the qubit. Thus, electrons are natural candidates as physical qubits to be exploited for quantum computing and information processing (QC/QIP).

The computation system in a quantum computer makes direct use of quantum-mechanical phenomena, such as superposition and entanglement, to perform operations on data; see Appendices 4 and 5 for more details. In quantum computation, one uses qubits (quantum bits), which can be in a superposition of states, giving scalable predictable outcomes. In contrast, digital computers require data to be encoded into binary digits (bits), each of which is always in one of two definite states (0 or 1). Spins are natural qubits, and therefore magnetic resonance techniques, consisting of EPR and NMR (nuclear magnetic resonance) are among the most appropriate techniques to be exploited for quantum computing. NMR has already been exploited to some extent, but EPR is still in its infancy as a QC technique due to some inherent drawbacks as compared to NMR, especially in context with electron decoherence time, which is three orders of magnitude shorter than nuclear decoherence time. This caused a delay in exploiting EPR for quantum computing. It is similar to the late arrival of the development of the technique of pulsed EPR because of the intrinsic technical restrictions, as compared to that of pulsed NMR. (The same applies to EPR imaging as compared to NMR imaging, which was developed later.) Hopefully, these drawbacks will be overcome in the not-too-distant future with further efforts to exploit EPR as an efficient QC technique.

Theoretically, quantum information processing and quantum computation have been put on firm footing during the last decades [6]. One can solve problems with QC/QIP technology that are impossible on currently available digital classical computers. Quantum algorithms can reduce the CPU time for some important problems by many orders of magnitude. An important merit of QC is the rapid parallel execution of logic operations carried out by quantum entangled (superposition) states. For example, given the same input and output, the quantum processing of given information data represents an exponential speedup for factorization by the Shor algorithm [1] and quadratic speedup for search problems using Grover algorithm [2]. Also, by the implementation of the quantum information algorithms such as quantum teleportation [7] and quantum super-dense coding [8], some intrinsic advantages can be achieved over the classical information processing. A quest toward the goal of building practical quantum computers (QCs) encounters problems to be solved, such as (i) establishment and possible utilization of the entangled states, (ii) implementation of quantum simulators (digital or analog), (iii) preparation of scalable qubits, (iv) creation and storage of quantum-data bases, and (v) implementation of novel QC algorithms.

Among matter qubits, molecular electron spin qubits, fulfilling the requirements for present-stage QCs/QIPs in the context of EPR, are the latest to be exploited for the implementation of scalable QCs/QIPSs [9]. To this end, one needs to design and implement electron spin qubits and nuclear spin qubits. This is feasible in organic-based molecular frames, with extremely stable radicals. They are synthetic qubits, well defined in terms of matter spin qubits in ensemble, to which one can apply the established general guidelines for the molecular designs of synthetic spin qubits. The synthetic qubits enable generation of quantum entanglements between the electron spin and proton nuclear spins. Both pulsed Electron-Nuclear-DOuble Resonance (ENDOR) and Electron-Electron DOuble Resonance (ELDOR) techniques can be used as the most useful spin manipulation technology in implementing QCs/QIPSs. Organic molecular frames are hybrid spin qubit system along with a nuclear spin-1/2 qubit, termed molecular electron-bus qubits. Electron spin qubits such as synthetic electron spin systems, i.e., unpaired electron spins in molecular frames, are promising candidates for QC/QIP from the materials science, and have the potential to be exploited for QC/QIP. There is a linkage between QC/QIP and pulsed electron magnetic resonance as enabling ensemble-spin manipulation technology. The linkage between QC/QIP and chemistry, or materials science, provides insights into the quest for practically scalable spin qubits. Pulsed EPR enables manipulation of electron spin and nuclear spin qubits in an equivalent manner. Super-dense coding (SDC) experiments by the use of pulse ENDOR are helpful to understand QC-ENDOR and how it differs from QC-NMR, based on modern nuclear spin technology. Direct observation of the spinor inherent in an electron spin, detected for the first time, demonstrates the entanglement of an electron-nuclear hybrid system, which is the simplest electron-bus system.

This chapter will briefly outline the pulsed EPR and/or ENDOR techniques as applied to quantum computing and the EPR systems that are suitable for this purpose, along with a review of relevant jargons. Section 2, mainly based on the material described by Sato et al. [10], discusses the various enabling technologies for spin manipulation for QC/QIP. This will include (a) Pulse-Based Fourier-Transform (FT) EPR/ENDOR Spectroscopy as Enabling Spin Technology; (b) Spin manipulation by pulsed EPR; (c) Two Types of Pulse-Based ENDOR Electron-Spin-Echo Detected ENDOR Spectroscopy: (i) Generation of a Pseudo Pure State for Electron-Nuclear Spin Qubit Systems by pulsed ENDOR, (ii)Pulse-Based ENDOR Spin Technique Generation and Identification of Quantum

Entanglement between an Electron and One Nuclear Spin Qubit; (e) Time-Proportional-Phase-Increment (TPPI) technique in pulsed ENDOR; (f) Inter-Conversion of Entangled States by Pulsed ENDOR; and (g) TPPI Detection of the Entanglement between Electron-Nuclear Hybrid Spin Qubits by Pulsed ENDOR. In Sect. 3 are presented two ideas for constructing QCs. The appendices outline explanations of concepts/jargons relevant to QC/QIP: (i) qubits, (ii) quantum gates, (iii) DiVincenzo's five criteria, (iv) the Bell states, (v) quantum entanglement.

2   Spin Manipulation Technology for QC/QIP in EPR

2.1   Pulse-Based Fourier-Transform (FT) EPR/ENDOR Spectroscopy as Enabling Spin Technology

One needs to carry out spin manipulation in time domain, i.e. to manipulate both electron and nuclear spins in molecular frames in terms of their time evolution and phases. This enables one to discriminate between any quantum spin states against decoherence. To this end, one uses Fourier-transform techniques in pulsed EPR, utilizing intense pulses of MW (microwave) and RF (radiofrequency) radiations in order to generate a coherent superposition of the relevant spin states in the ensemble so that the pulses link EPR to matter spin qubit-based QC/QIP. Macroscopic magnetic moments precessing at frequencies ω_k, ($k = 1$ to K), with amplitudes A_k emit free induction decay (FID) signals. They are coherently detected and digitized for further processing by Fourier-transform (FT) analyses. Both MW and RF pulses are used in pulse-based ENDOR spectroscopy, in which MW radiation signals in FID or electron spin-echo (ESE) scheme after on-resonance MW excitations are monitored when pulse-based NMR events occur. Macroscopic moments of electron and nuclear spin qubits have to be manipulated in required orientations in the Bloch sphere, in any QC/QIP ENDOR experiments, as shown in Fig. 1.

Under the operation of the $\pi/2$ pulse about the x-axis on the $|0\rangle$ state, a superposition of the $|0\rangle$ and $|1\rangle$ states with equal weights is generated, as shown in Fig. 2(1), whereas the representation of the direct product composed of the two superpositions in the macroscopic magnetization qubit scheme is shown in Fig. 2(2). Thus, Fig. 2(1) illustrates why the phase manipulation between the qubits is essential for QC/QIP experiments. Transformation of the $|0\rangle$ to the $|1\rangle$ state by π pulse is the NOT gate (Appendix 2) operation. In terms of the pulse-based spin technology, NMR spin technology is much advanced and matured, but pulse-based FT EPR manipulation of electron spins has not yet been efficiently developed due to technical difficulties.

In order to illustrate the entanglement between an electron spin qubit and nuclear spin qubits, quantum phases belonging to the spin states are exploited. QC types of experiments, in which the quantum phases are controlled and manipulated, have never been carried out in the past, as they have neither been necessary nor useful for ordinary pulsed EPR spectroscopy. Further development of pulse ENDOR QC/QIP is required to provide new directions to EPR spectroscopy.

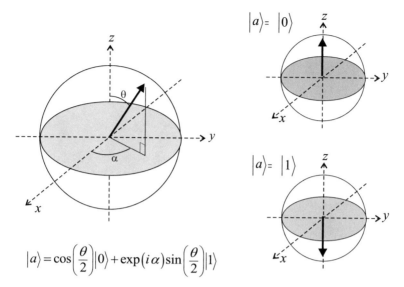

$$|a\rangle = \cos\left(\frac{\theta}{2}\right)|0\rangle + \exp(i\alpha)\sin\left(\frac{\theta}{2}\right)|1\rangle$$

Fig. 1 Representation of magnetic moments as qubits in the Bloch sphere, where the *thick arrow* denotes the moment. In the *xy* plane of the Bloch sphere, the moment is a superposition of the $|0\rangle$ and $|1\rangle$ states with equal weights (Adapted from [10])

2.2 *Spin Manipulation by Pulsed EPR*

For use in QC, the direction of a spin (magnetization) must be rotated. The direction of the magnetization, aligned originally along the *z*-axis, can be rotated by MW or RF pulses in resonance, as shown in Fig. 3. Such rotation produces superposition of spin states, known as "quantum gate". The pulse operations are applied in the rotating frame of the radiation field. In Fig. 3a, the state $|\psi\rangle$ is represented by two variables, θ and ϕ. For $\theta = \pi/2$, the choices of $\phi = 0$ and $\pi/2$ generate superpositions of the states, distinguishable in terms of the phase. These situations can be achieved by an on-resonance $\pi/2$ pulse radiation along the *y* or *x*-axis. It is noted that for a spin-1/2 qubit, the twofold rotation of the magnetization around the *x*-axis does not recover the original state, but rather changes the sign of its phase. The original state is achieved only by the fourfold rotation as shown in Fig. 3, demonstrating the spinor property of spin-1/2 qubit, manifesting the fact that the double-rotation group is not equivalent to the single-rotation group for a half-integral spin.

The bold arrow along a particular axis denotes the axis about which the radiation pulse is applied in Fig. 3b, and all the descriptions are exhibited in the rotating frame of the oscillating MW or RF radiation, with the static magnetic field orientation being along the *z*-axis. In practice, it is important, to use stable, narrow, and strong pulses of good shapes in spin manipulation by pulsed EPR. In EPR, unlike NMR, the MW high-frequency technology still suffers from technical difficulties in (i) power, (ii) multiple-frequency production, and (iii) relative-phase control between multiple frequencies.

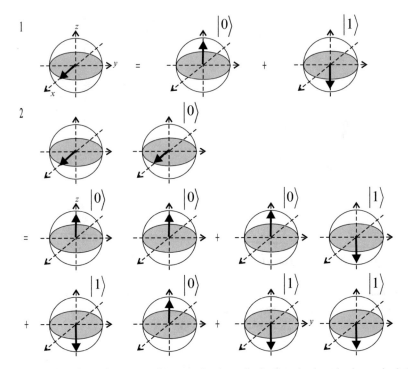

Fig. 2 The orientations of macroscopic magnetizations of spins in pulse-based spin manipulation technology. (*1*) A superposition of the $|0\rangle$ and $|1\rangle$ states as generated by the $\pi/2$ pulse applied along the *x*-axis in pulsed magnetic resonance. *Thick arrows* denote macroscopic magnetization of spins. (*2*) A schematic representation of the direct product of the two superpositions in terms of the macroscopic magnetizations. The coefficients associated to the states have been omitted for clarity in both (*1*) and (*2*) (Adapted from [10])

Quantum logic gates, transformation of the states after the operation, and the corresponding EPR pulses are exhibited in Fig. 4. The Hadamard gate in Fig. 4b is achieved by the use of the first $\pi/2$ pulse applied along the *y*-axis, followed by the second, π, pulse about the *x*-axis. The Hadamard transformation is effected by a π-rotation around the particular axis, rotated by $\pi/4$ from the *z*-axis in the *zx* plane. The operation around this particular rotation axis corresponds conventionally to the combination of the two above-mentioned pulses in pulsed EPR. In Fig. 4, the gate (c) is a controlled-not (CNOT) gate constituted by two qubits, consisting of an electron-nuclear hybrid system with one electron spin qubit and one nuclear spin-1/2 qubit. The corresponding CNOT gates in molecular frames composed of electron two qubits have not yet been accomplished. In (c) are shown the electron-nuclear spin energy level diagram and the labeling of the designation of states. The transition between levels 3 and 4 is an ENDOR transition, which converts the populations of the level 3 and 4 by a RF pulse applied about the *x*-axis. It is noted that all the quantum operations for EPR in Fig. 4 are achieved in the on-resonance rotating frame of the oscillating radiation field.

a

Bloch-sphere representation

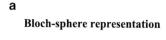

$$|\Psi\rangle = \cos\frac{\theta}{2}|\uparrow\rangle + e^{i\phi}\sin\frac{\theta}{2}|\uparrow\rangle$$

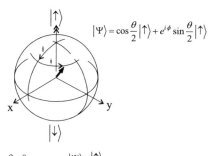

$\theta = 0 \qquad\qquad |\Psi\rangle = |\uparrow\rangle$

$\theta = \dfrac{\pi}{2}, \phi = 0 \qquad |\Psi\rangle = \dfrac{1}{\sqrt{2}}\left(|\uparrow\rangle + |\downarrow\rangle\right)$

$\theta = \dfrac{\pi}{2}, \phi = \dfrac{\pi}{2} \qquad |\Psi\rangle = \dfrac{1}{\sqrt{2}}\left(|\uparrow\rangle + i|\downarrow\rangle\right)$ $\Bigg\}$ superposition

$\theta = \pi, \phi = 0 \qquad |\Psi\rangle = |\downarrow\rangle$

$\theta = 2\pi \qquad\qquad |\Psi\rangle = -|\uparrow\rangle$

property of spinor

$\theta = 4\pi \qquad\qquad |\Psi\rangle = |\uparrow\rangle$

b

Manipulation of spin in the rotation frame by pulsed radiation field on resonance.

Generation of quantum gates by pulses

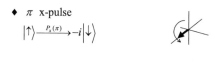

♦ $\pi/2$ x-pulse

$$|\uparrow\rangle \xrightarrow{P_x(\pi/2)} \frac{1}{\sqrt{2}}\left(|\uparrow\rangle + i|\downarrow\rangle\right)$$

♦ $\pi/2$ y-pulse

$$|\uparrow\rangle \xrightarrow{P_y(\pi/2)} \frac{1}{\sqrt{2}}\left(|\uparrow\rangle + |\downarrow\rangle\right)$$

♦ π x-pulse

$$|\uparrow\rangle \xrightarrow{P_x(\pi)} -i|\downarrow\rangle$$

Fig. 3 Figure showing the macroscopic magnetization on the Bloch sphere and the effect of on-resonance pulses generating various superpositions of the states $|\uparrow\rangle$ and $|\downarrow\rangle$ and generation of quantum gates. All the operations by the pulses are applied in the rotating frame of the oscillating radiation field. The magnetization is shown by the *thick arrow* in (**a**); this arrow was originally aligned along the *z*-axis in (**b**). It is noted that for a spin-1/2 qubit the twofold rotation of the magnetization around the *x*-axis does not recover the original state, but rather it is the fourfold rotation that does it, exhibiting the spinor property of spin-1/2 qubit (Adapted from [10])

2.3 Two Types of Pulse-Based ENDOR Electron-Spin-Echo Detected ENDOR Spectroscopy

Davies-type ENDOR and Mims-type ENDOR are typically two types of Electron-Spin-Echo (ESE) detected ENDOR techniques, exhibited in Fig. 5 with regard to their pulse sequences and timing. Here MW and RF pulse radiations induce EPR and NMR transitions, respectively. ENDOR signals are detected (D monitored) by an ESE technique. Figure 5a shows Davies-type ENDOR. Here P_{0S} and P_{2S} are MW π-pulses and P_{1S} is a MW $\pi/2$-pulse: P_{0S} possesses an irradiation strength $\omega_1 \ll A$ (converted to the corresponding frequency), where A is the hyperfine interaction (hf) constant, and P_I denotes the RF pulse applied during the waiting period T. P_{0S} pulse interchanges the populations of levels 1 and 3, as shown in Fig. 5c so that at 1–2 or 3–4 NMR resonance, the population change of level 1 with

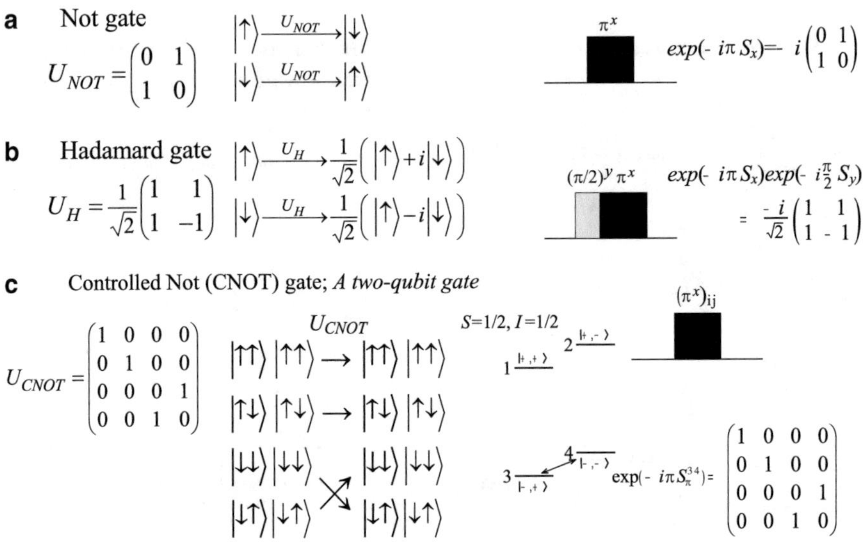

a   Not gate

$$U_{NOT} = \begin{pmatrix} 0 & 1 \\ 1 & 0 \end{pmatrix}$$

$|\uparrow\rangle \xrightarrow{U_{NOT}} |\downarrow\rangle$

$|\downarrow\rangle \xrightarrow{U_{NOT}} |\uparrow\rangle$

π^x

$exp(-i\pi S_x) = i\begin{pmatrix} 0 & 1 \\ 1 & 0 \end{pmatrix}$

b   Hadamard gate

$$U_H = \frac{1}{\sqrt{2}}\begin{pmatrix} 1 & 1 \\ 1 & -1 \end{pmatrix}$$

$|\uparrow\rangle \xrightarrow{U_H} \frac{1}{\sqrt{2}}\left(|\uparrow\rangle + i|\downarrow\rangle\right)$

$|\downarrow\rangle \xrightarrow{U_H} \frac{1}{\sqrt{2}}\left(|\uparrow\rangle - i|\downarrow\rangle\right)$

$(\pi/2)^y \pi^x$

$exp(-i\pi S_x)exp(-i\frac{\pi}{2} S_y)$
$= \frac{-i}{\sqrt{2}}\begin{pmatrix} 1 & 1 \\ 1 & -1 \end{pmatrix}$

c   Controlled Not (CNOT) gate; *A two-qubit gate*

$$U_{CNOT} = \begin{pmatrix} 1 & 0 & 0 & 0 \\ 0 & 1 & 0 & 0 \\ 0 & 0 & 0 & 1 \\ 0 & 0 & 1 & 0 \end{pmatrix}$$

U_{CNOT}

$|\uparrow\uparrow\rangle|\uparrow\uparrow\rangle \rightarrow |\uparrow\uparrow\rangle|\uparrow\uparrow\rangle$

$|\uparrow\downarrow\rangle|\uparrow\downarrow\rangle \rightarrow |\uparrow\downarrow\rangle|\uparrow\downarrow\rangle$

$|\downarrow\downarrow\rangle|\downarrow\downarrow\rangle \xrightarrow{\times} |\downarrow\downarrow\rangle|\downarrow\downarrow\rangle$

$|\downarrow\uparrow\rangle|\downarrow\uparrow\rangle \xrightarrow{\times} |\downarrow\uparrow\rangle|\downarrow\uparrow\rangle$

$S=1/2, I=1/2$

$(\pi^x)_{ij}$

$exp(-i\pi S_\pi^{34}) = \begin{pmatrix} 1 & 0 & 0 & 0 \\ 0 & 1 & 0 & 0 \\ 0 & 0 & 0 & 1 \\ 0 & 0 & 1 & 0 \end{pmatrix}$

Fig. 4 The various quantum logic gates, the transformation of the states after the operations of the gates, and the corresponding EPR pulses. The NOT (**a**) and CNOT (**c**) gates are constituted by the operations of the corresponding single pulses. The Hadamard gate is constructed by the first $\pi/2$ pulse applied about the *y*-axis, followed by the second, π pulse, about the *x*-axis. The CNOT (**c**) gate is a two-qubit one, for which the corresponding energy level diagrams with the state labeling is specified. In (**c**), an electron-nuclear hybrid system with one electron spin qubit and one nuclear spin-1/2 is exploited. The state $|+-\rangle$ designates $|M_s = -1/2, M_s = +1/2\rangle$, etc. (Adapted from [10])

respect to 3 is detected as an increase in the amplitude of the electron spin echo (ESE) signal. When the sublevel population of the NMR transition 1–2 or 3–4 are inverted, i.e., for the nuclear flip angle $\theta_1 = \omega_r t_p = \pi$, where ω_r is the effective nuclear Rabi-frequency (nutation frequency), and t_p is the RF pulse length, the effect is maximum. An EPR excitation has to be hyperfine nuclear-level selective, which is essential for generating entanglement composed of electron-nuclear spin qubits for QC/QIP ENDOR experiments. Mims-type ENDOR spectroscopy is shown in Fig. 5b with regard to the pulse and timing sequences. Here the MW three-pulse ESE scheme is utilized for the preparation and detection periods. Mims-type ENDOR spectroscopy is particularly useful to study molecular information on nuclei with small hyperfine interactions and small nuclear Zeeman splitting. The two pulses in the preparation period produce a periodic pattern $M_{zi} = M_0 \cos(\Delta\omega_i\tau)$ in the frequency domain. The M_z component of a spin packet "i" is determined by how its precession frequency in the rotating frame ($\Delta\omega_i$) "fits" in the waiting period τ. The whole pattern refocuses at the time t after the third pulse in the standard stimulated echo. The polarization transfer shifts the whole M_z pattern up and down in frequency by an amount of A, when the RF pulse is resonant with a transition matching a hyperfine interaction, A. As a consequence, the pattern of M_z-components becomes blurred, and thus the intensity of the echo is reduced. In that

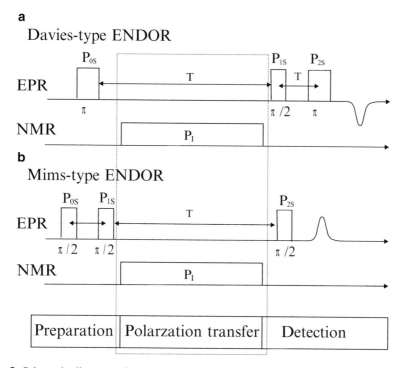

Fig. 5 Schematic diagrams of two typical Electron-Spin-Echo (ESE) detected ENDOR techniques: (**a**) Davies type ENDOR and (**b**) Mims-type ENDOR, showing their pulse sequences and timing charts. Here MW and RF pulse radiations induce EPR and NMR transitions, respectively. The transfer of polarization between particular electron-nuclear sublevels takes place during the period T. Any change of an ESE (Electron Spin Echo) signal during the NMR transition driven by the RF pulse is monitored in the detection period of the gate (Adapted from [10])

case, only the $A = n/\pi$ ($n = 0, 1, 2,...$) pattern is retained and the stimulated echo amplitude is unaffected. This implies that the echo amplitude is modulated by a factor $\cos(2\pi A\tau)$.

2.3.1 Generation of a Pseudo Pure State for Electron-Nuclear Spin Qubit Systems by Pulsed ENDOR

ENDOR spectroscopy using pulses, as described in the rotating frame of applied coherent radiation fields, consists of three main operation periods: preparation, polarization transfer, and detection, as shown in the last row of Fig. 5. They correspond to those in QC/QIP processes in time in pulse-based EPR. In pulse-EPR-based QC/QIP experiments the first, second, and third periods are initialization, manipulation/computing, and readout (D detection), respectively. The initialization operation prepares an either pure or a pseudo-pure spin state required for executing any quantum computation. The manipulation/computing is

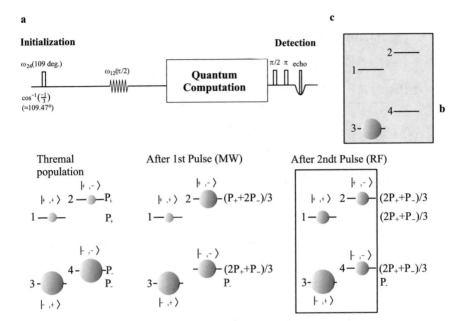

Fig. 6 Figure showing the initialization of an electron-nuclear spin qubit system by pulse ENDOR spin technique. (**a**) A pulse sequence based on ENDOR for preparing the initial state of an electron-nuclear system with one electron and one nuclear spin-1/2. (**b**) The change in the population among the state on each pulse operation of resonance. (**c**) Level 3 is shown here as a pseudo-pure state of the electron-nuclear hybrid system (Adapted from [10])

carried out for selective/nonselective excitation among the allowed or forbidden transitions between the spin states. For particular purposes, the time evolution of the states involved is carried out. Quantum phases are manipulated in phase-controlled experiments for QC/QIP in the second period. Electron-spin-based detection, e.g. Hahn ESE, three-pulse stimulated echo, refocused echo, and FID are parts of the readout.

An ENDOR-based pulse sequence for preparing the initialization of an electron-nuclear system with one electron and one nuclear spin-1/2 and the population change among the states involved on each pulse operation on resonance are shown in Fig. 6a, b, respectively. The first MW pulse effects population inversion between the levels 3 and 4 for selective excitation, assuming an equal Boltzmann distribution for the nuclear spin states belonging the same electron-spin sublevel M_S. The populations of the nuclear sublevels, 1 and 2 of the electron-spin $M_S = +1/2$ level are equalized by the second RF $\pi/2$-pulse. The populations $2P^+$ and P^- are redistributed equally among the levels, 1, 2, and 4, making only the level 3 more populated by $2(P^- - P^+)/3$ by the two pulses of the MW and RF radiations at resonance. After the action of the second RF $\pi/2$ pulse in Fig. 6b, a pseudo-pure state of the electron-nuclear hybrid system with the four spin states is generated as level 3, shown in Fig. 6c. Any quantum computing with operations is carried out during the second period as shown in Fig. 6a, and the readout is exhibited in a Hahn ESE scheme.

2.3.2 Pulse-Based ENDOR Spin Technique Generation and Identification of Quantum Entanglement Between an Electron and One Nuclear Spin Qubit

Quantum entanglement plays an important role in QC/QIP. The generation of quantum entanglement between an electron and one nuclear spin-1/2 qubit in a molecular entity was achieved by Mehring et al. [11] by pulse ENDOR technology for QC/QIP experiments. The establishment of entanglement was identified by invoking TPPI (Time-Proportional-Phase-Increment) technique, enabling detection of quantum phases belonging to particular spin states in the hybrid system. Generation of entangled state in an electron-nuclear spin qubit system by the use of the pulse ENDOR technique is illustrated in Fig. 7, according to which, after the initialization of an electron-nuclear spin qubit system, e.g., level 3 as an initialized state, called pseudo-pure state, a sequence of RF2 and MW pulses on-resonance are applied for generating entangled states. The resulting state-transformation by the pulses are schematically shown in Fig. 7a, where the role of each pulse is indicated. In order to entangle the electron-nuclear spin states, MW pulses are inevitably utilized, which force electron spin sublevels to become involved in the entanglement process. In the present pulse scheme, levels 2 and 3 are entangled. The four spin states involved and their population changes by the pulses are shown in Fig. 7b, level 1 being apparently not involved during the processes. Relaxations are not explicitly considered here. The pulse sequence in time for establishing the entanglement between an electron and one nuclear spin-1/2 is schematically shown in Fig. 7c, as discussed above, and the RF2 π/2-pulse and π-MW pulses generate a pair of the entangled states during the first period, which is used for the preparation of the pseudo-pure state. Manipulation of the spin qubits involved in any quantum operation is carried out during the second period. The readout of the manipulation shown as the light gray part in Fig. 7c is performed in the third period. Illustration of QC/QIP experiments in terms of quantum phase is the highlighted third part. Quantum logic gates for generating the entanglement between one spin qubit and another spin qubit are shown in Fig. 7d, with S and I being electron and nuclear spin qubits, respectively.

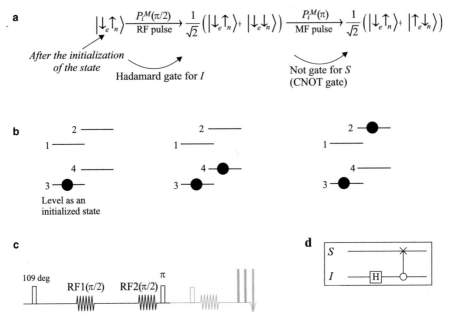

Fig. 7 Pulse ENDOR generation of entanglement between an electron and one nuclear spin-1/2 qubit by pulse technique. (**a**) Subsequent to the initialization of an electron-nuclear spin qubit system, e.g., level 3 as an initialized state (pseudo-pure state), a sequence of RF2 and MW on-resonance pulses is required for generating entangled states and the resulting state transformation by the pulses. The role of each pulse is indicated. Levels 2 and 3 are entangled in the present pulse scheme. (**b**) The four spin states involved and their population changes by the pulses. Level 1 is apparently not involved during the processes. Any relaxations are not explicitly considered. (**c**) The pulse sequence in time for establishing the entanglement between an electron and one nuclear spin-1/2. The first period is for the preparation of the pseudo-pure state and the RF2 $\pi/2$-pulse and π-MW pulse generate a pair of the entangled states. (**d**) Quantum logic gates for generating the entanglement between one spin qubit and another spin qubit. Here, S and I denote electron and nuclear spin qubits, respectively (Adapted from [10])

2.4   Time-Proportional-Phase-Increment (TPPI) Technique in Pulsed ENDOR

To enhance spectroscopic information by increasing the number of spectral dimensions, TPPI technique was introduced to pulse ENDOR technique for QC/QIP experiments by Mehring et al. [11] to identify the establishment of entanglement between an electron and one nuclear spin-1/2 qubit. This technique really convinces one of the occurrences of entanglement between the matter spin qubits, which can be achieved by introducing multiple phases for the pulses, i.e. the MW and/or RF radiations relevant to the magnetic transitions. The phase increment is described in terms of the angular frequency by time increment. This frequency is composed of the difference between two relevant frequencies introduced in an arbitrary manner. Using TPPI, one can make spectroscopic

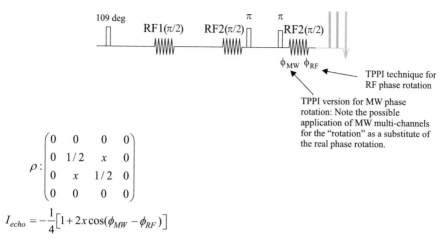

$$\rho : \begin{pmatrix} 0 & 0 & 0 & 0 \\ 0 & 1/2 & x & 0 \\ 0 & x & 1/2 & 0 \\ 0 & 0 & 0 & 0 \end{pmatrix}$$

$$I_{echo} = -\frac{1}{4}\left[1 + 2x\cos(\phi_{MW} - \phi_{RF})\right]$$

Fig. 8 Detection of establishment of entanglement between an electron and nuclear spin-1/2 qubit by Enabling pulse ENDOR spin technology. The schematics of the pulse sequence enabling manipulation of quantum phases of matter spin qubits is shown. There are two variants of the phase rotations of MW and/or RF pulses. One of these is a variant of the real MW phase rotation termed "MW-phase quasi-rotation," as a technique for substitute rotation when the real rotation of the MW pulse phase is technically difficult. In the quasi-rotation variant, different MW channels are utilized, to achieve quasi-rotation of the MW pulse (Adapted from [10])

information multidimensional, e.g. TPPI has been applied to allow on-resonance excitation with the spreading of n-quantum-transition spectra by $n\Delta\omega$. Each time the evolution time is incremented by δt_1, the phase of the pulse is shifted by $\Delta\phi = \delta\omega\Delta t_1$, i.e., $\delta\phi = 2\pi\Delta\nu\delta t_1$, thereby resolving multiple-quantum coherence in pulse-based ENDOR spectroscopy in solution [11].

Experimental approaches to the evolution of quantum entanglement between the electron-nuclear hybrid systems are shown in Fig. 8. This is based on the technique for rotating an MW phase when the real MW rotation is not applicable, wherein MW pulse channels can be utilized as a substitute "quasi-rotation" technology for the MW part. This variant has been used for identifying the occurrence of entanglement between an electron and one nuclear spin-1/2 qubit. For the entangled (Bell) states generated by an electron and one nuclear spin-1/2 qubit, each Bell state is characterized by its own quantum phase originally described by the two quantum numbers, M_S and M_I. Thus, the introduction of the corresponding two phases, ϕ_{MW} and ϕ_{RF} for the MW π-pulse and the RF $\pi/2$-pulse, respectively, enables discrimination between the Bell states. The required phase shift is controlled by the above-mentioned time increment. One can experimentally acquire any possible quantum phase-interference between an electron and nuclear spin qubit in time via interferograms transformed into the frequency domain. The ESE intensity is given by the equation inscribed in Fig. 8. It depends on the difference between the two phases when entanglement occurs. If not, the ESE signal remains constant during the time increment.

2.5   Inter-Conversion of Entangled States by Pulsed ENDOR

The pulse ENDOR technique enables one to interchange the entangled states
between an electron and one nuclear spin-1/2 qubit by manipulating the nuclear
spin sublevels by RF pulses once they are generated by a particular pulse protocol,
using the procedures schematically depicted in Fig. 9, where attention should be
paid to the difference in the phase belonging to each Bell state. Inter-conversion
between the entangled (Bell) states is achieved by one of the unitary transformations denoted by X, Y, and Z, each of which corresponds to the curved thick
arrows, shown in Fig. 9a. The 2π rotation for a half-integral spin qubit is
designated by Z operations. In this manner, the inter-conversion between the
electron-nuclear hybrid spin qubit systems is implemented by pulse ENDOR
spin technique. The procedures depicted in Fig. 9a are represented by a quantum
logic gate. In Fig. 9b, wherein a unitary operation U_i is applied after generating an
entangled state.

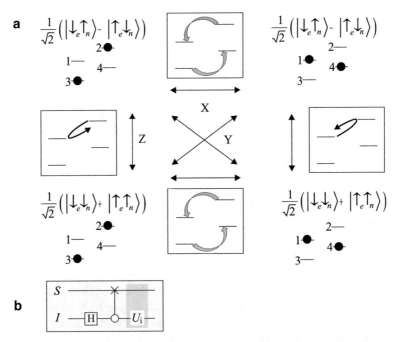

Fig. 9 Figure showing the inter-conversion between entangled (Bell) states by unitary transformations denoted by X, Y and Z, each of which is described by *curved arrows*. (**a**) The
Z operations describe 2π rotation for a half-integral spin qubit. The inter-conversion between the
Bell states is achieved by pulse ENDOR. (**b**) The procedures shown in (**a**) are equivalent to a
quantum logic gate, wherein a unitary operation U_i is applied after generating the entangled state
(Adapted from [10])

2.6 TPPI Detection of the Entanglement Between Electron-Nuclear Hybrid Spin Qubits by Pulsed ENDOR

TPPI detection of the entanglement between an electro and one nuclear spin-1/2 qubits by the pulse ENDOR technique is outlined in Fig. 10. The TPPI pulse sequence is shown at the top along with the role of the three periods. During the second period of quantum operation/manipulation of the qubits, the TPPI procedure is carried out, where the phases of the MW π-pulse and the RF2 $\pi/2$-pulse are controlled in time in pulse ENDOR. The corresponding phase-control technique for two electron qubits with non-equivalent g-factors in molecular frames had to be introduced in order to manipulate genuine electron spin qubits in contrast to the hybrid qubit system. Current MW spin technology for QC/QIP requires two MW sources with their relative phases locked electronically, unlike that for ordinary pulse-based EPR. The phase information on which an electron-nuclear sublevel is entangled with another sublevel corresponds to the TPPI frequency, ν_{TPPI}. This is outlined in the table in Fig. 10, where it is seen that the two pairs among the four Bell states give the same ν_{TPPI}. The ENDOR transition frequencies are ω_{12} and ω_{34}, between the levels 1 and 2 and the levels 3 and 4, respectively. The TPPI frequency is either the simplest combination of addition or the one of subtraction in the Bell states composed of an electron and one nuclear spin-1/2 qubit. The M_S manifolds involved in the MW transitions appear explicitly in the ν_{MW}, in case the sublevels of an electronic high-spin qubit are utilized with the spin quantum number S.

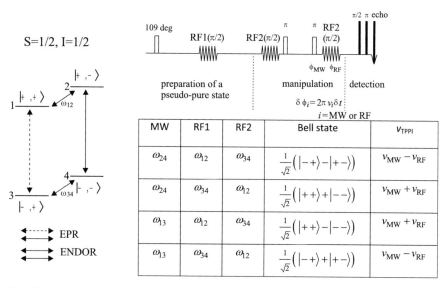

Fig. 10 Detection of the entanglement between an electron and one nuclear spin-1/2 qubit by the pulse ENDOR technique by TPPI. The TPPI pulse sequence is shown at the *top* along with the role of the three periods. ω_{ij} denote the transitions. The longer *solid* and *dotted arrows* show the EPR transitions. The two pairs among the four Bell states give the same ν_{TPPI} as seen in the table (Adapted from [10])

3 Designing QC: Two Proposals

3.1 Using Molecular Magnets

An implementation of Grover's algorithm that uses molecular magnets was proposed by Leuenberger and Loss [12]. Molecular magnets [13] are solid-state systems with a large spin. Their spin eigenstates make them natural candidates for single-particle systems. It has been shown theoretically that molecular magnets can be used to build dense and efficient memory devices based on the Grover algorithm. In fact, one single crystal can serve as a storage unit of a dynamic random access memory device. Fast EPR pulses are proposed to be used to decode and read out stored numbers of up to 105, with access times as short as 10^{-10} s. This proposal was shown to be feasible using the molecular magnets Fe_8 and Mn_{12}.

3.2 Using Endohedral Fullerenes

Pulsed EPR was used to assess the possibilities for processing quantum information in the electronic and nuclear spins of endohedral fullerenes [14]. It was shown that 15 N@C60 could be used for universal two-qubit quantum computing. First, the nuclear and electron spins were initialized by applying resonant RF and microwave radiation with a magnetic field of 8.6 T at 3 K so that each can store one qubit. This is a dynamic nuclear polarization technique, which made it possible to show that the nuclear T_1 time of 15 N@C60 is on the order of 12 h at 4.2 K. The electronic T_2 was, however, the limiting decoherence time for the system. By using amorphous sulfur as the solvent, this was extended to 215 μs at 3.7 K. Pulse sequences that could perform all single-qubit gates to the two qubits independently, as well as CNOT gates, were used. Two techniques were exploited to measure the value of the qubits after these manipulations. Another fullerene, Sc@C82, was also found useful for quantum computation. By comparing EPR measurements with density functional theory calculations, it was shown how the orientation of a Sc@C82 molecule affects the molecule's Zeeman and hyperfine coupling in an applied magnetic field. This is accomplished by expressing the g- and A-tensors in the coordinate frame of the molecule. The decoherence time was determined by pulsed EPR to be 13 μs at 20 K, which is 20 times longer than that previously reported. The arrangement of filling carbon nanotubes with endohedral fullerenes, forming 1D arrays, can lead to a scalable quantum computer. To this end, N@C60 and Sc@82 were used for filling in various concentrations. EPR measurements of these samples were found to be consistent with simulations based on the dipolar coupling.

4 Concluding Remarks

This chapter provides an outline of how pulsed EPR can be used for quantum computing, based on existing literature. To this end, some of the techniques for electron and nuclear spin manipulation using pulse EPR and ENDOR are briefly described. In addition, the various technical jargons that are relevant in QC are elaborated in the various appendices. This is not a thorough coverage, but rather as the title indicates, it is a brief review of quantum computing as accomplished by EPR. The various references included here should lead the reader to a more thorough knowledge of the subject.

Appendix 1: Qubits

This description is abstracted from Steane [15]. The elementary unit of quantum information is the *qubit* [16]. A single qubit can be envisaged as a simple two-state system, e.g. a spin-half or a two-level atom, but it should be mentioned that when measuring quantum information in qubits something more abstract is really being done. A quantum system possesses n qubits if it has a Hilbert space of $2n$ dimensions so that it has $2n$ mutually orthogonal quantum states available to it. (Note that n classical bits can represent only up to $2n$ different things).

The two orthogonal states of a single qubit can be written as $\{|0\rangle, |1\rangle\}$. More generally, $2n$ mutually orthogonal states of n qubits can be written as $\{|i\rangle\}$, where i is an n-bit binary number. For example, three qubits have eight: $\{|000\rangle, |001\rangle, |010\rangle, |011\rangle, |100\rangle, |101\rangle, |110\rangle, |111\rangle\}$ states available to it.

Appendix 2: Quantum Gates

This description is abstracted from Steane [15]. Simple unitary operations on qubits are called quantum "logic gates" [17, 18]. For example, if a qubit evolves as $|0\rangle \rightarrow |0\rangle$, $|1\rangle \rightarrow e^{i\omega t}|1\rangle$, then after time t, one would say that the operation, or "gate"

$$P(\theta) = \begin{pmatrix} 1 & 0 \\ 0 & e^{i\theta} \end{pmatrix}$$

Has been applied to the qubit, where $\theta = \omega t$. This can also be expressed as $P(\theta) = |0\rangle\langle 0| + e^{i\theta}|1\rangle\langle 1|$. Some other elementary quantum gates, with their notations, are:

$$I \equiv |0\rangle\langle 0| + |1\rangle\langle 1| = \text{identity}$$
$$X \equiv |0\rangle\langle 1| + |1\rangle\langle 0| = \text{NOT}$$

$$Z \equiv P(\pi)$$

$$Y \equiv XZ$$

$$H \equiv \frac{1}{\sqrt{2}}[(|0\rangle + |1\rangle\langle 0|) + (|0\rangle - |1\rangle\langle 1|)]$$

The last gate is denoted as H because its effect is a Hadamard transformation. All these gates act on a single qubit, and can be achieved by the action of some Hamiltonian operator in Schrodinger's equation, since they are all unitary operators. There are an infinite number of single-qubit quantum gates, in contrast to classical information theory, where only two logic gates are possible for a single bit, namely, the identity and the logical NOT operation. The quantum NOT gate carries $|0\rangle$ to $|1\rangle$ and vice versa, and so it is analogous to a classical NOT. This gate is also called X since it is effected by the Pauli spin σ_x operator. Note that the set $\{I, X, Y, Z\}$ is a group under multiplication. Of all the possible unitary operators acting on a pair of qubits, an interesting subset is $|0\rangle\langle 0| \otimes I + |1\rangle\langle 1| \otimes U$, where I is the single-qubit identity operation, and U is some other single-qubit gate. Such a two-qubit gate is called a "controlled U" gate, since the action of I or U on the second qubit is controlled by whether the first qubit is in the state $|0\rangle$ or $|1\rangle$. For example, the effect of controlled-not (CNOT) is

$$|00\rangle \rightarrow |00\rangle$$
$$|01\rangle \rightarrow |01\rangle$$
$$|10\rangle \rightarrow |11\rangle$$
$$|11\rangle \rightarrow |10\rangle$$

Here the second qubit undergoes a NOT if and only if the first qubit is in the state $|1\rangle$. This list of changes of states is the analogue of the truth table for a classical binary logic gate. The effect of controlled-NOT acting on a state $|a\rangle|b\rangle$ can be written as $a \rightarrow a$, $b \rightarrow a \oplus b$, where $\oplus$ denotes the exclusive or (XOR) operation. For this reason, this gate is also called the XOR gate. Other logical operations require more qubits. For example, the AND operation is achieved by use of the 3-qubit "controlled-controlled-not" gate, in which the third qubit experiences not if and only if both the others are in the state $|1\rangle$. This gate is named a Toffoli gate [19], which showed that the classical version is universal for classical reversible computation. The effect of Toffoli gate on a state $|a\rangle|b\rangle|0\rangle$ is $a \to a$, $b \to b$, $0 \to a \cdot b$. In other words, if the third qubit is prepared in $|0\rangle$, then this gate computes the AND of the first two qubits. The use of three qubits is necessary in order to permit the whole operation to be unitary, and is thus allowed in quantum-mechanical evolution.

Table 1 QC-ENDOR spin qubit systems fulfilling DiVincenzo's five criteria

	DiVincenzo's criteria	ENDOR spin qubit systems
Qubit	Identifiable; well characterised and scalable qubits are required	Molecule-based electrons and nuclear spins in molecular open-shell entities, in which hyperfine couplings play an essentially important role for selective excitations of both the electron spin- and nuclear spin qubits. Molecular designs, syntheses, and identifications of spin properties are required. The scalability of client nuclear spin qubits in electron spin bus quantum computers is limited from the synthetic view point. Proto-types of 1D periodic electron spin qubit system have been designed and synthesised
Initialisation	Any possibility for qubits to be initialised to simple and fiduciary states is necessary	Pseudo-pure states can be used in this context, whereas in order to avoid pseudo-pure states high polarisations of the electron spin can be coherently transferred to the nuclear spin by applying relevant pulse sequences followed by proper waiting time
Decoherence time	Long relevant decoherence times, much longer than the gate operation time are necessary	Long decoherence times of nuclear spins and an electron spin in organic radical qubits in solid state have been available for the demonstration of quantum operations between the bi- or tri-partite qubits. Proper molecular entities with long decoherence times for multi-qubit operations are not out of reach, for which stable isotope-labelled open-shell molecules have been designed and synthesised. QC-ENDOR experiments in solution also are not out of reach
Quantum operation	A universal set of quantum gates is required	Quantum gates between a single electron and a single nuclear spin have been demonstrated experimentally. Multi-qubits operation in terms of ENDOR spin Hamiltonians are underway. Particularly, a protocol for tripartite QC operations has been implemented
Measurement	The capability of measurements on quantum qubits to obtain the result of the computation is required	The current measurement scheme is ensemble-based, in which an individual client nuclear spin qubit is read out via the electron but spin qubit. A field gradient approach for the readout is proposed. On the other hand, single electron spin detections may be available in the future by the use of STM-base electron magnetic resonance detection

Appendix 3: DiVincenzo's Five Criteria

There are some fundamental criteria, namely, DiVincenzo's five criteria [20], listed below in Table 1 (reproduced from [10]), which should be satisfied by a physical system for its realization as a QC [9]. Molecular spin qubit QC-ENDOR is emerging as novel electron-spin manipulation technique. The high frequency versions are preferable for true QC/QIP, in particular, but need further technological developments for QC/QIP purposes. Molecule-based ENDOR system satisfies DiVincenzo's criteria, so that it is a realistic physical system for QC/QIP, as seen from Table 1 below, outlining DiVincenzo's five criteria and the corresponding properties of the ENDOR system. In the ENDOR-based QC/QIP, molecular electron spins are introduced as qubits in conjunction with nuclear spins. Electron qubits play the role of "bus" spins, while the nuclear spins act as "client" qubits. In thermal equilibrium, the ground states populations of the molecular electron spins are more than 103 times larger than those in the corresponding excited states with different M_s-manifolds in the presence of a static magnetic field or those with zero-field splittings, as compared with QC-NMR. Therefore, by using ground-state ENDOR systems, the required experimental conditions for preparing the initial state for QC/QIP becomes substantially easier to achieve with the help of the current EPR technology. On the other hand, for exact and complete preparation of pure initial states, possible manipulation of single-molecule-based systems, using EPR or Larmor precession detection, is rather difficult to achieve. It appears quite feasible in the near future to realize the experimental setup using electric detection schemes.

Appendix 4: The Bell States

The **Bell states** is a concept in quantum information science. (This discussion is extracted from Wikipedia, as found by a Google search. See also [6, 21, 22].) They represent the most simple examples of entanglement. Named after John S. Bell, being the subject of his famous Bell inequality, an **EPR pair** is a pair of qubits which are in a Bell state together. That means that they are entangled with each other. Unlike classical phenomena, entanglement is invariant under separation of distance, and is not subject to relativistic limitations. Bell states are maximally entangled *specific* quantum states of two qubits. Although usually spatially separated, they exhibit perfect correlation which can only be explained by quantum mechanics. In order to understand this, it is important to first examine the Bell state $|\Phi^+\rangle$:

$$|\Phi^+\rangle = \frac{1}{\sqrt{2}}\left(|0\rangle_A \otimes |0\rangle_B + |1\rangle_A \otimes |1\rangle_B\right)$$

This state implies that the qubit held by Alice (subscript "A") can be 0 as well as 1. If Alice measured her qubit in the standard basis the outcome would be perfectly random, either possibility having probability 1/2. But if Bob (subscript B) then measured his qubit, the outcome would be the same as that of Alice. So, if Bob measured, he would also get a random outcome on first sight, but if Alice and Bob communicated they would find out that, although the outcomes appear random to each one individually, they are correlated. One may say that maybe the two particles "agreed" in advance, when the pair was created (before the qubits were separated), which outcome they would show in case of a measurement. To address this, Einstein, Podolsky, and Rosen in their famous "EPR paper" in 1935, explained that there is something missing in the description of the qubit pair given above. Specifically, this "agreement" maybe called more formally a hidden variable.

On the other hand, quantum mechanically qubits can be in quantum superposition, implying that they can be in the states 0 and 1 simultaneously, or, a linear combination of the two classical states, e.g. the states $|+\rangle = \frac{1}{\sqrt{2}}(|0\rangle + |1\rangle)$, or $|-\rangle = \frac{1}{\sqrt{2}}(|0\rangle - |1\rangle)$.

If Alice and Bob chose to measure in this basis, that is, checking whether their qubits were $|+\rangle$ or $|-\rangle$, they would find the same correlation result as above. That is because the Bell state can be formally expressed as:

$$|\Phi^+\rangle = \frac{1}{\sqrt{2}}\left(|+\rangle_A \otimes |+\rangle_B + |-\rangle_A \otimes |-\rangle_B\right)$$

Note that this is still the *same* state, as described above for $|\Phi^+\rangle$.

Specifically, there are three other states of two qubits which are also regarded as Bell states. The four together are known as the four *maximally entangled two-qubit Bell states*:

$$|\Phi^+\rangle = \frac{1}{\sqrt{2}}(|0\rangle_A \otimes |0\rangle_B + |1\rangle_A \otimes |1\rangle_B)$$

$$|\Phi^-\rangle = \frac{1}{\sqrt{2}}(|0\rangle_A \otimes |0\rangle_B - |1\rangle_A \otimes |1\rangle_B)$$

$$|\Psi^+\rangle = \frac{1}{\sqrt{2}}(|0\rangle_A \otimes |1\rangle_B + |1\rangle_A \otimes |0\rangle_B)$$

$$|\Psi^-\rangle = \frac{1}{\sqrt{2}}(|0\rangle_A \otimes |1\rangle_B - |1\rangle_A \otimes |0\rangle_B)$$

Bell-State Measurement

The Bell measurement is an important concept in QIS. It is a joint quantum-mechanical measurement of two qubits that determines which of the four Bell states the two qubits are in. If the qubits were not in a Bell state before, they would get projected into a Bell state, due to the projection operation inherent in quantum measurements. Furthermore, as Bell states are entangled, a Bell measurement becomes an entangling operation.

Appendix 5: Quantum Entanglement

Quantum entanglement occurs when pairs or groups of particles are generated or interact in ways such that the quantum state of each particle cannot be described independently, rather, a quantum state may be given for the system as a whole. (This discussion is extracted from Wikipedia, as found by a Google search. See also, [23–25]). Measurements performed on entangled particles of physical properties such as position, momentum, spin, polarization, are found to be appropriately correlated, in the context of quantum measurement, giving rise to effects that can appear paradoxical. Apparently, one particle of an entangled pair "knows" what measurement has been performed on the other, and with what outcome. This happens even though there is no known means for such information to be communicated between the particles, which may be separated by arbitrarily large distances at the time of measurement. These phenomena, known as EPR paradox, were the subject of a paper by Einstein et al. [23], and two by Schrödinger and Born [24] and Schrödinger and Dirac [25].

Applications of Quantum Entanglement

In quantum information theory, entanglement has many applications, so that with the aid of entanglement, otherwise impossible tasks may be achieved. Super-dense coding and quantum teleportation are among the best-known applications of entanglement.

References

1. P. Shor, in *Proceedings of the 35th Annual Symposium on Foundations of Computer Science*, IEEE Computer Society Press, Los Alamitos, 1994, pp. 124–134, ed. by S. Goldwasser
2. L.K. Grover, Quantum computers can search arbitrarily large databases by a single query. Phys. Rev. Lett. **79**, 4709–4712 (1997)

3. S. Lloyd, Quantum search without entanglement. Phys. Rev. A **61**, R010301-1-010301-4 (1999)
4. A.K. Ekert, R. Jozsa, Quantum computation and Shor's factoring algorithm. Rev. Mod. Phys. **68**, 733–753 (1996)
5. J. Ahn, T.C. Weinacht, P.H. Bucksbaum, Information storage and retrieval through quantum phase. Science **287**, 463–465 (2000)
6. M.A. Nielsen, I.L. Chuang, *Quantum Computation and Quantum Information* (Cambridge University Press, Cambridge, 2000), p. 25. ISBN 978-0-521-63503-5
7. C.H. Bennett, G. Brassard, C. Crepeau, R. Jozsa, A. Peres, W. Wootters, Phys. Rev. Lett. **70**, 1895 (1993)
8. C.H. Bennett, S.J. Wiesner, Phys. Rev. Lett. **69**, 2881 (1992)
9. K. Sato, S. Nakazawa, R. Rahimi, T. Ise, S. Nishida, T. Yoshino, N. Mori, K. Toyota, D. Shiomi, Y. Yakiyama, Y. Morita, M. Kitagawa, K. Nakasuji, M. Nakahara, H. Hara, P. Carl, P. Hoefer, T. Takui, Molecular electron-spin quantum computers and quantum information processing: pulse-based EPR spin technology applied to matter spin-qubits. J. Mater. Chem. **19**, 3739–3754 (2009)
10. K. Sato, S. Nakazawa, S. Nishida, R.D. Rahimi, T. Yoshino, Y. Morita, K. Toyota, D. Shiomi, M. Kitagawa, T. Takui, Chapter 4: Novel applications of ESR/EPR: quantum computing/ quantum information processing, in *EPR of Free Radicals in Solids II, Progress in Theoretical Chemistry and Physics*, ed. by A. Lund, M. Shiotani, vol. 25 (Springer, Dordrecht, 2012). doi:10.1007/978-94-007-4887-34
11. M. Mehring, J. Mende, W. Scherer, Entanglement between an electron and a nuclear spin 1/2. Phys. Rev. Lett. **90**, 153001 (2003)
12. M.N. Leuenberger, D. Loss, Nature **410**, 789 (2001)
13. S.K. Misra, in *Multifrequency EPR: Theory and Applications*, ed. by S.K. Misra (Wiley-VCH, Weinheim, 2011)
14. G.W. Morley, Wolfson College, thesis submitted for the degree of Doctor of Philosophy at the University of Oxford, Hilary, 2005
15. A. Steane, Rep. Prog. Phys. **61**, 117 (1998). doi:10.1088/0034-4885/61/2/002. (Cond mat/9612126) 1/2. Phys. Rev. Lett. **90**, 153001
16. B. Schumacher, Quantum coding. Phys. Rev. A **51**, 2738–2747 (1995)
17. D. Deutsch, Quantum theory, the Church-Turing principle and the universal quantum computer. Proc. Roy. Soc. Lond. A **400**, 97–117 (1985)
18. D. Deutsch, Quantum computational networks. Proc. Roy. Soc. Lond. A **425**, 73–90 (1989)
19. T. Toffoli, Reversible computing, in *Automata, Languages and Programming*, ed. by J.W. de Bakker, J. van Leeuwen. Seventh Colloquium, Lecture Notes in Computer Science, vol. 84 (Springer, Berlin, 1980), pp. 632–644
20. D.P. Divincenzo, Topics in quantum computers, in *Mesoscopic Electron Transport*, ed. by L. Sohn, L. Kouwenhoven, G. Schon. NATO ASI Series E, vol. 345 (Kluwer, Dordrecht, 1997) (Cond mat/9612126)
21. Bell System Technical Journal, On the Einstein Podolsky and Rosen paradox, 1964
22. P. Kaye, R. Laflamme, M. Mosca, *An Introduction to Quantum Computing* (Oxford University Press, New York, 2007), p. 75. ISBN 978-0-19-857049-3
23. A. Einstein, B. Podolsky, N. Rosen, Can quantum-mechanical description of physical reality be considered complete? Phys. Rev. **47**(10), 777–780 (1935). doi:10.1103/PhysRev.47.777
24. E. Schrödinger, M. Born, Discussion of probability relations between separated systems. Math. Proc. Cambridge Philos. Soc. **31**(4), 555–563 (1935). doi:10.1017/S0305004100013554. Bibcode:1935PCPS...31..555S
25. E. Schrödinger, P.A.M. Dirac, Probability relations between separated systems. Math. Proc. Cambridge Philos. Soc. **32**(3), 446–452 (1936). doi:10.1017/S0305004100019137. Bibcode:1936PCPS...32..446S

Exploiting Quantum Effects in Electron-Nuclear Coupled Molecular Spin Systems

Robabeh Rahimi Darabad, Kazunobu Sato, Patrick Carl, Peter Höfer, Raymond Laflamme, and Takeji Takui

Abstract Molecular spin systems coupled with nuclear spins are introduced as promising matter spin qubits in quantum information processing and quantum computing (QC). Introductory remarks are given for nonspecialists. For this purpose, NMR-based QC is described and an approach to QC exploiting electron-nuclear coupled molecular systems is given. Requisites for qubits are described as DiVincenzo's criteria. Since Shor's quantum algorithm appeared, the first successful QC experiment was carried out by highly sophisticated pulsed NMR techniques, and this very attempt brought quantum computers down to earth. It has been claimed, nevertheless, that quantum entanglement as the heart of QC has not been established in any experiments in solution. Thus, advantages of QC experiments with molecular spins over the counterparts of NMR QC are described. Quantum computing (QC) experiments with molecular spins are exemplified for a few qubits.

R. Rahimi Darabad (✉)
Institute for Quantum Computing, University of Waterloo, 200 University Avenue West, Waterloo, ON, Canada, N2L 3G1

Department of Physics, Science and Research Branch of Azad University, University Sq., Tehran, Iran

Departments of Chemistry and Molecular Materials Science, Graduate School of Science, Osaka City University, Sumiyoshi-ku, Osaka 558-8585, Japan
e-mail: robabehrahimi@gmail.com

K. Sato • T. Takui
Departments of Chemistry and Molecular Materials Science, Graduate School of Science, Osaka City University, Sumiyoshi-ku, Osaka 558-8585, Japan

P. Carl • P. Höfer
Bruker BioSpin GmbH, Silberstreifen 4, Rheinstetten 76287, Germany

R. Laflamme
Institute for Quantum Computing, University of Waterloo, 200 University Avenue West, Waterloo, ON, Canada, N2L 3G1

Department of Physics, University of Waterloo, 200 University Avenue West, Waterloo, ON, Canada, N2L 3G1

Perimeter Institute, 31 Caroline Street North, Waterloo, ON, Canada, N2L 2Y5

© Springer New York 2016
T. Takui et al. (eds.), *Electron Spin Resonance (ESR) Based Quantum Computing*, Biological Magnetic Resonance 31, DOI 10.1007/978-1-4939-3658-8_2

1   Introduction

The enormous impact of computers on everyday life cannot be underestimated. The current technology of computers, classical computers, is based on the technology of transistors, which is an appreciated synergy between computer science and quantum physics. Smaller transistors work with less power; they are highly dense and can be switched on and off very fast. While miniaturization is necessary to increase the computation power, it provides us with an intuitive way of understanding why quantum laws are becoming important for computation and information processing.

Moore [1] in 1965 codified his law, known as Moore's law, on the growth of computers. It states that the power of computers will double for constant cost roughly once every two years. This statement amazingly has come to be true for decades, since the 1960s. The growth is achieved by shrinking the size of the processors, which is reaching a fundamental physical limit: the size of atoms where quantum effects will become important. In fact, we have already reached the limit in some devices [2] where quantum effects have become important. For classical computing, these effects are a hindrance but the goal of quantum information science is to take advantage of them.

Alan Turing drew the blue print of what we know today as the programmable computer [3]. Assessing the power of this model of computation has lead to the strong Church Turing thesis [4, 5].

> "Any model of computation can be simulated on a probabilistic Turing machine with at most a polynomial increase in the number of elementary operations required."

Although the polynomial difference in speed can be still significant, the above statement verifies the equivalency of all the computers, from the most pioneer ones to today's supercomputers. In practical settings, the thesis gives a robust definition of what types of problems that might or might not be solved by today's computers. These sets of problems define computational complexity classes which have been taken as assumptions of computer science. Transforming information using the laws of quantum mechanics suggests a new type of complexity classes which is different from the ones using the classical rules of physics.

An important milestone in quantum computing has been established by Feynman in 1980s [6]. He suggested that a quantum computer based on quantum logics would be ideal for simulating quantum-mechanical systems by making a hint on how to get involved to these problems. Feynman said that [6]:

> "So, as we go down and fiddle around with the atoms down there, we are working with different laws, and we can expect to do different things. We can manufacture in different ways. We can use, not just circuits, but some system involving quantized energy levels, or the interactions of quantized spins, etc."

A priori, using the quantum laws of nature could be an obstacle to information processing. After all, the uncertainty principle might suggest that we cannot compute as precisely as we desire. Surprisingly, what we have learned is the opposite: the quantum mechanics allows to solve algorithms for interesting problems efficiently where no efficient classical algorithms are known.

Physical realization of a quantum computer is a major goal for research activities in the field of quantum computing. An important guideline to assess the viability of proposed modalities for quantum computing devices is the so-called DiVincenzo criteria. These criteria are: (1) having access to well-defined qubits, (2) initialization of the qubits to a pure state, (3) availability of a universal set of quantum gates, (4) having qubit-specific measurements, and (5) long coherence times.

In this contribution, we study molecular electron and nuclear spins in spectroscopic systems, namely, electron paramagnetic resonance, EPR, and EPR-like systems for realizing quantum computing and quantum information processing. There are appreciated facts about EPR-like systems for quantum information processing and quantum computing. EPR-like systems are good since almost pure states could be generated with reasonable amount of efforts. Spin manipulations are faster due to fast microwaves in comparison to radio frequencies (in NMR). More importantly, quantum error correction (QEC) codes are implementable with an EPR-like system since the purity of the qubits that are needed for QEC codes can be, in principal, achieved in EPR-like systems, at least after performing some sort of spin polarization enhancement techniques.

In order to understand EPR and EPR-like systems for quantum information processing and quantum computing, we will give some examples that are better known from NMR. NMR system has been historically the first and foremost used physical system to implement quantum information processing. But, despite its successes in having exquisite control, NMR suffers from the difficulty of having relatively slow gates (compared to decoherence time) and to lack having a practical way to extract entropy during QEC.

Our goal is to explore EPR with the aim of keeping NMR's superb control with introducing the ability of purifying NMR quantum states for quantum computing and quantum information processing. Thus, we start with NMR and its characteristics for quantum computing and quantum information processing but will gradually switch from NMR to EPR-like systems. We will emphasize spin polarization enhancement of nuclear spins that are involved in quantum processing by getting contacted to an electron. We will show that the achievable spin polarization is indeed enough for a successful implementation of QEC. Finally, we will demonstrate the good control over the entire electron-nuclear coupled spins system by presenting experimental results on exploiting quantum effects such as superposition and nonclassical correlated states that have been generated with Electron Nuclear DOuble Resonance (ENDOR).

2 Experimental Requisites

Quantum computers have been defined through a set of criteria known as the DiVincenzo's five criteria. We will first describe them and comment on how NMR fulfills them. Here, we assume (if not otherwise mentioned) NMR system is in liquid state for implementing quantum information processing since solid-state

NMR has somewhat different properties. According to the presented discussion, we will admit advantages of including electron spins in the nuclear spin systems. Thus, we will approach systems of EPR and will evaluate their practicality, advantages, and difficulties, in terms of being used for realizing quantum computing and quantum information processing. EPR-like systems will give easier and more forgivable experimental difficulties for satisfying the criteria; however, still there are theoretical and experimental challenges remaining as to be solved so that making the EPR-like systems is the best fit for engineering a fully controllable quantum processor.

2.1   DiVincenzo's Criteria

The minimal requirements for a quantum computer have been originally introduced by DiVincenzo [7] (there are some additional criteria for communications but here we explain only the original list).

2.1.1   A Scalable Physical System with Well-Characterized Qubits

A set of physical system is required in order to give a representation of quantum bits (qubits). The physical system should have two distinct levels (e.g. energy levels) for being a good representation of a two-level quantum bit (qubit). The famous examples are spin-1/2 particles and polarized photons. It is also important to evaluate if the system of interest is practically scalable in the sense that the number of qubits can be increased freely and on-demand and with an error rate that is smaller than the relevant fault tolerant error threshold.

2.1.2   A Universal Set of Quantum Gates

Operations on qubits are defined in terms of quantum gates. Any realization of quantum computing must have access to a universal set of quantum gates so that even an elaborated and advanced operation can be realized with an affordable cost and reasonable effort. The time evolution of a quantum system is determined by its Hamiltonian. In order to realize quantum logic gates, it must be abilities to control the Hamiltonian over time. In other words, the resulting time evolutions of the total Hamiltonian (initial system Hamiltonian plus the control Hamiltonian) should be corresponding to the computational steps for an algorithm that is supposed to be realized in the physical system. Theoretically, this can be done by simplifying and rearranging the required steps and making them based on the existing terms or those available to be added through the control Hamiltonian in the total Hamiltonian of the system. Experimentally, engineering the Hamiltonian meaning that refinement of the control Hamiltonian is of practical importance.

2.1.3   Ability to Initialize the State of Qubits to a Simple Fiducially State

In fact, if the starting initial state for any computation or information processing is not well defined and known, the output will be useless. Thus, for any credited implementation of quantum computing and quantum information processing, it is an inevitable task to find access to well-defined well-known input states. For a classical computer, it is generally an easy task to initialize all the bits; however, for a quantum computer somewhat this task can be very challenging such that for some particular physical systems, the initialization criterion can be one of the most challenging criteria. Indeed, it is generally the one serious obstacle for ensemble systems such as NMR.

2.1.4   A Qubit-Specific Measurement Capability

Computation is useful only if we can read out the results. Because of the postulates of quantum physics, it is impossible to get all the information about the state of a qubit by measurement. However, quantum algorithms make it possible to extract the required information through the projective measurements. For ensemble systems, such as NMR and EPR-like systems, this criterion sometimes seems to be challenging because that all the measurements give averages on the states. Therefore, quantum algorithms need to be, and in fact have been, adapted to be implementable on ensemble systems.

2.1.5   Long Relevant Coherence Times

Coherence time of a physical system should be much longer than the gate operation time in order to have possibility to perform several operations in a computational process before the quantum state disappears. For matter spin qubits, coherence time is relevant to spin relaxation times. This criterion is not a trivial one to be satisfied by majority of the physical systems since a quantum system is typically very fragile against environmental noise.

3   NMR Quantum Information Processing and Quantum Computation

Nuclear Magnetic Resonance, NMR, is a well-established field in physics, originally, and in chemistry, widely. NMR technology goes back to 1940s and constantly has been used largely for varieties of purposes. In chemistry, NMR is a major tool to study the structures and properties of solids, liquids, and gases [8–11].

NMR has been used extensively for implementing even relatively complicated quantum algorithms [12–17]. There are several good reasons why NMR has been one of the foremost physical systems used for realizing quantum computing and quantum information processing [18–21]. NMR naturally satisfies part of the criteria mentioned, as explained in the followings. However, some of the important factors are still missing with NMR. Despite those still remaining challenges, NMR has been determined to be yet useful since it employs available special techniques and knowledge that overall make NMR an excellent system for being controllable (see the chapter in this book on "NMR Quantum Information Processing"). Therefore, it is worth trying to solve the important issues with NMR, e.g. by adding an electron spin to the system of nuclear spins and improving the polarization of the whole system.

3.1 Scalable and Well-Characterized Physical System of Qubits

The qubit system used in NMR quantum computing and quantum information processing is an n-spin molecular system. The molecule involves n magnetically distinct nuclear spins. Usually, the spins are spin-½ particles, though the higher spins are also workable. Characterizations of spins are possible by considering the resonance frequencies for each different spins.

The challenges for NMR, in this regard, are its scalability, large decoherence, and hard control over the currently available twelve qubits. The number of nuclei in each molecule is restricted and cannot be increased freely. The idea of cellular automata has been proposed by Lloyd [22], which might be useful in this context. However, the scalability problem, in its real meaning, as it should be possible to extendedly increase the number of qubits while the computation is yet fault tolerant, for liquid state NMR still is an open problem.

3.2 Universal Set of Quantum Gates

From a theoretical point of view, gates or operations are fixed and qubits are introduced to the gates. However, in NMR quantum computing, qubits are being represented by spins that are fixed in molecular structures and gates are introduced by pulses that are selectively applied on each spins. Generally speaking, spins are manipulated by applying radio-frequency pulses in the $x - y$ plane to excite the spins on their resonance frequencies. Other techniques such as pulse shaping or GRAPE pulses are used for this purpose (see the "NMR Quantum Information Processing" chapter in this book). Two-qubit gates are implemented by using the pairwise interactions between spins in the same molecule.

Arbitrary single qubit operations in addition to a CNOT gate make a universal set of gates. NMR has the ability to construct any arbitrary single qubit operation (radio-frequency pulses on resonance with each spins) and the CNOT gate (by using the couplings in between the spins). Therefore, any arbitrary operation (single- or multi-qubit operations) can be performed on the selected spins as far as we have known how to make a universal set of gates. "Identity" operation is a rather challenging operation in NMR since evolutions of spins are naturally never turned off. Identity operation is performed by using a common NMR technique known as refocusing.

The good point is that NMR is an already rich field of research going back to about 70 years ago. Then, occasionally, the advanced techniques discovered by the NMR community are proved to be useful for quantum computing and quantum information processing purposes specially for designing quantum operations and control operators.

3.3 Initialization of the State

Quantum computing and quantum information processing with liquid-state NMR have been done conventionally and mostly at thermal equilibrium condition. The thermal equilibrium state of NMR is described by a density matrix as follows

$$\rho = \frac{e^{-\frac{H}{k_B T}}}{\mathrm{Tr}\left(e^{-\frac{H}{k_B T}}\right)}.$$

At room temperature, $k_B T$ is much larger than the differences between the energy levels, typically 10^5 times larger. Then, the state is approximated, with a very good accuracy, as follows

$$\rho \sim 1 - \frac{H}{K_B 2^n},$$

where n is the number of spins. For example, $n = 2$ and suppose that $\omega_A \sim 4\omega_B$ then

$$\rho \sim 1 - \frac{\hbar \omega_B}{4 k_B T} \begin{pmatrix} 5 & 0 & 0 & 0 \\ 0 & 3 & 0 & 0 \\ 0 & 0 & -3 & 0 \\ 0 & 0 & 0 & -5 \end{pmatrix}.$$

This is a mixture of all possible pure states in the computational basis.

Recall the fact that NMR observables are traceless. Then, the identity term in the above equation is not detectable. What remains detectable is the difference in the populations of different states. Microscopic states for NMR might be in large varieties of states; however, as far as only the ensemble averages are measured, there is no way to distinguish them.

Pseudo-pure state has been a useful concept defined for NMR and other ensemble physical systems for quantum computing and quantum information processing. A pseudo-pure state is a state which practically resembles a pure state, particularly because of the NMR specifications. Pseudo-pure state generally has been introduced in different ways. Preparation of pseudo-pure state inherently requires some non-unitary operations, such as summation of different experiments.

Under the executed experimental conditions, the states are mixed rather than pure [23–26]. Even with a pseudo-pure state, an NMR state with an initial low spin polarization will not be useful because that for controlling and correcting the error effects on the NMR system (using QEC) generally initial pure states or very close to pure states are required.

3.3.1 QEC and NMR

Even in a classical scheme, states are supposed to be robust against the environmental, systematic, and any sort of imposed errors since otherwise the final outcome from the computation or the whole processing will not be reliable. For a quantum system this requirement is even more critical since a quantum system will easily leave its quantum state by any minor error effects; therefore, it is of priority in any practices to be able to detect and refine the quantum states affected by errors. QEC is one of the approaches taking care of such important job. There are other approaches for controlling errors or making a quantum system robust against noise but we are not aiming in reviewing this topic here.

QEC is for controlling and correcting the noises and errors that are occurring on the physical system. A properly designed QEC code should be in operation, in multiple rounds, all during that a computation or quantum processing is in progress. Therefore, as first and the most important experimental testing, it is inevitable to check the successful implementation of multiple rounds of QEC with the corresponding physical system. If it turns out to be a successful implementation, then the system will get enough credibility for being assigned for quantum implementation purposes.

In this context, NMR has a serious challenging situation. NMR initial states are largely mixed and for QEC we need to have access to fresh ancillary qubits. Criger et al. [27] showed that the required purity for ancilla qubits for QEC can be somewhat less than an absolute purity but still a specific QEC might be successful as far as the purity of the ancillary qubits are larger than a threshold value. Therefore, if the purity of qubits bypasses the given threshold value, in principle the noise effects on the system can be controlled and corrected.

As an example, for a conventional 3-qubit phase-flip error, the minimum polarization of the ancilla qubits has to be larger than 0.41. This polarization is clearly far beyond an achievable value for NMR. Direct purification of NMR mixed states requires very strict experimental conditions of the temperature down to milli-Kelvin and a very high magnetic field. Therefore, instead of getting involved in preparation of the experimental conditions for making a pure state, it has been considered to follow indirect approaches. Dynamic nuclear polarization (DNP) and heat-bath algorithmic cooling (HBAC, see the chapter Heat Bath Algorithmic Cooling with Spins: Review and Prospects in this book) are some of the techniques that have been used for improving the polarization of the NMR states [28–30]. These techniques may not give a perfect pure initial state but at least the enhanced purity of the final state would be high enough so that a QEC code may be executed. Therefore, one may still need to run some form of pseudo-pure state for having a clear and distinct starting initial state for the processing and/or computation after having access to a reasonably high spin polarization, as much as needed for implementing a genuine quantum processing.

By considering what we have just mentioned in the above sections, with an electron involved molecule in an EPR-like system, e.g. ENDOR/ELDOR, 0.41 is indeed an accessible polarization even with a commercially available spectrometer without very much modifying the default settings. Suppose we work with a fully labeled malonic acid [31]. In a W-band system (95 GHz) at 4 K, the electron spin polarization is about 0.60. This polarization can be exchanged with nuclear spins such that finally all the involved nuclear and electron coupled spins end up with the electron initial polarization. Note that this can be done, basically with swap gates without applications of any further advanced methods. In the end, QEC with polarized ancillary qubits can be implemented and repeated in multiple rounds assuming that the electron is on duty for refreshing the nuclear spins on-demand, in between the rounds.

This is actually a very powerful side of using high field ENDOR/ELDOR for quantum computing and quantum information processing purposes. Eventually, shaped pulses, GRAPE, can be used for optimizing the whole process but what has been explained in the above section is based on generally available square and Gaussian pulses, hence it has its credibility of being feasible with less interrupting the initial set up of the spectrometers. By upgrading and customizing an available commercial spectrometer and equipping it with Arbitrary Waveform Generator (AWG), even further advanced and interesting applications will be possible. A large number of microwave frequencies with their amplitude and relative phase controlled at a desired manner have been prepared at X-band or higher bands for QC experiments on molecular spins.

3.3.2 Exchange Polarization in Between an Electron and a Nuclear Spins

It is indeed an advantage of electron involved systems that a higher polarized nuclear spin can be achieved with reasonable efforts since a highly polarized electron spin is readily available in the system therefore by applying appropriate radio-frequency and microwave pulses the nuclear spin polarization can be enhanced to an electron initial polarization. One possible approach to achieve

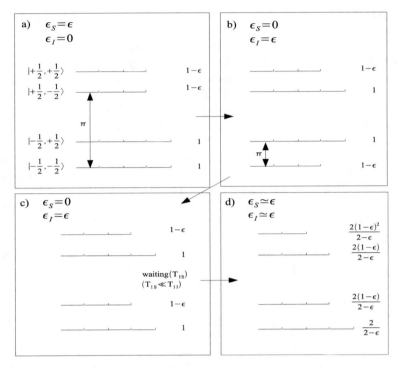

Fig. 1 A scheme on how to make nearly equal spin polarizations on nuclear spin and electron spin, equal to the initial electron spin polarization. The horizontal length of each energy level refers to the corresponding population of that level (the differences are exaggerated). The spin polarizations are shown as ϵ_S for the electron and ϵ_I for the nuclear spin. The initial spin polarization (thermal equilibrium) for the electron is equal to ϵ. Nuclear spin polarization is neglected in comparison with the electron spin polarization

nuclear spin polarization as almost equal to an electron spin polarization is shown in Fig. 1.

The spin polarizations are shown as ϵ_S for the electron and ϵ_I for the nuclear spin. The initial spin polarization for the electron is equal to ϵ. In the end of the process, the two spins pertain spin polarizations as almost same as the initial one, ϵ. The initial nuclear spin polarization is neglected in comparison with the electron spin polarization.

$$\frac{N_4}{N_1} = \exp\left(\frac{-g\beta H}{k_B T}\right) \equiv 1 - \frac{g\beta H}{k_B T}$$
$$= 1 - \epsilon.$$

Firstly, an on-resonance microwave (ω_{13}) π pulse is applied. The state after the pulse would be as shown in Fig. 1b. The polarizations are interchanged to $\epsilon_S = 0$ and $\epsilon_I = \epsilon$. The radio-frequency π pulse (ω_{12}) is applied so that it interchanges the populations between two energy levels, 1 and 2. Now, we make an assumption that is usually satisfied by carefully choosing a proper molecular sample. Suppose that spin-lattice relaxation time for electron, T_{1e}, is less than the relaxation time for nuclear spin, T_{1n} (this is usually satisfied). Therefore, after a waiting time of T_{1e} the system goes back to equilibrium on electron spin level and may yield the energy levels as shown in Fig. 1d. Finally, we will have electron and nuclear spin polarizations equal to $\frac{2\epsilon}{2-\epsilon}$ and $\frac{2}{2-\epsilon}(1-\epsilon)$. Hence, we have

$$\epsilon_S \cong \epsilon,$$
$$\epsilon_I \cong \epsilon.$$

The above simplified approximation for calculating the population is based on a rate-equation method.

Although the explained approach is an experimentally easy and accessible approach, it has some drawbacks. It can only enhance the nuclear spin polarization up to the electron spin polarization. If we work with a high field spectrometer and at low temperature, the achievable polarization might be good enough, but in a generally available X-band (9.5 GHz) and at higher temperatures, we may not be satisfied by the final polarization since the electron initial polarization is low. Also, a careful sample preparation is necessary. Other approaches might be used for a better enhancement of spin polarization, such as HBAC which is good because it can bypass the polarization of the bath (electron in our examples). We should however admit that HBAC also has its own challenges and issues. In this contribution, we keep doing experiments and increasing the nuclear spin polarization with techniques close to what is just explained here. We will prove our good control on the nuclear and electron coupled molecular systems in EPR-ENDOR machines of X-band and Q-band (35 GHz) by exploiting quantum properties such as superposition and nonclassical correlation.

3.4 Readout

Measurement in NMR is done with a radio-frequency coil placed close to the sample. Free induction decay, FID, from the sample is captured by the pickup coil. Then, FID is Fourier transformed to obtain the spectrum. In the obtained spectrum, different spins (qubits) in the molecule are spectrally distinguishable via their Larmor frequencies. The amplitude and phase of different spectral lines give information about the corresponding spin states. The extracted information depends on the convention; typically, a positive absorptive line is due to a $|0\rangle$ state and negative absorptive line is due to the spin in the state $|1\rangle$.

The magnetic signal of a single nuclear spin is too weak to be directly detected. Therefore, NMR experiments should be running by using a large ensemble of identical molecules, typically on the order of 10^{18}, dissolved in a liquid solvent (in a case of liquid-state NMR, however, for solid state also we should have an ensemble system of molecular spins). In fact, the system is an ensemble system, rather than a single n-spin molecule.

Suppose an NMR implementation of a particular quantum algorithm. The final read out information should be given by the distribution of random numbers detected through the measurement. Signals coming from the NMR states are averaged over the ensemble state. Averages of random numbers clearly are useless. This looks like a problem but in fact it has been shown that it does have solutions that are by slightly modifying quantum algorithms in a way that the averaged result gives meaningful outcome.

The density matrix representing the state of an ensemble system is completely determined if all the elements are detected and known. NMR measurements only selectively address specific entries in the density matrix, called single quantum coherence elements. Single quantum coherence elements connect basis states, which differ by only one quantum of energy. Therefore, in order to get the total density matrix elements, several 90° pulses are systematically applied in order to rotate each spin around the x and y axes then to observe all the terms in the deviation of the density matrix from the identity. The process to get the total density matrix through the measurement is called "state tomography." In a general scheme, without any prior knowledge on the state, state tomography involves many experiments and then it is impractical for experiments involving a large number of qubits.

3.5 Decoherence

The decoherence process of spins is well described by a combination of two phenomena, longitudinal and transverse relaxations. These two processes are closely related to generalized amplitude damping and phase damping, respectively. In QEC, also there are different errors assumed to be imposed to a quantum system and among them are the two important ones, amplitude damping and phase damping. In other words, theory has already established a nice framework in learning the above-mentioned errors in NMR and more importantly has given some techniques to suppress the relevant errors effects.

Relaxations of nuclear spins can be caused by fluctuations in the magnetic field experienced by the spins. Whether the magnetic field fluctuations contribute to energy exchange with the bath or only undergo a phase randomization depends on the timescale of the fluctuations. Roughly speaking, two processes are happening. Fluctuations at resonance frequencies of the nuclear spins lead to efficient energy exchange with the spins and slow fluctuations or fluctuations at zero or very small frequencies give rise to phase randomization. The extended discussions on decoherence in NMR might be found in literature [9, 28, 29].

4 Electron-Nuclear Coupled Spin Molecular Systems for Implementing Quantum Information Processing; Practical Examples

For quantum computing and quantum information processing implementations, the electron involved molecular spin systems should be in the solid state. Liquid-state systems are not appropriate since by any techniques for polarization enhancement, the achievable polarization would not be as large as the critical value that is required for QEC.

In order to use any solid-state sample in EPR-like systems, for implementations of quantum information processing and quantum computing, the first step is characterizing the spin Hamiltonian because from this information the entire quantum control will be designed. For a particular molecular sample that is picked up for realizing an algorithm, it is typical to have different final fidelities if the Hamiltonian is somewhat different. In terms of experimental practices, this statement is translated to the specific orientation that the crystal sample is positioned with respect to the external magnetic field.

By measuring all continuous wave EPR and ENDOR/TRIPLE spectra, an accurate form of the Hamiltonian can be found. Then, an optimal orientation of the sample is detected. Next, T_1 and T_2 are measured. We assume that the terms of the Hamiltonian are well resolved and they are accessible in experiment with reasonable operational complexities. Also, T_1 and T_2 are assumed to be long enough for realizing particular quantum processing.

Special care should be on preparing high polarized states, at least as high polarized as needed for using QEC. The absolute forms of quantum operations for the particular quantum algorithm would be calculated based on the determined Hamiltonian. For these quantum operations, pulse sequences are designed with respect to available laboratory tools and machines. Finally, pulses (operations) are applied on the states and the resultant state is measured by the available techniques from EPR and EPR-like systems. In the following, these steps and techniques are reviewed by giving some experimental examples.

4.1 Sample Studies

Any sample that is determined for quantum practices should be chemically stable all during the processing. Malonic acid (X- or γ-irradiated single crystal) has been proved as a good candidate for the case of small numbers of qubits. Synthetic organic open-shell entities, which are robust against long and high-power irradiations of radio-frequency and microwave pulses even at ambient temperature, are also good candidates, for example Diphenyl Nitroxide (DPNO) embedded in a proper diamagnetic lattice. In this section, we give an overview on the profiles of the above-mentioned two samples, malonyl radical and DPNO.

4.1.1 Malonyl Radical

Malonyl radicals are incorporated in the single crystal of malonic acid (HOOC)CH (COOH), as depicted in Fig. 2. Spin Hamiltonian parameters of non-labeled malonyl radical have been reported [32, 33]. For a central carbon labeled malonyl radical, $(HOOC)^{13}CH(COOH)$, the spin Hamiltonian is known [34, 35]. We have recently studied this sample and found the spin Hamiltonian for a fully carbon labeled sample that is a better sample for quantum information processing practices because of the larger number of accessible spin qubits, compared to a non-labeled malonyl radical [31].

Figure 3 shows the energy levels of malonyl radical for X-band (9.5 GHz) and Q-band (35 GHz) experiments. In Fig. 3, ω_{13} and ω_{24} denote EPR transitions, and ω_{12} and ω_{34} denote ENDOR transitions. The magnetic field for Q-band is more than three times larger than X-band. The NMR frequency becomes three times lager in Q-band thus its corresponding relation with the hyperfine coupling yields different patterns for ENDOR spectra. Figures 4 and 5 show the experimental results of malonyl radical at X-band and Q-band. Since, the corresponding energy levels are different, in case of pulsed ENDOR for X-band and Q-band the experimental results are different. Relaxation times are measured for malonyl radical. T_1 was 91.5 ms at 10 K, and T_2 about 5.200 µs [36].

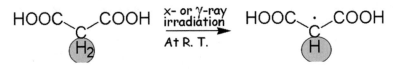

Fig. 2 Stable malonyl radicals are produced by X- or γ-irradiating malonic acid

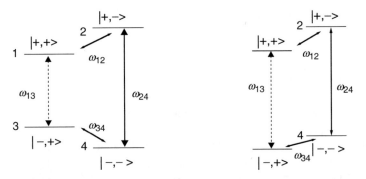

Fig. 3 $S = 1/2$ and $I = 1/2$. Energy levels and corresponding EPR/ENDOR resonance transitions in the presence of a static magnetic field. The levels of energy are $|++\rangle$: $|M_S = +1/2, M_I = +1/2)$, $|-+\rangle$: $|M_S = -1/2, M_I = +1/2)$, $|+-\rangle$: $|M_S = +1/2, M_I = -1/2)$ and $|--\rangle$:$|M_S = -1/2, M_I = -1/2)$; *Left*: X-band. *Right*: Q-band

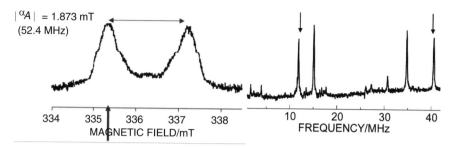

Fig. 4 *Left*: Pulsed EPR spectrum of malonyl radical in the single crystal, X-band. The *arrow* indicates the static magnetic field for the ENDOR measurements. *Right*: Pulsed ENDOR X-band spectrum from malonyl radical at 20 K. The *arrows* separate for $2\mathcal{V}_n$ (twice the proton Larmor frequency) and the central frequency is $\left|\frac{A}{2}\right| = 26.2\,\mathrm{MHz}$ to the first order, where A is the hyperfine coupling at the measured orientation of the sample with respect to the magnetic field

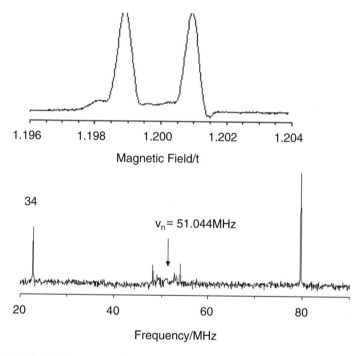

Fig. 5 *Up*: Pulsed EPR spectrum of malonyl radical in the single crystal, Q-band. *Bottom*: Pulsed ENDOR spectrum at Q-band from malonyl radical at 50 K. The central frequency is the nuclear Larmor frequency to the first order and the separation of the peaks corresponds to the hyperfine coupling

The available number of qubits: The unlabeled malonyl radical has one electron and one nuclear spin which is the α-proton. We usually do not count the γ protons, but one may work with them as extra qubits if an excellent control is achieved. By labeling carbons in malonic acid, the number of possibly available qubits can increase up to one electron and four nuclear spins, all spin $\frac{1}{2}$. Since the lateral carbons are very close, at least in some specific orientations, we may also use them as a single spin-1 nucleus. Therefore, the number of the available qubits will be one electron and two nuclear spins, $\frac{1}{2}$, and one nucleus with spin-1.

4.1.2 Diphenyl Nitroxide

DPNO is an open-shell molecular entity that we study as a molecular spin for exploiting quantum effects. Open-shell molecular systems have emerged in inter-disciplinary areas such as molecular spin science for giving us new aspects of quantum functionality [37]. DPNO is potentially a good candidate for applications relevant to molecular quantum technologies since its coherence time is typically very long. It is also possible to control the relaxation time of DPNO by controlling the concentration of DPNO in the diamagnetic lattice.

DPNO has been studied previously by several groups. To our knowledge, the first pioneering work has been done by Deguchi, 1961 [38]. This work is an EPR work both on pure DPNO single crystals and on DPNO diluted in benzophenone single crystals, even before the X-ray structural analysis of the host molecule appeared in 1968. The exchange line broadening was analyzed in this work. Then, later high-resolution hyperfine EPR spectra in solution were analyzed by Yamauchi et al., 1967 [39]. The **g** tensor for DPNO diluted in the benzophenone lattice and the hyperfine tensor of the nitrogen nucleus of the nitroxide site were determined by conventional EPR spectroscopy as early as 1970s by Lin [40]. The principle values for **g** tensor for DPNO and hyperfine tensor **A** for nitrogen have been reported to be, $g_{xx} = 2.0092$, $g_{yy} = 2.0056$, $g_{zz} = 2.0022$, $A_{xx} = 1.9$ G, $A_{yy} = 3.6$ G, $A_{zz} = 23.8$ G. Brustolon's group [41] revisited DPNO in the benzo-phenone lattice by cw ENDOR spectroscopy in 1988. According to their paper, the **g** tensor has the principle values of $g_{xx} = 2.0079$, $g_{yy} = 2.0040$, $g_{zz} = 2.0014$. Only preliminary results of the nitrogen hyperfine coupling and quadrupole tensors were given in [41] without giving the tensor analysis. Also, ^{1}H ENDOR/TRIPLE spec-troscopy was carried out in isopropanol at 210 K and radical pairs were detected from the concentrated mixed crystals. In between the two latter introduced works, Yamauchi et al. measured proton ENDOR in ethylbenzene at 203 K, 1987 [42]. The substituted ortho-methyl effect was influential. Nevertheless, complete analyses of the magnetic tensors of DPNO from the experimental side have never been documented yet because of inhomogeneously broadened EPR lines in the solid state due to the existence of protons.

There are several reasons on our interest in DPNO. The relaxation time of DPNO can be controlled by controlling the dilution (DPNO is a very easy-to-dilute molecular spin in the diamagnetic molecular lattices). DPNO is selected because it is a stable molecular-spin physical system allowing us to characterize the magnetic tensors under strong microwave and radio frequency irradiations. The irradiation in this regard is sometimes required for quantum information processing and quantum computing. DPNO is also selected because it is feasible to have measurements in a wide range of temperature from ambient to liquid helium temperature.

For sample preparation, DPNO has been magnetically diluted in benzophenone single crystals. Benzophenone molecule is isostructurally substituted by DPNO at a desired concentration, see Fig. 6.

The crystal symmetry of the benzophenone crystal is orthorhombic with $a = 1.030$ nm. $b = 1.215$ nm and $c = 0.800$ nm, see Fig. 7.

In each unit cell, benzophenone has four molecules. All the angular dependencies of EPR and ENDOR spectra were carried out in the crystallographic abc coordinate system at ambient temperature with a Bruker ESP300/350 spectrometer (a TM mode cavity and helical coil for RF irradiation) [36]. In each crystallographic plane, two of the molecules are equivalent. Therefore, two sets of molecules exist

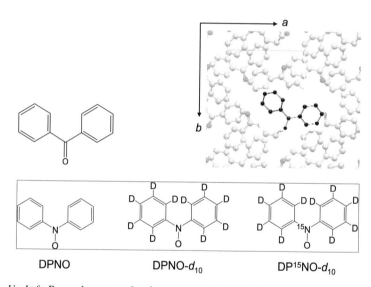

Fig. 6 *Up Left*: Benzophenone molecular structure. *Up Right*: Benzophenone is isostructurally substituted by DPNO. *Bottom left to right*: DPNO, deuterated DPNO and nitrogen labeled deuterated DPNO [36]

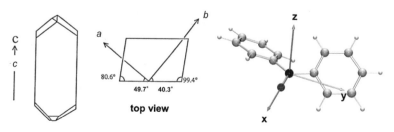

Fig. 7 *Left*: Benzophenone crystal. *Right*: DPNO in the principal *xyz*-axes system

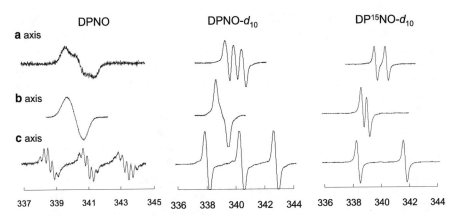

Fig. 8 Single crystal EPR spectral of DPNO, DPNO-d_{10}, and DP15NO-d_{10} in the benzophenone single crystal. The horizontal axes are magnetic field in units of mT

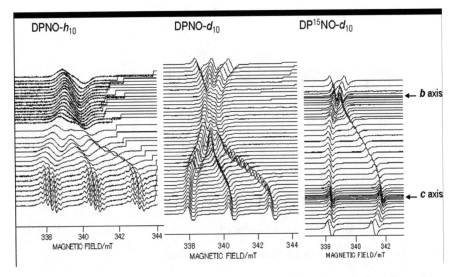

Fig. 9 Angular dependencies of single crystal EPR spectra of DPNO, DPNO-d_{10}, and DP15NO-d_{10} in the crystallographic bc plane

while for measurements along the axis, all the four molecules of a unit cell are equivalent. Therefore, there is not any site splitting due to the different sites. This property is used in order to define the axis, Fig. 8. For DPNO, we cannot detect the site splitting because of the proton broadening of the spectra, while this fact for each plane is clearer in case of the nitrogen labeled deuterated sample. ENDOR spectra can be observed in the temperature range of 350 K to liquid helium temperature.

In Fig. 9, angular dependencies of the three DPNO samples are shown in the crystallographic bc plane, as an example. Figure 10 shows ENDOR spectra of DPNO with the static magnetic field along the crystallographic a axes.

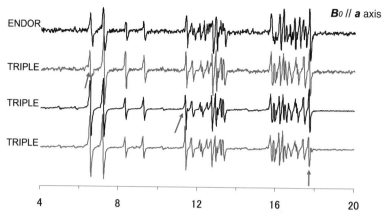

Fig. 10 Typical ENDOR and TRIPLE spectra of DPNO in the benzophenone single crystal. *Arrows* indicate the second frequencies for the TRIPLE experiments

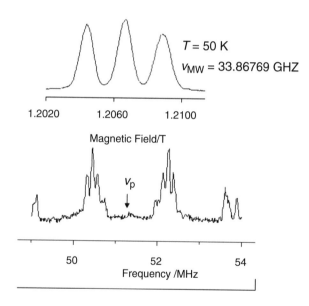

Fig. 11 DPNO pulsed *Up*: EPR, *Bottom*: ENDOR spectra

From this study, the **g** tensor is derived and the principal values are as follows: $g_{iso} = 2.0069$, $g_{xx} = 2.0110$, $g_{yy} = 2.0065$, and $g_{zz} = 2.0033$ [36].

Pulsed ENDOR measurements on DPNO have been done at X-band and Q-band, at different temperatures. At Q-band, pulsed EPR and pulsed ENDOR measurements were run at 50 K. Figure 11 shows the results for DPNO. Results for DP^{15}NO-d_{10} are shown in Fig. 12.

Spin-lattice relaxation time, T_1, for DPNO is measured to be 392 ms and for DP^{15}NO-d_{10} is 42.5 ms, at 10 K. Measurements on spin-spin relaxation time T_2 give 0.777 μs for DPNO, and 0.489 μs for DP^{15}NO-d_{10}.

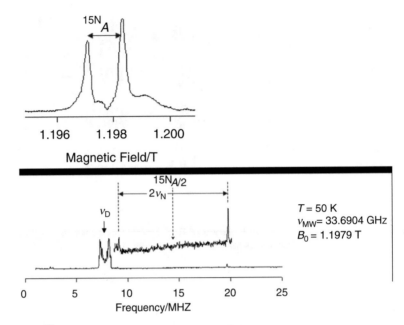

Fig. 12 DP^{15}NO-d_{10} pulsed *Up*: EPR, *Bottom*: ENDOR spectra

The available number of qubits: In the liquid state, DPNO and its derivatives provide up to six different qubits, each selectively controllable [43]. In the solid state, the number of qubits, in principle, can be up to the existing protons and nitrogen with the static magnetic field along arbitrary orientation, in addition to an electron. DPNO is specifically a strong candidate for realizing HBAC since its large number of involved qubits can make it hard for a general quantum processing scheme (at least for the near future), however for the algorithmic cooling, the ENDOR control on protons and nitrogen with an electron bath qubit should be enough.

4.2 Generating Pseudo-Pure State

Pseudo-pure states are acquired by applying particular pulse sequences and waiting time for equalizing different populations. Mehring et al. [44] gave one particular approach for producing pseudo-pure states for molecular systems such as malonyl radical.

In a rather similar approach, we implemented pseudo-pure states. Figure 13 gives the pseudo-pure state in comparison to the initial state after applying the pulse sequence, as shown in Fig. 14.

It is clear that the state corresponding to ω_{34} is suppressed demonstrating the pseudo-pure state on the state corresponding to ω_{12}. It should be noted that in the pulse sequence, Fig. 14, the first 109° microwave pulse of ω_{24} and $\pi/2$ radio-

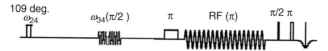

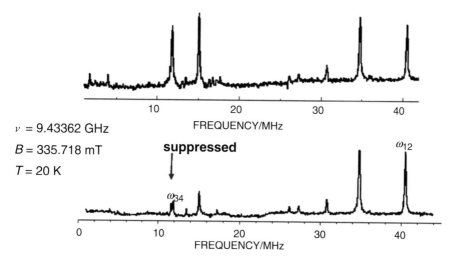

Fig. 13 Pseudo-pure state; ENDOR results before (*up*) and after (*bottom*) applying the pulse sequence given in Fig. 14

Fig. 14 The pulse sequence for generating pseudo-pure state

frequency pulse of ω_{34} are for pseudo-pure state generation and the other pulses are applied for (Davies) ENDOR detection. Pseudo-pure states to the other energy levels, shown in Fig. 5, would be acquired by applying other forms of pulse sequences.

This experiment demonstrates our control on the electron-nuclear coupled molecular spin systems because as evidenced by the experimental results the operations and the required waiting times have been implemented successfully. Next, in the following section, we show the experimental results on enhancing the nuclear spin polarizations by an electron spin. As an example and in order to demonstrate the built-up polarization on the nuclear spins, we have studied the generation of nonclassical correlations between the electron and the nuclear spins as a result of the larger nuclear spin polarization.

4.3 Polarization Built Up on Nuclear Spins and Generating Nonclassical Correlations

The following experiments demonstrate our control over the electron-nuclear coupled spin systems. Nuclear spins polarizations are enhanced by applying the pulses, as explained in the above sections. One physical property that is changing as the result, after building up polarization on the nuclear spins, is nonclassical correlations between the coupled spins. For a matter of demonstrating the experimental outcome and to check its closeness to the expected results, we use some nonclassical/quantum coherence measure and investigate if the corresponding values are enhanced by the nuclear spin polarizations enhancements. We run the experiments at X-band and Q-band.

It is worth mentioning that if we run the experiment at W-band, the required spin polarization for starting to generate entanglement between an electron and a nuclear spin is achieved in a magnetic field for 95 GHz at a temperature of 0.83 K or lower. However, if a transfer of spin polarization, as explained above, from electron spin to nuclear spin is performed the required temperature is 5.17 K, or lower, which is well in reach with current technology with a W-band ENDOR spectrometer operating at liquid helium temperature. The experimental conditions are given for two cases of the experiments without and with transfer of spin polarization.

We may use some sort of witness operators for detecting non-classical correlation and entanglement [18, 45]. Here we use another technique available from EPR. The technique is called Time Proportional Phase Incrementation, TPPI [46]. TPPI is a technique for separating multiple quantum coherences. The technique gives global information on the total state of electron and nuclear spins. TPPI is an essential tool for detecting and resolving the correlated states from the simple superposition states. In TPPI, the phase shifts are implemented by incrementing the phase frequencies of the individual detection pulses in consecutive experiments. Detection pulses are unitary back operations applied in accordance to the expected state for detecting the coherences. Detection pulses are applied with arbitrary phase frequencies, v_j on jth spin. Therefore, we have

$$\Delta\omega_j = 2\pi v_j.$$

Consecutive experiments are performed for a time Δt. We have

$$\phi_j = \Delta\omega_j \Delta t.$$

The phase shifts are detected through the experiment and give information on the state.

Let us give an example. Suppose that the state in the experiment is a Bell state of the following form

$$|\psi\rangle = \frac{1}{\sqrt{2}}(|01\rangle - |10\rangle).$$

Detection pulses that we apply are a microwave π pulse followed by a radio-frequency $\pi/2$ pulse, with phases of ϕ_1 and ϕ_2, respectively, Fig. 16. Then the detection unitary operation might be written as

$$U_d = \omega_{34}\left(\frac{\pi}{2}, \phi_2\right)\omega_{24}(\pi, \phi_1).$$

The first pulse is a microwave π pulse, $\omega_{24}(\pi)$ and the second pulse is a $\pi/2$ radiofrequency pulse, $\omega_{34}(\pi/2)$. Then, the measurement is performed with the detection of electron spin echo. The intensity would be as follows

$$S_d^{\psi}(\phi_1, \phi_2) = \text{Tr}\{S_z^{24}U_d|\psi\rangle\langle\psi|U_d^{\dagger}\}$$
$$= -\frac{1}{2}[1 - \cos(\phi_1 - \phi_2)].$$

Therefore, through the detection by TPPI, we would get the phase shift as follows

$$\phi_1 - \phi_2 = \Delta(\omega_1 - \omega_2)\Delta t.$$

Here, for the angular frequencies, ω_j, we have

$$\Delta(\omega_1 - \omega_2) = 2\pi(\nu_1 - \nu_2).$$

Detection of a pulse with a phase shift of $\phi_1 - \phi_2$ demonstrates that the state has been $|\psi\rangle$. If the state under measurement is a superposition of the state then after applying the detection unitary operations with ν_1 and ν_2, the results will be only ϕ_1 and ϕ_2 and not the coherences, $\phi_1 - \phi_2$. After applying phase-dependent pulses, π microwave ω_{24} with phase ϕ_1 followed with a $\pi/2$ radiofrequency ω_{34} with phase ϕ_2, the phase-dependent echo intensity of the following form is given

$$I = -\frac{1}{4}[1 - \cos(\phi_1 - \phi_2)].$$

Table 1 shows possible choices of microwave and radiofrequencies for the pulse sequence for generating different coherences (Fig. 15).

The artificial phase frequencies in our experiments are $\Delta\omega_j = 2\pi\Delta\nu_j$, $\nu_1 = 1.0$ MHz and $\nu_2 = 5.2$ MHz, as arbitrary values. The resultant spectrum is a 2D spectra, the TPPI frequency against time. The phase interferogram against time is Fourier transformed. The combination of the phases, whether to be addition or subtraction, gives evidence of the phase of the coherence state. See Fig. 16 for the results that have been achieved from experiments with malonyl radical.

Table 1 Different coherent states derived by different pulse sequences

Microwave	Radio frequency 1	Radio frequency 2	State	ν_{TPPI}
ω_{24}	ω_{12}	ω_{34}	$\frac{1}{\sqrt{2}}(|10\rangle - |01\rangle)$	$\phi_1 - \phi_2$
ω_{24}	ω_{34}	ω_{12}	$\frac{1}{\sqrt{2}}(|00\rangle + |11\rangle)$	$\phi_1 + \phi_2$
ω_{13}	ω_{12}	ω_{34}	$\frac{1}{\sqrt{2}}(|00\rangle - |11\rangle)$	$\phi_1 + \phi_2$
ω_{13}	ω_{34}	ω_{12}	$\frac{1}{\sqrt{2}}(|10\rangle + |01\rangle)$	$\phi_1 - \phi_2$

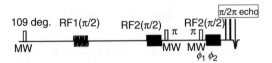

Fig. 15 The pulse sequence that has been used for generation of coherences between an electron spin and a nuclear spin

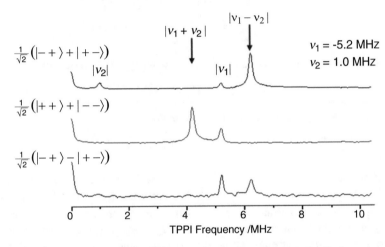

Fig. 16 Experimental results demonstrating the coherences with malonyl radicals

Similar experiments have been carried out on DPNO. Fourier-transformed experimental results showed that three-partite coherence among one electron and two proton spins is acquired for the first time. However, because of the small gyromagnetic ratio of nitrogen and the fact that we didn't have access to a high-power radio-frequency amplifier, we were unable to appropriately manipulate nitrogen. Here, nitrogen is a basis for discriminating proton energy levels. However, we are planning to use this molecule for more elaborated quantum computing and quantum information processing such as implementing multiple rounds of HBAC and QEC. From the experimental side, another approach will be the usage of multiple and strong microwave frequencies allowing us to manipulate nitrogen nuclei.

5 Conclusion

Electrons (in addition to nuclear spins) involved in molecular spin systems have intrinsic properties important for exploiting quantum effects, in which the electron plays the role of a bus qubit. Nuclear spins with typically long coherence times play the role of quantum memories. Fast electron spin manipulations are achieved by applying on-resonance microwave pulses. Couplings between spins make it plausible to speed up nuclear spin manipulations by using the electron spins as quantum actuators. In addition, flexibilities are offered by synthetic chemistry for designing new open-shell molecular materials for quantum applications such as high-resolution imaging, molecular sensors, and quantum information processing.

One of the main challenges in utilizing the spin systems for quantum practices is the thermal fluctuations of spins. In principle, a highly pure initial state should be prepared in order to establish a clean start-up. The idea is to employ the coupled spins and take advantage of the electron high spin polarization. Polarizations of nuclear spins are enhanced to the electron spin polarization by applying direct pulses, DNP methods, or HBAC.

Extracting reliable processing outcome, i.e. robust against noise, is the ultimate goal for every effort relating to engineering a processing system. In quantum context, only few examples are applicable since generally quantum systems are fragile against noise. The electron-nuclear coupled molecular spin systems are useful since extra spins can be introduced by appropriate molecular optimization; spins are refreshed by different techniques and algorithms, and they are controlled by using varieties of advanced tools and knowledge from ESR/ENDOR/ELDOR [47]. In addition, NMR paradigm-based electron magnetic spin technology has already been emerging in this field.

Acknowledgments We thank Prof. Lawrence Berliner for proofreading the manuscript. We have appreciated the synthetic work on DPNOs by Shinsuke Nishida and Yasushi Morita, Osaka University. This work has been supported by Grants-in-Aid for Scientific Research on Innovative Areas "Quantum Cybernetics" and Scientific Research (B) from MEXT, Japan. The support for the present work by the FIRST project on "Quantum Information Processing" from JSPS, Japan and by the AOARD project on "Quantum Properties of Molecular Nanomagnets" (Award No. FA2386-13-1-4030) is also acknowledged. RRD would like to thank Howard Halpern and members of the Center for EPR Imaging in Vivo Physiology, for warm hospitality while the last stage of this work was conducted.

References

1. G.E. Moore, Electron. Mag. **38**(8), 114 (1965)
2. R.P. Peering, Nature **406**, 1023 (2000)
3. A.M. Turing, Proc. Lond. Math. Soc. 2 **42**, 230 (1936)
4. A. Church, Am. J. Math. **58**, 345 (1936)
5. M.D. Davis, *The undecidable* (Raven Press, New York, 1965)
6. R.P. Feynman, Int. J. Theor. Phys. **21**, 467 (1982)
7. D.P. DiVincenzo, Fortschr. Phys. **9**, 771 (2000)
8. R.R. Ernst, G. Bodenhausen, A. Wokaun, *Nuclear Magnetic Resonance in One and Two Dimensions* (Oxford University Press, Oxford, 1994)
9. A. Abragam, *The Principles of Nuclear Magnetism* (Clarendon Press, Oxford, 1961)
10. M. Golden, *Quantum Description of High-Resolution NMR in Liquids* (Oxford Scientific Publication, London, 1998)

11. C.P. Slichter, *Principles of Magnetic Resonance* (Springer, Berlin, 1996)
12. X. Fang, X. Zhu, M. Feng, X. Mao, F. Du, Phys. Rev. A **61**, 022307 (2000)
13. R. Rahimi, K. Takeda, M. Ozawa, M. Kitagawa, J. Phys. A: Math. Gen. **39**, 2151 (2006)
14. J.A. Jones, M. Mosca, R.H. Hansen, Nature **393**, 344 (1998)
15. I.L. Chuang, L.M.K. Vandersypen, X. Zhou, D.W. Leung, S. Lloyd, Nature **393**, 143 (1998)
16. M.A. Nielsen, E. Knill, R. Lafflamme, Nature **396**, 52 (1998)
17. L.M.K. Vandersypen, M. Steffen, G. Breyta, C.S. Yannoni, M.H. Sherwood, I.L. Chuang, Nature **414**, 883 (2001)
18. I.L. Chuang, N. Gershenfeld, M.G. Kubinec, D.W. Leung, Proc. R. Soc. Lond. A. **454**, 447 (1998)
19. D.G. Cory, R. Lafflamme, E. Knill, L. Viola, T.F. Havel, N. Boulant, G. Boutis, E. Fortunato, S. Lloyd, R. Martinez, C. Negrevergne, M. Pravia, Y. Sharif, G. Teklemariam, Y.S. Weinstein, W.H. Zurek, Fortschr. Phys. **48**, 875 (2000)
20. D.G. Cory, M.D. Price, T.F. Havel, Physica D **120**, 82 (1998)
21. D.G. Cory, A.F. Fahmy, T.F. Havel, Proc. Natl. Acad. Sci. U. S. A. **94**, 1634 (1997)
22. S. Lloyd, Science **273**, 1073 (1996)
23. G. Vidal, Phys. Rev. Lett. **83**, 1046 (1999)
24. K. Zyczkowski, P. Horodecki, A. Sanpera, M. Lewenstein, Phys. Rev. A **58**, 883 (1999)
25. S.L. Braunstein, C.M. Caves, R. Jozsa, N. Linden, S. Popescu, R. Schack, Phys. Rev. Lett. **83**, 1054 (1999)
26. R. Schack, C.M. Caves, Phys. Rev. A **60**, 4354 (1999)
27. B. Criger, O. Moussa, R. Laflamme, Phys. Rev. A **85**, 044302 (2012)
28. H.K. Lo, S. Popescu, T. Spiller, *Introduction to Quantum Computation and Information* (World Scientific Publication, Singapore, 1998)
29. L.M.K. Vandersypen, PhD Dissertation arXiv:quant-ph/0205193, 2002
30. K. Takeda, K. Takegoshi, T. Terao, J. Phys. Soc. Jpn. **73**, 2313 (2004)
31. D. Park, G. Feng, R. Rahimi, T. Shibata, T. Takui, J. Baugh, R. Laflamme, to be published
32. R. Bergene, T.B. Melø, Biophysik **9**, 1 (1972)
33. H.M. McConnell, C. Heller, T. Cole, R.W. Fessenden, J. Am. Chem. Soc. **82**, 766 (1960)
34. M. McConnell, W. Fessenden, J. Chem. Phys. **31**, 1688 (1959)
35. T. Cole, C. Heller, J. Chem. Phys. **34**, 1085 (1960)
36. R. Rahimi, PhD thesis, Osaka University, Japan, arXiv: 0609063
37. K. Sato, S. Nakazawa, S. Nishida, R. Rahimi, T. Yohsino, Y. Morita, K. Toyota, D. Shiomi, M. Kitagawa, T. Takui, Novel applications of ESR/EPR: quantum computing/quantum information processing, in *EPR of Free Radicals in Solids II: Trends in Methods and Applications*, ed. by A. Lund, M. Shiotani (Springer, Dordrecht, 2013). ISBN 978-94-007-4886-6
38. Y. Deguchi, Bull. Chem. Soc. Jpn. **34**, 910 (1961); Y. Deguchi, Bull. Chem. Soc. Jpn. **35**, 260 (1962)
39. J. Yamauchi, H. Nishiguchi, K. Mukai, Y. Deguchi, Bull. Chem. Soc. Jpn. **40**, 2512 (1967)
40. T.-S. Lin, J. Chem. Phys. **57**, 2260 (1972)
41. A.L. Maniero, M. Brustolon, J. Chem. Soc. Faraday Trans. 1 **84**, 2875 (1988)
42. J. Yamauchi, K. Okada, Y. Deguchi, Bull. Chem. Soc. Jpn. **60**, 483 (1987)
43. T. Yoshino, S. Nishida, K. Sato, S. Nakazawa, R. Rahimi, K. Toyota, D. Shiomi, Y. Morita, M. Kitagawa, T. Takui, J. Phys. Chem. Lett. **2**, 449 (2011)
44. M. Mehring, J. Mende, W. Scherer, Phys. Rev. Lett. **90**, 153001 (2003)
45. R. Rahimi, A. SaiToh, Phys. Rev. A **82**, 022314 (2010)
46. M. Mehring, P. Hoefer, A. Grupp, Phys. Rev. A **33**, 3523 (1986)
47. S. Nakazawa, S. Nishida, T. Ise, T. Yoshino, N. Mori, D.R. Rahimi, K. Sato, Y. Morita, K. Toyota, D. Shiomi, M. Kitagawa, H. Hara, P. Carl, P. Höfer, T. Takui, Angew. Chem. **124**, 9998 (2012)

Molecular Spins in Biological Systems

Hideto Matsuoka and Olav Schiemann

Abstract Quantum effects in biological systems have recently been studied extensively in the fields of quantum computing (QC) and quantum information processing (QIP). The focus of this review is on quantum coherences and entanglement properties created in natural photosynthesis, whose understanding may be crucial for achieving the remarkable efficiency of its excitation energy transfer. In the beginning, an overview of electron and energy transfer in photosynthetic reaction centers (RCs) and light-harvesting complexes (LHCs) is given. Then the physical aspects of spin-correlated radical pairs (SCRPs) are described, which are ubiquitous intermediates in a wide range of biochemical reactions. Examples are given mainly with relation to quantum coherences in RCs and LHCs, which persist at room temperature, since such long-lived quantum coherences are crucial for quantum information storage and manipulation. Where appropriate, experimental observations of quantum coherences in artificial molecular assemblies are also briefly surveyed. In the second part, site-directed spin-labeling and pulsed electron-electron double resonance (PELDOR or DEER) are described, which are becoming important techniques in QC/QIP.

1 Introduction

In addition to solid-state materials [1–4], biological systems have attracted much attention in the field of quantum computing and quantum information processing (QC/QIP), which is called "Quantum Biology" [5–8]. Within Quantum Biology, photosynthesis has been one of the main research subjects [5–8]. In part, because photosynthetic organisms harvest sunlight with near unity quantum efficiency and recent theoretical studies have suggested that a coherent superposition of

H. Matsuoka • O. Schiemann (✉)
Institute of Physical and Theoretical Chemistry, University of Bonn,
Wegelerstrasse 12, Bonn 53115, Germany
e-mail: schiemann@pc.uni-bonn.de

© Springer New York 2016   51
T. Takui et al. (eds.), *Electron Spin Resonance (ESR) Based Quantum Computing*,
Biological Magnetic Resonance 31, DOI 10.1007/978-1-4939-3658-8_3

delocalized excited states (quantum coherence) may be crucial for achieving the remarkable efficiency of the excitation energy transfer [6–22].

In 2007, Graham Fleming and his coworkers showed the existence of coherent quantum beating in bacterial reaction centers (RCs) at 77 and 180 K [12, 13]; and in 2010, Gregory S. Engel and his coworkers provided clear evidence for the existence of quantum coherence in the bacterial complex at ambient temperature [14]. Those pioneering works proved that the observation of quantum coherence is not due to an artifact under cryogenic laboratory conditions but that quantum coherences are preserved in photosynthetic systems for up to a picosecond at ambient and cryogenic temperatures [11–15, 17, 19–21]. These findings have raised questions concerning the utilization of quantum coherence in the solar energy conversion because one had expected that the coherence between the excited states is immediately destroyed at ambient temperature in the biological environment composed of thermally fluctuating water and amino acids. Persistent electronic coherences were also observed in a series of rigid synthetic heterodimers [23]. A very recent study of a photoexcited supramolecule demonstrated that the driving mechanism of the primary photoinduced event is a correlated wavelike motion of electrons and nuclei [24]. Even in conjugated polymer samples, coherent electronic energy transfer has been observed at room temperature [25, 26]. In addition, a coherent charge-transfer model related to the motion of charges has been discussed in blend films of organic photovoltaic materials [26, 27].

Fleming et al. proposed a particular quantum computation algorithm called a quantum search, in which an exciton finds its destination (RC) by using quantum coherences [12]. Seth Lloyd and his coworkers suggested a different quantum algorithm called a quantum walk [16], in which a quantum particle walks coherently toward its destination. Creating a practical quantum computer requires that the surrounding environment is prevented from affecting the coherence of the quantum bits (qubits). Thus, a better understanding of quantum coherence in the biological systems under ambient conditions would be of significant importance to achieve practical quantum computing. The long-lived quantum coherences in the biological systems also stimulated the construction of artificial molecular systems, which can be used either for direct electric power generation (photovoltaic approach) [28] or solar fuel production (photosynthetic approach) [5]. Quantum teleportation across a photosynthetic membrane using SCRPs is another example for direct utilization of biological systems in QC/QIP [29–31]. In addition, SCRPs are ubiquitous in a wide range of biochemical reactions and spatially separated, non-interacting SCRPs can be considered as entangled objects, which have been extensively investigated by time-resolved electron paramagnetic resonance (TR-EPR) [32–41].

A different example is to use spin-labeled biological systems as scalable qubits for electron spin-based QC/QIP [42–44]. Site-directed spin labeling (SDSL), which has been employed to determine the structures of membranes, proteins, and nucleic acids [45], is becoming an ever more important technique in QC/QIP. For example, Takeji Takui and his coworkers have suggested that scalable electron spin-qubits can be constructed by incorporating spin labels with spatially different orientations of magnetic tensors into DNA [44]. A pulsed electron–electron double resonance (PELDOR) technique was employed to evaluate the spin dipolar and exchange interactions between the spin labels [46], which are necessary information for implementing quantum gate operations in open shell compounds. Beyond using PELDOR merely as an analytical technique, it has been recognized that it is also a powerful tool for the coherent manipulations of electron spins [47].

2 Photosynthesis

2.1 Reaction Centers and Light-Harvesting Complexes

Light-induced electron transfer reactions in membrane-bound proteins called reaction centers (RCs) play a crucial role in the primary energy conversion steps of photosynthesis. The RCs are found in large pigment-protein complexes called photosystems. Two types of photosystems can be distinguished in all oxygen evolving photosynthetic organisms (plants, cyanobacteria, algae), which are referred to as photosystem I and II (PS I and PS II). The RCs contain chlorophyll dimers referred to as P_{700} and P_{680} in PS I and PS II, respectively. When a thylakoid membrane is exposed to sunlight, pigment-protein antennas known as LHCs absorb solar energy and transfer it to the RCs.

The chlorophyll dimer P_{700} locates on the electron transfer chain in PS I, which contains six chlorophylls (Chls), two phylloquinones (A_1), and three Fe_4S_4 clusters (F_x, F_A, F_B) arranged in two similar branches related by a pseudo-C_2 symmetry axis, as shown in Fig. 1 [48]. The Chls are separated into three groups: the special pair P_{700}, the accessory Chls (A), and the primary electron acceptors (A_0). The cofactors (A, A_0, A_1) are part of either branch A or branch B. Extensive studies have been performed to reveal the route of the electron transfer from the special pair to the iron cluster. Especially, TR-EPR [49–51] has been extensively employed to investigate the electron transfer pathway [32, 33, 52]. It was initially thought that the electron transfer is unidirectional in PS I, by analogy with the type II reaction centers of purple bacteria and PS II, where only one cofactor branch is active for the electron transfer. However, during the past decade, it has been recognized that both cofactor chains in PS I are functionally relevant (bidirectional mechanism) [32, 33].

Within PSII, molecular oxygen is produced from water by the water-oxidizing complex [53–57], which is composed of four exchange-coupled manganese (Mn) atoms and one calcium (Ca) atom (Fig. 2a, b). EPR techniques have provided detailed information on the electronic and molecular structures of redox-active molecules in PSII [55–57]. Very recently, the crystal structure of PSII was disclosed at a resolution of 1.9 Å [53]. The crystal structure also revealed the presence of a vast number of water molecules, as shown in Fig. 2c. Obviously, photosynthetic proteins are situated in the warm, wet, and noisy conditions due to thermally fluctuating water, which is expected to destroy quantum coherence immediately.

Fig. 1 Arrangement of the
cofactors in the RCs of PS I
(PDB entry 1JB0)

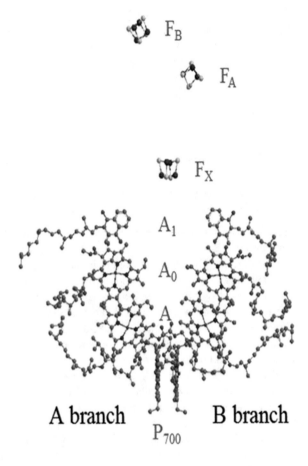

Two types of LHCs called LHC-I and -II are found in higher plants and green
algae, which are associated with PS I and PS II, respectively. In purple bacteria, two
types of LHCs are distinguished: the peripheral light harvesting (LH2) [58] and the
core light-harvesting antenna complexes (LH1). Until recently, the main mechanism of energy transfer in the LHCs has been interpreted by the classical hopping
mechanism assumed in Förster theory [59]. However, recent theoretical and experimental studies have proposed wavelike energy migration through quantum coherence as an alternative to the classical model, revealing the presence of long-lasting
quantum coherence in the warm, wet, and noisy biological systems [10–16].

2.2 Spin-Correlated Radical Pair in an Entangled State

After the chlorophyll dimers absorb light in photosystems, an electron is transferred
from the excited singlet state of each pigment to a primary electron acceptor in the

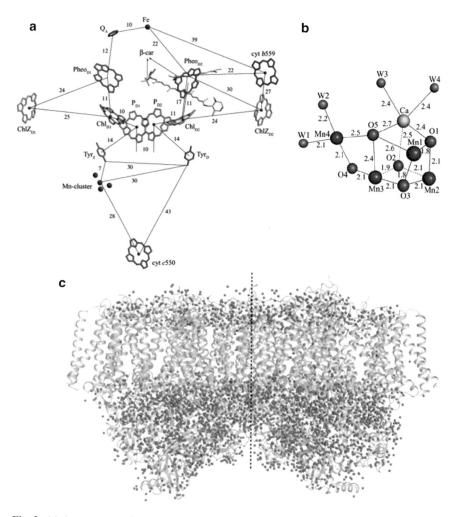

Fig. 2 (**a**) Arrangement of the cofactors in the RCs of PS II (adapted from [54]). (**b**) Geometric structure of the Mn_4CaO_5 cluster (adapted from [53]). (**c**) Structure of PSII dimer from *Thermosynecoccus vulcanus* at a resolution of 1.9 Å. Arrangement of water molecules is shown by *orange circle*. The *broken lines* represent the noncrystallographic twofold axes relating the two monomers (adapted from [53])

pico- to subnanosecond time range. After losing their electrons, the chlorophyll dimers become positively charged pigments and higher plants, and the acceptor becomes negatively charged. The positively charged pigments are normally termed as P_{700}^+ or P_{680}^+ in cyanobacteria, green algae, and higher plants. Through a specific pathway, electrons are transferred via intermediate electron carriers to a terminal electron acceptor, which is the iron cluster and quinone in PS I and II, respectively. Generally, the electron transfer reactions in RCs can be described as

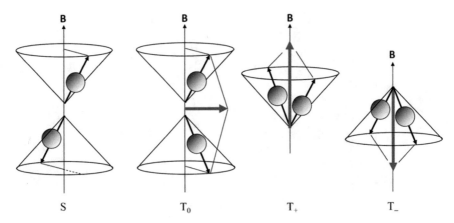

Fig. 3 A vector model of the four possible spin states in a radical pair consisting of two unpaired electrons: one singlet state (S) and three triplet (T_+, T_0, T_-)

$$P\ A_0A_IA_T \xrightarrow{h\nu} {}^1P^*\ A_0A_IA_T \rightarrow P^+A_0{}^-A_IA_T$$

$$\rightarrow P^+A_0A_I{}^-A_T \rightarrow P^+A_0A_IA_T{}^-$$

where P, A_0, A_I, and A_T are referred to as the chlorophyll dimers, primary, intermediate, and terminal electron acceptors, respectively. The photoinduced cation (P^+) and anion ($A_i{}^-$) are radicals, and thus, the charge separation state forms the radical pair $P^+A_i{}^-$ that can be detected by TR-EPR [32–41, 52].

A radical pair consisting of two unpaired electrons forms one singlet state (S) and three triplet (T_+, T_0, T_-) illustrated by a vector model in Fig. 3. At high magnetic fields, the eigenstates of the four possible electron spin states can be described as

$$
\begin{aligned}
|S\rangle &= \frac{1}{\sqrt{2}}(|\alpha_1\beta_2\rangle - |\beta_1\alpha_2\rangle)\\
|T_+\rangle &= |\alpha_1\alpha_2\rangle\\
|T_0\rangle &= \frac{1}{\sqrt{2}}(|\alpha_1\beta_2\rangle + |\beta_1\alpha_2\rangle)\\
|T_-\rangle &= |\beta_1\beta_2\rangle
\end{aligned}
\tag{1}
$$

where α_i and β_i are referred to as the "spin-up" and "spin-down" states of a radical i. A radical pair consisting of two radicals with their respective spins, S_1 and S_2, has the total spin $S = S_1 + S_2$. Since spin multiplicity is conserved in electron transfer processes, the total spin S is the same as the spin multiplicity of the precursor molecule (spin correlation): $S = 0$ for an excited singlet precursor and $S = 1$ for a triplet precursor. Thus, such a radical pair is often called a SCRP. The two radicals are physically separated by a large distance rapidly after the absorption of light, so that SCRPs can be practically considered as a non-interacting species. Since SCRPs are generated from the singlet precursor in photosynthesis, the initial state of SCRPs is a spin singlet, which can be regarded as a maximally entangled Bell state under this condition. A pair of quantum systems in an entangled state can be used as a resource for quantum teleportation. It is well known that SCRPs play a crucial role not only in photosynthesis but may also be important in the bird's navigation system [60, 61].

2.3 TR-EPR of Spin-Correlated Radical Pair

The singlet radical pairs give rise to high electron spin polarization, which is often called either CIDEP (chemically induced dynamic electron polarization) or ESP (electron spin polarization). Due to CIDEP/ESP, the radical pairs can be monitored by TR-EPR with high-time resolution and high sensitivity [32–41, 52, 62]. In the charge separation, the electron and the hole are separated rapidly by a large distance. For example, the transfer of an electron from the excited singlet state of P_{700} to the primary and secondary electron acceptors (A_0 and A_1) occurs within 10 and 100 ps, respectively. If the distance between two radicals is sufficiently large, the exchange interaction J between the spins becomes essentially negligible, so that the S and T_0 states are nearly degenerate. In such a condition, the singlet state can interact only with the T_0 state (S – T_0 mixing). When the S – T_0 mixing is considered, the possible four spin states can be described as [34, 36, 38, 40]

$$
\begin{aligned}
|1\rangle &= |T_+\rangle \\
|2\rangle &= \cos\phi|S\rangle + \sin\phi|T_0\rangle \\
|3\rangle &= -\sin\phi|S\rangle + \cos\phi|T_0\rangle \\
|4\rangle &= |T_-\rangle
\end{aligned}
\tag{2}
$$

where

$$
\begin{aligned}
\tan 2\phi &= \frac{2Q}{2J+d}, \\
Q &= \frac{1}{2}(\omega_1 - \omega_2), \\
d &= D\left(\cos\xi - \frac{1}{3}\right).
\end{aligned}
\tag{3}
$$

Here, ω_i stands for the electron Zeeman interaction of an electron i. J and D are referred to as the exchange and electron-spin dipolar interactions, respectively. The angle ξ represents the orientation of the dipolar axis with respect to the magnetic field direction. Under this condition, coherent interconversion (intersystem

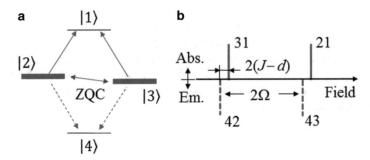

Fig. 4 (**a**) Energy levels, EPR allowed transitions, and zero quantum coherence for a SCRP. (**b**) A stick diagram of an EPR spectrum for a SCRP, in which absorption and emission signals are illustrated by *red solid* and *dashed lines*, respectively

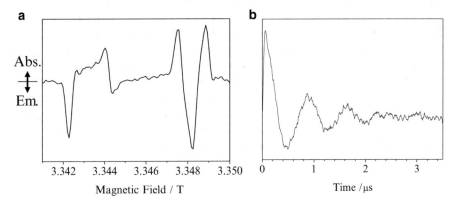

Fig. 5 (**a**) Transient W-band EPR spectrum of the light-induced radical pair, $P_{700}{}^+A_1{}^-$, in PS I from cyanobacteria *S. lividus* at 80 K. (**b**) Nutation signal (Torrey oscillation) at the field position of 3.3475 T

cross-ing) between the S and T_0 states can be occurred with time, and thus, only the S and T_0 states are populated, giving CIDEP/ESP. As a result, either absorptive (positive) signals from the two states, $|2\rangle$ and $|3\rangle$, to $|1\rangle$ or emissive (negative) ones to $|4\rangle$ are observed, as shown in Fig. 4.

In addition to TR-EPR, electron spin transient nutation (ESTN) spectroscopy also enables one to identify weakly interacting radical pairs [34–36, 38, 40, 63, 64]. In ESTN spectroscopy, the nutation frequency, which is proportional to the transition moment of an EPR transition, is monitored as a function of the microwave irradiation strength [63, 64]. Figure 5 shows the transient W-band EPR spectrum of the light-induced radical pair, $P_{700}{}^+A1^-$, in PS I from cyanobacteria *Synechococcus lividus* (*S. lividus*) [52]. The nutation frequency is given for an EPR allowed transition between $|S, M_S\rangle \leftrightarrow |S, M_S + 1\rangle$ sublevels by

$$\omega_N = \sqrt{S(S+1) - M_S(M_S+1)}\,\omega_1 \tag{4}$$

with $\omega_N = g\beta B_1$. For short distances between the two radicals (strongly interacting radical pairs), the exchange interaction J splits the singlet and triplet levels, which can be described by the eigenstates in (1). In this condition, only transitions between the triplet levels can be detected by EPR spectroscopy. Since the EPR transitions for $|1, -1\rangle \leftrightarrow |1, 0\rangle$ and $|1, 0\rangle \leftrightarrow |1, 1\rangle$ are allowed in the strong-coupling limit, the nutation frequency is given by

$$\omega_N = \sqrt{1.2 - 0.1}\ \omega_1 = \sqrt{2}\omega_1 \tag{5}$$

In the weak-coupling limit, which is expected for SCRPs in photosynthesis, the nutation frequency is given by ω_1 [34–36, 38, 40]. The ESTN spectroscopy is a novel technique to identify weakly or strongly interacting radical pairs based on the transition moment.

As described above, there is zero quantum coherence (ZQC) between the eigenstates $|2\rangle$ and $|3\rangle$ in weakly interacting radical pairs, which manifests itself as quantum beat oscillations in an EPR experiment with adequate time resolution [32, 37, 39, 41, 52, 62]. Gerd Kothe and coworkers have extensively studied ZQCs. A high-time resolution X-band study was performed for the $P_{700}^+A1^-$ radical pairs at room temperature [37, 41]. Very recently, Kothe et al. have explored the electron transfer pathways of PS I in fully deuterated green alga *Chlamydomonas reinhardtii* using high-time resolution EPR, in which quantum oscillations were clearly observed at different field positions, as shown in Fig. 6 [32]. Surprisingly, analysis of the quantum oscillation in fully deuterated *S. lividus* revealed that the spin coherence time T_2 was 500 ns, even at room temperature despite the warm, wet, and noisy biological environment [41]. The coherence time extended to microsecond range at 70 K [62]. In nondeuterated *Chlamydomonas reinhardtii*, the coherence time was around 500 ns at 100 K [33], indicating that the coherence time is affected by the nuclear spins of protons. However, the mechanism of causing the long-lived spin coherence at ambient temperature is still an open question. The ZQC studies in PS I have been very recently extended to the W-band (94 GHz) regime, in which the excellent spectral resolution is realized [52]. No significant magnetic field dependence of the coherence time was observed from the high-field/high-frequency EPR study [66].

2.4 Quantum Teleportation Using Spin-Correlated Radical Pairs

An exciting application of entanglement is quantum teleportation, which plays an important role in QIP [65]. Quantum teleportation provides a way for transporting a quantum state between two separated parties, the sender (Alice) and receiver (Bob). Imagine that Alice possesses a qubit labeled A that is in an unknown state:

$$|\Psi_A\rangle = C_1|\uparrow_A\rangle + C_2|\downarrow_A\rangle \tag{6}$$

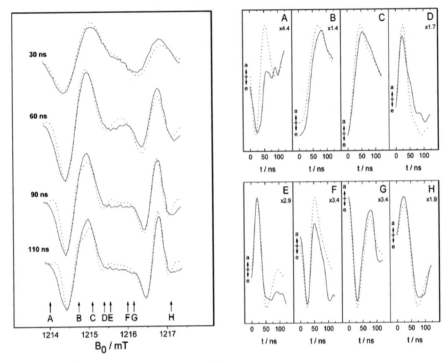

Fig. 6 Transient Q-band EPR spectra of the light-induced radical pair $P_{700}^+A_1^-$ on the B branch in PS I at various times after the laser pulse, and time evolution of the EPR signals at different field positions (adapted from [26])

Here, $|\uparrow_A\rangle$ and $|\downarrow_A\rangle$ represent eigenstates of the qubit in the measurement basis, which correspond to the spin-up and spin-down states in SCRPs. In addition, Alice and Bob each share one partner of a two-qubit entangled pair, which can be described in a singlet state as

$$|S_{BC}\rangle \equiv |\uparrow_B\downarrow_C\rangle - |\downarrow_B\uparrow_C\rangle \tag{7}$$

where normalization factors are omitted here, for simplicity. In this condition, Alice possesses qubits A and B, while Bob possesses qubit C. In quantum teleportation, the state of qubit A is transported to Bob's qubit. The essential elements of this protocol are shown in Fig. 7. Kev. M Salikhov and his coworkers have proposed quantum teleportation across a photosynthetic membrane using SCRPs. In Fig. 7, the scheme is arranged in such a way as to represent the photosynthetic RC complex, where the upper and lower sides of the figure correspond to the lumen and stroma sides in the photosynthetic systems, respectively. The Salikhov's proposal is as follows [29–31]:

1. The first process is to incorporate a stable anion radical as qubit A into the photosynthetic systems by using a different light-induced reaction, chemical

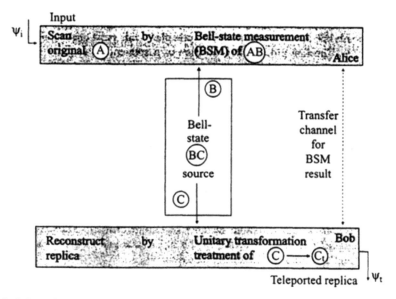

Fig. 7 Schematic representation of quantum teleportation (adapted from [30])

reduction, or spin labeling. And then, a coherent state of qubit A is prepared by a short microwave pulse.

2. The second process is to generate an entangled pair composed of qubits B and C. As described above, the initial state of SCRPs generated in photosystems is the spin singlet, which can be regarded as the maximally entangled Bell state. Thus, this process can always be realized in natural photosynthesis, where qubits B and C correspond to the positively charged special pair and negatively charged electron acceptor, respectively.

3. The third process is the so-called Bell state measurement, which is the crucial step in quantum teleportation. Charge recombination to a singlet state between qubits A and B is required. In order to avoid the singlet-triplet conversion, the charge recombination should be completed within a nanosecond. Thus, the incorporation of the stable radical, A, must be engineered properly in such a way as to satisfy the condition. Due to the fixed spin correlation in SCRPs, the spin state of qubit C is the same as that of qubit A created by the first MW pulse. As a result, the input (spin) quantum state is teleported from the lumen side to the stroma side across the photosynthetic membrane.

Quantum teleportation using SCRPs in biological systems has been extensively studied from the theoretical side, but the proposed processes are very demanding experimentally. However, as described above the maximally entangled Bell state is naturally created in the photosynthetic systems by the primary charge separation. Thus, utilization of SCRPs in biological systems for quantum teleportation is still of great interest.

2.5   Wavelike Energy Transfer Through Quantum Coherence in Photosynthetic Systems

Nature harvests solar energy with a remarkably high quantum efficiency, followed by rapid and highly efficient transport of excitation energy to a RC [17]. Until recently, a classical random hopping assumed in the Förster model has been considered as the main mechanism of energy transfer in the LHCs. However, emerging experimental and theoretical results have revealed that coherent (wavelike) motion of the electronic excitations through photosynthetic complexes may be responsible for such a remarkably high quantum yield [6, 7, 10, 12–14, 16–22]. The classical incoherent hopping and quantum coherent transfer mechanisms are illustrated in Fig. 8 [22]. In 2007, Graham Fleming and his coworkers demonstrated the existence of coherent quantum beating in the Fenna-Matthews-Olson (FMO) complex [12, 13]. In 2010, Gregory S. Engel et al. [14] and Gregory D. Scholes et al. [15] independently provided clear evidences of the existence of quantum coherence at ambient temperature in the bacterial complex and in cryptophyte algae, respectively. As shown in Fig. 9 [21], long-lived electronic coherence was directly observed at room temperature between two rings, called B800 and B850, of the bacteriochlorophyll *a* pigments in single LH2 complexes, where B800 and B850 have the distinct electronic absorption bands in the infrared region.

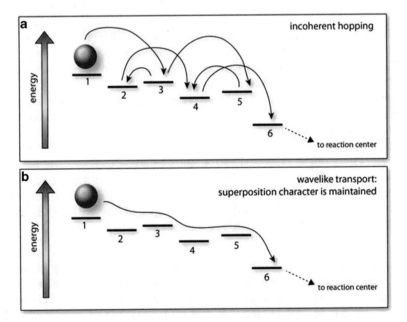

Fig. 8 The classical hopping and quantum coherent energy transfer mechanisms (adapted from [22])

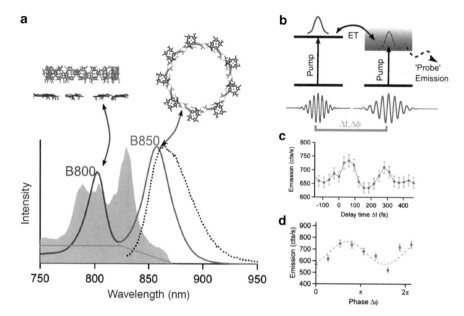

Fig. 9 Ultrafast phase-coherent excitation of the peripheral light-harvesting (LH2) complexes at room temperature. (**a**) The bacteriochlorophyll *a* molecules in LH2 are arranged in two concentric rings termed B800 (*blue*) and B850 (*red*). The emission spectrum is depicted in a *dotted line*. (**b**) Schematic representation of the experiment, in which the first pulse (*blue*) excites the B800 band, the second pulse (*red*) resonant with the B850 band modulates the population transfer to the B850 excited states, and the emission is monitored as a function of Δt or $\Delta \phi$. Emission monitored in the single LH2 complexes as a function of (**c**) the interpulse delay time and (**d**) phase shift (Adapted and modified from [21])

The dynamics of energy transfer is commonly interpreted in terms of the evolution of populations and coherence [5, 14, 19]. Here, imagine a two-site system with a single excitation spread coherently over both sites:

$$|\Psi(t)\rangle = c_1|e_a, g_b\rangle + C_2|g_a, e_b\rangle = c_1|\phi_1\rangle + C_2|\phi_2\rangle \tag{8}$$

where "e_i" and "g_i" represent the excited and ground states of a system i, respectively. In quantum mechanics, populations and coherences are described by the density matrix. The time evolution of the density matrix is given by [14]

$$
\begin{aligned}
|\Psi(t)\rangle\langle\Psi(t)| = {} & |c_1|^2|\phi_1\rangle\langle\phi_1| + |c_2|^2|\phi_2\rangle\langle\phi_2| \\
& + c_1 c_2^* e^{-i(E_1 - E_2)t/\hbar}|\phi_1\rangle\langle\phi_2| + c_1^* c_2 e^{-i(E_1 - E_2)t/\hbar}|\phi_2\rangle\langle\phi_1|
\end{aligned}
\tag{9}
$$

The first two terms represent the diagonal elements of the density matrix describing populations and the latter two represent the off-diagonal elements describing coherences. The coherence dynamics of the photosynthetic systems has been manifested in two-dimensional electronic spectra by the presence of quantum

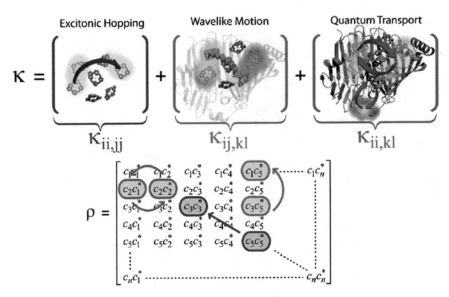

Fig. 10 The three types of transfer of the density matrix elements. The transfer between the diagonal elements (population transfer) corresponds to the classical hopping mechanism (*blue*), the transfer between the off-diagonal elements (coherence transfer) to the wavelike motion (*green*), and the transfer between a population and a coherence to quantum transport (*red*) (Adapted and modified from [19])

beats due to the phase factors of the coherence terms. The transfer between the diagonal elements (population transfer) corresponds to the classical hopping mechanism for energy transfer, in which energy is transferred from one state to the next. The transfer between off-diagonal elements (coherence transfer) corresponds to the wavelike motion. As shown by Gregory S. Engel and his coworkers, quantum transport of energy can be described as coherent population transfer, in which coherences couple to populations [13–15, 19, 30]. The three types of transfer are schematically illustrated in Fig. 10 [19].

The role of quantum coherence to enhance the quantum efficiency for the energy transfer is still an open and intriguing question. To understand the origins of such long-lived coherences and their role in the high efficient photosynthetic property will inspire the development of new energy technologies.

3 Quantum Coherence in Artificial Energy Conversion Systems

Carlo A. Rozzi et al. evidenced that the photoinduced process is triggered by a wavelike motion of electrons and nuclei on a timescale of few tens of femtoseconds in a prototypical artificial RC [24]. Very recently, a series of rigid synthetic heterodimers were engineered by Gregory S. Engel and his coworkers, which exhibited quantum beating in two-dimensional electronic spectra [23]. Compared with the complicated photosynthetic systems, the synthetic heterodimers are the smaller and simpler systems that can be a model system to investigate the fundamental physics underlying the persistent electronic coherences.

4 Site-Directed Spin-Labeling and Pulsed Dipolar Spectroscopy

SDSL in combination with Pulsed Dipolar Spectroscopy (PDS) is an important tool for obtaining structure and dynamics information of biomacromolecules [45]. However, SDSL in biological systems may also become an important technique in QC/QIP. For example, the incorporation of organic radicals at designed positions might be useful for building up scalable qubits of electron-spin-based quantum computing and spin labels with narrow spectral widths may enable selective excitation of EPR transitions, which would additionally be supported if the label is rigid. In addition, molecular spin-based QC/QIP requires stable radicals with long phase memory times, also for this new types of labels are available. Such radicals could then be attached to the biomolecule in a way that they have different orientations. For example, nitroxide spin labels with spatially different orientations of the magnetic tensors were incorporated into DNA to construct scalable electron spin-qubits [42–44]. Here, several SDSL techniques with different types of labels are surveyed, and a small selection of PDS methods will be introduced, especially PELDOR.

4.1 Labeling of Proteins with Nitroxides

Based on the seminal work of Hubbell, proteins are usually labeled at cysteines [67]. In order to achieve the site specificity, the label carries a functional group that reacts selectively with the SH group of the cysteine. If the protein carries several cysteines or a cysteine at an unwanted site, these are exchanged for other amino acids, e.g. alanine, via site-directed mutagenesis. In turn, site-directed mutagenesis is also used to incorporate a cysteine at the wanted site. Thus, the label contains a spin-bearing moiety, commonly a five- or six-membered nitroxide ring, the functional group that reacts specifically with the SH side chain of the cysteine, and a linker connecting both. For example, maleimide [68] (Fig. 11a), iodoacetamide [69] (Fig. 11b), or methanethiosulfonate [70] (Fig. 11c) has been used as functional groups. The latter one, the so-called MTSSL label, is the most selective and most used one.

However, one would have to make sure that the mutagenesis and the label itself do not lead to structural changes, e.g. via testing the proteins function. If the function is inhibited or if the protein precipitates upon mutagenesis, labeling via cysteines

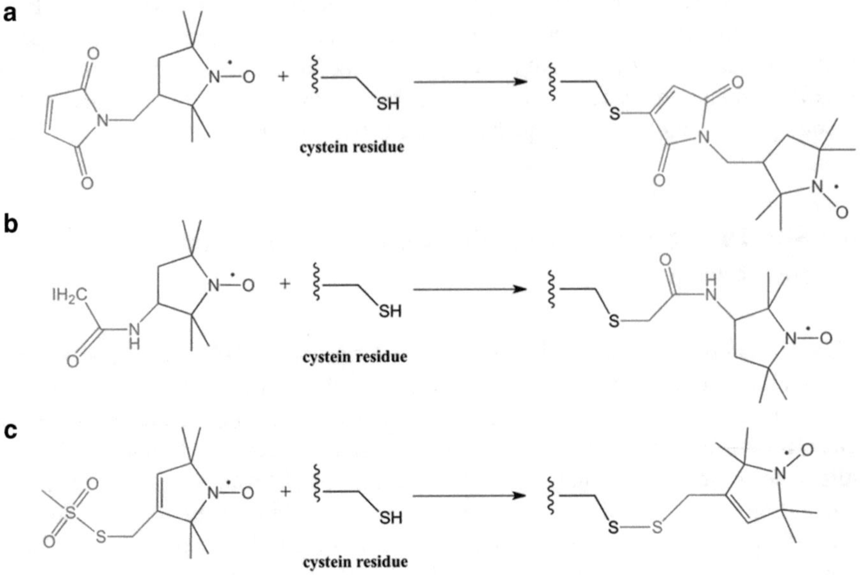

Fig. 11 Nitroxides used to label cysteines in proteins. (**a**) A maleimide label, (**b**) a iodoacetamide label, and (**c**) the methanethiosulfonate label MTSSL. All labels can be obtained from Toronto Research Chemicals

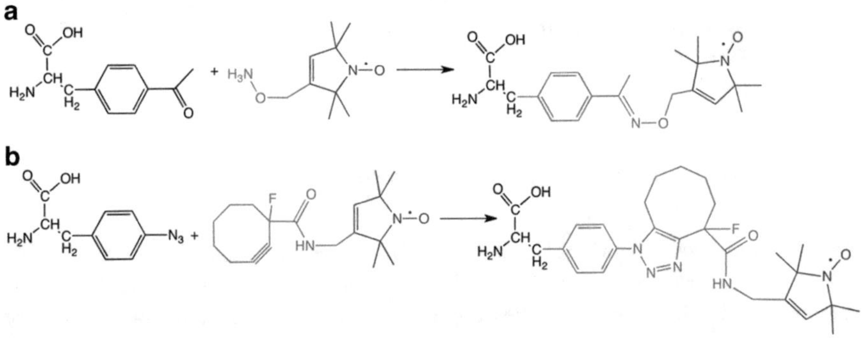

Fig. 12 Labeling of unnatural amino acids. (**a**) Labeling with the *p*-acetyl-phenylalanine/hydroxylamine couple and (**b**) labeling via "click"-chemistry

might not be feasible. In this case, labeling via unnatural amino acids can be used [71, 72]. Here, the idea is to introduce an amino acid that carries a functional group that is unique in the protein and to react this with a compatible functional group at the label. An example for this is the para-acetylphenylalanine/hydroxylamine couple [71] (Fig. 12a), which has been used successfully by several labs [73, 74].

Under reducing conditions, as encountered for example within cells, the disulfide bridge formed between MTSSL and the cysteine will be cleaved. In such cases,

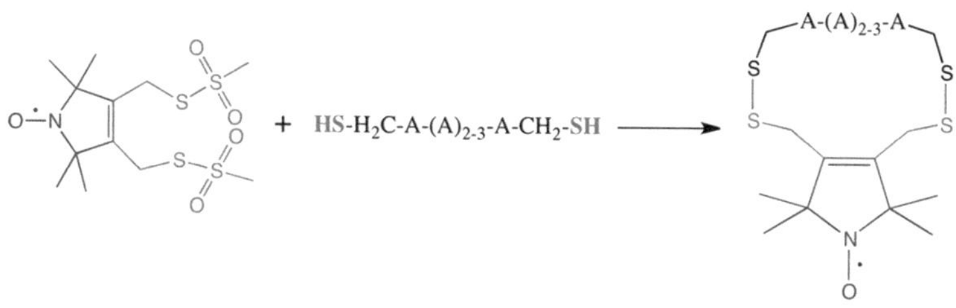

Fig. 13 Labeling with the two-legged nitroxide R_X

labels with other functional groups have to be employed. One possibility is to use click chemistry. This requires again the incorporation of an unnatural amino acid carrying a terminal alkyne group and a nitroxide with an azide group or the other way round [75] (Fig. 12b).

Beyond the linker cleavage, the nitroxide group itself is instable under reducing conditions. Studies showed that five-membered nitroxides are more stable than six-membered and that steric shielding with bulkier alkyl groups then methyl can increase the lifetime of nitroxides [76–78].

With respect to the linker, one should also keep in mind that both, structural studies and QC/QIP, will usually benefit from linker groups that are rather rigid because this reduces the label flexibility and thus structural ambiguity. Possibilities to achieve this are (a) making the linker as short as possible e.g. TOAC [79], (b) by e.g. non-covalent interactions with the protein [80, 81] or to use labels with two functional groups that bind covalently to two sites in the proteins as demonstrated by the Hubbell lab with the label R_X [82]. R_X binds to two cysteines, which are separated by 2–3 amino acids between them (Fig. 13).

4.2 Labeling of Proteins with Trityl Radicals

In order to overcome the short lifetime under reducing conditions, short phase memory times and low spectral sensitivity other spin-bearing moieties than nitroxides are thought after. Currently, there are efforts made to establish the carbon centered trityl radicals as spin labels. These have line widths as narrow as 3 Gauss, which enables the selective excitation of a particular spin state; and the phase memory times at ambient temperature are up to several microseconds, which is longer than those of radicals in photosynthetic proteins. In addition, the trityl radicals are stable under reducing conditions. Double Quantum Coherence (DQC) and PELDOR measurements on bis-trityl and trityl/nitroxide model systems showed that such labels also yield higher sensitivity in these experiments and that exchange and dipolar coupling can be separated [83, 84] (Fig 14a). Application of trityls as labels for proteins has been shown by the Hubbell lab (Fig. 14b), which permitted DQC measurements at room temperature [85].

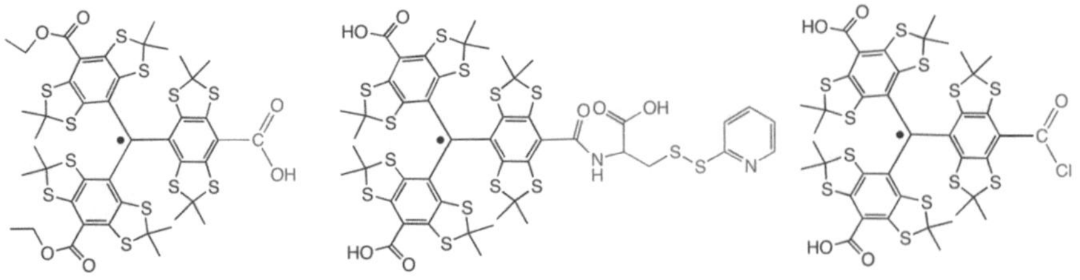

Fig. 14 Trityl labels for (**a**) hydroxyl groups in materials, yielding ester linkages, (**b**) for cysteines in proteins, yielding disulfide bridges, and (**c**) for oligonucleotides, yielding together with *N,N'*-carbonyldiimidazole and 1,4-piperazine a Trityl conjugated to the 5'-end of an oligonucleotide via an ester-piperazine linker

4.3 Labeling of Proteins with Metal Centers

The limitations of the nitroxide labels might also be overcome by using paramagnetic metal complexes. Well-studied examples are the Gd^{3+}-labels pioneered by the Goldfarb lab [86]. Such labels are stable under in-cell conditions [87], have at high field/high frequency a narrow $m_s = \pm 1/2$ transition, and give in PELDOR experiments on model peptides [88] and on proteins [89] time traces with high signal to noise ratio and rather narrow distance distributions. Usually, these measurements are performed at Q- or W-band [86]. Recently, the Mn^{2+} analogue of the Gd^{2+}-DOTA has been reported and successfully used on model peptides to obtain distances up to 4.5 nm [90]. The lab of Saxena showed that a double histidine sequence enables to rigidly bind a Cu^{2+}-complex site specifically to this sequence in a protein. In this way, they were able to obtain a Cu-Cu distance of 2.5 nm in the B1 immunoglobulin-binding domain of protein G [91].

Instead of using artificial metal complexes, one can also make use of intrinsic paramagnetic ions or clusters within proteins. Examples for this are the Mn^{2+} ion in PSII, which has been studied with PELDOR as early as 1998 by the lab of Kawamori [92], FeS and NiFe clusters in a hydrogenase [93] and Cu^{2+} in the EcoRI endonuclease [94]. A combination of SDSL and PELDOR has recently been shown to enable the localization of a Cu^{2+} ion within the three-dimensional fold a protein, here azurin [95]. For metal centers with faster relaxation times, broad spectral width or a spectrum separated from $g = 2$ a pulsed EPR method called Relaxation Induced Dipolar Modulation Enhancement (RIDME) might be more useful especially in its dead-time free five pulse version [96], due to better sensitivity, weaker orientation selection, and because the metal center does not need to be excited by a microwave pulse but flips instantaneous by its T_1 relaxation. For metal centers in proteins, this has been demonstrated for example on the heme protein Cyp_{101} [97], other examples have been reviewed by Astashkin [98].

4.4 Labeling of Oligonucleotides

The DNA double helix contains only four different canonical nucleotides with the bases adenine, guanine, cytosine, and thymine. Thus, the uniqueness of chemical groups in DNA is even more limited than in proteins. However, unique groups can be introduced during the phosphoramidite synthesis of the DNA at the wanted position in the nucleotide sequence and this can then be reacted selectively with labels carrying a complementary functional group. Examples of site-specifically attached nitroxides are shown in Fig. 15.

Labeling at the phosphate backbone can be achieved with the thiol-reactive nitroxide 3-iodomethyl-(1-oxy-2,2,5,5-tetramethylpyrroline), which reacts with a phosphorothioate modification leading (**1**) in Fig. 15 [100]. One possibility of labeling the sugar group is to react isocyanate tetramethylpiperidinyl-*N*-oxy with 2'-amino modified uridine (**2**) [101]. Bases can be labeled for example via palladium catalyzed cross coupling between 2,2,5,5-Tetramethylpyrroline-1-oxyl-3-acetylene and iodo-modified bases e.g. 5-iodo-uridine (**3**) [102]. Another possibility is to react 4-Amino tetramethylpiperidinyl-*N*-oxy with a correspondingly modified cytidine phosphoramidite (**4**) [103] or to click Azidoisoindoline-*N*-oxy with an alkyne modified uridine (**5**) [104]. Instead of incorporating a matching modified nucleotide into the DNA and reacting it after the DNA synthesis with a spin label, one can also incorporate an already spin-labeled phosphoramidite into the DNA. Such an example is the very rigid spin label **Ç** (**6**), which has been successfully used in orientation selective PELDOR measurements on DNA [105]. The analogue of **Ç** shown in (**7**) has the advantage that it is still rigid but it avoids elaborate synthesis of the phosphoramidite because the label binds non-covalently to abasic sites opposite to a guanine in DNA duplexes [106]. The initialization, manipulation/computing, and readout of quantum information stored in spin systems are crucial for QC/QIP.

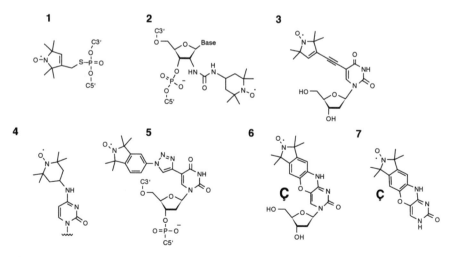

Fig. 15 Nitroxides used for spin labeling of nucleic acids (adapted from [99])

Orientation selective excitation becomes possible by rather rigid spin labels. Since the manipulation corresponds to the selective excitation between particular spin states, such rigid spin labels are necessary in QC/QIP. For more details on nitroxide labeling of oligonucleotides, see for example [107]. Highly excitingly, the lab of Bagryanskaya reported recently the labeling of oligonucleotides with trityl labels at the 5′-ends of the duplexes. This enabled, as for proteins, DQC-based distance measurements on immobilized DNA at ambient temperatures (Fig. 14c) [108].

4.5 EPR-Based Nanometer Distance Measurements

EPR spectroscopy provides various methods for measuring the dipolar coupling between unpaired electrons. Continuous wave (CW) EPR methods are usually restricted to distances below 2.5 nm [109] whereas pulsed EPR experiments have been shown to be applicable for distances of up to 8 nm [110].

Pulse sequences working with one microwave frequency are SIFTER, double-quantum coherence (DQC) EPR, and RIDME (Fig. 16). SIFTER is based on the solid echo sequence and has been shown to work nicely in combination with shaped broadband pulses using an arbitrary wave function generator [111]. DQC-EPR uses a double-quantum filter and works best if the whole spectrum is excited either by

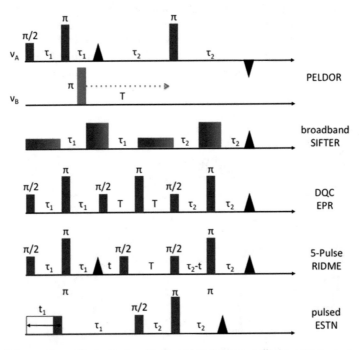

Fig. 16 Pulse sequences for measuring dipolar and exchange coupling constants

using hard (broadband) pulses or by using labels with narrow spectral widths, e.g. trityl radicals [85]. RIDME relies on one of the spin centers having a faster T_1 relaxation time than the other [97], although it has also been applied to bis-nitroxide systems [96]. An alternative strategy for removing unwanted hyperfine interactions is used in PELDOR [112–114]. Here, the detection pulses, applied at one microwave frequency (ν_A), excite spin A in a two-spin system and create a refocused Hahn-echo. In contrast, the pump pulse excites spin B in the same system using a different microwave frequency (ν_B) than for spin A. This requires two microwave sources, which are not phase correlated. If two identical spin labels are used, the differentiation between spin A and B can be done if the spectral width is larger than the excitation bandwidth of the pulses (orientation selection via the hyperfine and g-tensor). If in addition spin A and B are structurally correlated, meaning the labels are rigidly attached to a rigid biomolecule, the PELDOR time traces are orientation selective with respect to the dipolar tensor, which provides not only distance but also angular information [105]. Application of the pump pulse between the two π-pulses of the detection makes the PELDOR time traces dead-time free, like the 5-pulse RIDME sequence. Thus, the dipolar coupling frequencies and the distance distributions can be obtained very precisely. This also enables the separation of dipolar from exchange coupling as shown on several model systems [115]. If the dipolar and exchange coupling between the spin centers is very small, pulsed ESTN spectroscopy may be used to determine both contributions [116]. With respect to QC/QIP, especially the excitation with two different microwave frequencies, like in PELDOR, may become a key technology to manipulate particular spin states selectively.

Acknowledgments We gratefully acknowledge financial support of the Deutsche Forschungsgemeinschaft (DFG) through the Collaborative Research Center SFB813 "Chemistry at Spin Centers." This work was also supported by Grants-in-Aid for Scientific Research (C) and Scientific Research on Innovative Areas, "Quantum Cybernetics," MEXT, Japan.

References

1. S. Barz, E. Kashefi, A. Broadbent, J.F. Fitzsimons, Z. Zeilinger, P. Walther, Demonstration of blind quantum computing. Science **335**, 303–308 (2012)
2. B.P. Lanyon, C. Hempel, D. Nigg, M. Müller, R. Gerritsma, F. Zähringer, P. Schindler, J.T. Barreiro, M. Rambach, G. Kirchmair, M. Hennrich, P. Zoller, R. Blatt, C.F. Roos, Universal digital quantum simulation with trapped ions. Science **334**, 57–60 (2011)
3. K.C. Nowack, M. Shafiei, M. Laforest, G.E.D.K. Prawiroatmodjo, L.R. Schreiber, C. Reichl, W. Wegscheider, L.M.K. Vandersypen, Single-shot correlations and two-qubit gate of solid-state spins. Science **333**, 1269–1272 (2011)
4. X. Zhu, S. Saito, A. Kemp, K. Kakuyanagi, S. Karimoto, H. Nakano, W.J. Munro, Y. Tokura, M.S. Everitt, K. Nemoto, M. Kasu, N. Mizuochi, K. Semba, Coherent coupling of a superconducting flux qubit to an electron spin ensemble in diamond. Nature **478**, 221–224 (2011)

5. G.D. Scholes, G.R. Fleming, A. Olaya-Castro, R. van Grondelle, Lessons from nature about solar light harvesting. Nat. Chem. **3**, 763–774 (2011)
6. S. Lloyd, A quantum of natural selection. Nat. Phys. **5**, 164–166 (2010)
7. N. Lambert, Y.N. Chen, Y.C. Cheng, C.M. Li, G.Y. Chen, F. Nori, Quantum biology. Nat. Phys. **9**, 10–18 (2013)
8. P. Ball, The dawn of quantum biology. Nature **474**, 272–274 (2011)
9. E. Romero, R. Augulis, V.I. Novoderezhkin, M. Ferretti, J. Thieme, D. Zigmantas, R. van Grondelle, Quantum coherence in photosynthesis for efficient solar-energy conversion. Nat. Phys. **10**, 676–682 (2014)
10. A. Ishizakia, G.R. Fleminga, Theoretical examination of quantum coherence in a photosynthetic system at physiological temperature. Proc. Natl. Acad. Sci. U. S. A. **106**, 17255–17260 (2009)
11. G.S. Schlau-Cohen, A. Ishizaki, T.R. Calhoun, N.S. Ginsberg, M. Ballottari, R. Bassi, G.R. Fleming, Elucidation of the timescales and origins of quantum electronic coherence in LHCII. Nat. Chem. **4**, 389–395 (2012)
12. H. Lee, Y.C. Cheng, G.R. Fleming, Coherence dynamics in photosynthesis: protein protection of excitonic coherence. Science **316**, 1462–1465 (2007)
13. G.S. Engel, T.R. Calhoun, E.L. Read, T.K. Ahn, T. Mančal, Y.C. Cheng, R.E. Blankenship, G.R. Fleming, Evidence for wavelike energy transfer through quantum coherence in photosynthetic systems. Nature **446**, 782–786 (2007)
14. G. Panitchayangkoon, D. Hayes, K.A. Fransted, J.R. Caram, E. Harel, J. Wen, R.E. Blankenship, G.S. Engel, Long-lived quantum coherence in photosynthetic complexes at physiological temperature. Proc. Natl. Acad. Sci. U. S. A. **107**, 12766–12770 (2010)
15. E. Collini, C.Y. Wong, K.E. Wilk, P.M.G. Curmi, P. Brumer, G.D. Scholes, Coherently wired light-harvesting in photosynthetic marine algae at ambient temperature. Nature **463**, 644–647 (2010)
16. M. Mohseni, P. Rebentrost, S. Lloyd, A.A. Guzik, Environment-assisted quantum walks in photosynthetic energy transfer. J. Chem. Phys. **129**, 174106 (2008)
17. M. Sarovar, A. Ishizaki, G.R. Fleming, K.B. Whaley, Quantum entanglement in photosynthetic light-harvesting complexes. Nat. Phys. **6**, 462–467 (2010)
18. G.D. Scholes, Green quantum computers. Nat. Phys. **6**, 402–403 (2010)
19. G. Panitchayangkoon, D.V. Voronine, D. Abramavicius, J.R. Caram, N.H.C. Lewis, S. Mukamel, G.S. Engel, Direct evidence of quantum transport in photosynthetic light-harvesting complexes. Proc. Natl. Acad. Sci. U. S. A. **108**, 20908–20912 (2011)
20. E. Harel, G.S. Engel, Quantum coherence spectroscopy reveals complex dynamics in bacterial light harvesting complex 2 (LH2). Proc. Natl. Acad. Sci. U. S. A. **109**, 706–711 (2012)
21. R. Hildner, D. Brinks, J.B. Nieder, R.J. Cogdell, N.F. van Hulst, Quantum coherent energy transfer over varying pathways in single light-harvesting complexes. Science **340**, 1448–1451 (2013)
22. E. Collini, Spectroscopic signatures of quantum-coherent energy transfer. Chem. Soc. Rev. **42**, 4932–4947 (2013)
23. D. Hayes, G.B. Griffin, G.S. Engel, Engineering coherence among excited states in synthetic heterodimer systems. Science **340**, 1431–1434 (2013)
24. C.A. Rozzi, S.M. Falke, N. Spallanzani, A. Rubio, E. Molinari, D. Brida, M. Maiuri, G. Cerullo, H. Schramm, J. Christoffers, C. Lienau, Quantum coherence controls the charge separation in a prototypical artificial light-harvesting system. Nat. Commun. **4**, 1602 (2013)
25. E. Collini, G.D. Scholes, Coherent intrachain energy migration in a conjugated polymer at room temperature. Science **323**, 369–373 (2009)
26. S.M. Falke, C.A. Rozzi, D. Brida, M. Maiuri, M. Amato, E. Sommer, A. De Sio, A. Rubio, G. Cerullo, E. Molinari, C. Lienau, Coherent ultrafast charge transfer in an organic photovoltaic blend. Science **344**, 1001–1005 (2014)
27. S. Gélinas, A. Rao, A. Kumar, S.L. Smith, A.W. Chin, J. Clark, T.S. van der Poll, G.C. Bazan, R.H. Friend, Ultrafast long-range charge separation in organic semiconductor photovoltaic diodes. Science **343**, 512–516 (2014)

28. C.J. Brabec, N.S. Serdar Sariciftci, J.C. Hummelen, Plastic solar cells. Adv. Funct. Mater. **11**, 15–26 (2001)
29. K.M. Salikhov, Potential of electron paramagnetic resonance to study Einstein-Podolsky-Rosen-Bohm pairs. Appl. Magn. Reson. **25**, 261–276 (2003)
30. K.M. Salikhov, J.H. Golbeck, D. Stehlik, Quantum teleportation across a biological membrane by means of correlated spin pair dynamics in photosynthetic reaction centers. Appl. Magn. Reson. **31**, 237–252 (2007)
31. Y.E. Kandrashkin, K.M. Salikhov, Numerical simulation of quantum teleportation across biological membrane in photosynthetic reaction centers. Appl. Magn. Reson. **37**, 549–566 (2010)
32. T. Berthold, E.D. von Gromoff, S. Santabarbara, P. Stehle, G. Link, O.G. Poluektov, P. Heathcote, C.F. Beck, M.C. Thurnauer, G. Kothe, Exploring the electron transfer pathways in photosystem I by high-time-resolution electron paramagnetic resonance: observation of the B-side radical pair $P_{700}^+A_{1B}^-$ in whole cells of the deuterated green alga *chlamydomonas reinhardtii* at cryogenic temperatures. J. Am. Chem. Soc. **134**, 5563–5576 (2012)
33. S. Santabarbara, I. Kuprov, W.V. Fairclough, S. Purton, P.J. Hore, P. Heathcote, M.C.W. Evans, Bidirectional electron transfer in photosystem I: determination of two distances between P_{700}^+ and A_1^- in spin-correlated radical pairs. Biochemistry **44**, 2119–2128 (2005)
34. P.J. Hore, D.A. Hunter, C.D. McKie, A.J. Hoff, Electron paramagnetic resonance of spin-correlated radical pairs in photosynthetic reactions. Chem. Phys. Lett. **137**, 495–500 (1987)
35. R. Bitt, G. Kothe, Transient EPR of radical pairs in photosynthetic reaction centers prediction of quantum beats. Chem. Phys. Lett. **177**, 547–553 (1991)
36. M. Gierer, A. van der Est, D. Stehlik, Transient EPR of weakly coupled spin-correlated radical pairs in photosynthetic reaction centres: increased spectral resolution from nutation analysis. Chem. Phys. Lett. **186**, 238–247 (1991)
37. G. Kothe, S. Weber, R. Bitt, E. Ohmes, M.C. Thurnauer, J.R. Norris, Transient EPR of light-induced radical pairs in plant photosystem I: observation of quantum beats. Chem. Phys. Lett. **186**, 474–480 (1991)
38. G. Zwanenburg, P.J. Hore, EPR of spin-correlated radical pairs. Analytical treatment of selective excitation including zero-quantum coherence. Chem. Phys. Lett. **203**, 65–74 (1993)
39. G. Kothe, S. Weber, E. Ohmes, M.C. Thurnauer, J.R. Norris, High time resolution electron paramagnetic resonance of light-induced radical pairs in photosynthetic bacterial reaction centers: observation of quantum beats. J. Am. Chem. Soc. **114**, 1129–1134 (1994)
40. Z. Wang, J. Tang, J. Norris, The time development of the magnetic moment of correlated radical pairs. J. Magn. Reson. **97**, 322–334 (1992)
41. G. Kothe, S. Weber, E. Ohmes, M.C. Thurnauer, J.R. Norris, Transient EPR of light-induced spin-correlated radical pairs: manifestation of zero quantum coherence. J. Phys. Chem. **98**, 2706–2712 (1994)
42. K. Maekawa, S. Nakazawa, H. Atsumi, D. Shiomi, K. Sato, M. Kitagawa, T. Takui, K. Nakatani, Programmed assembly of organic radicals on DNA. Chem. Commun. **46**, 1247–1249 (2010)
43. H. Atsumi, K. Maekawa, S. Nakazawa, D. Shiomi, D. Sato, M. Kitagawa, T. Takui, K. Nakatani, Tandem arrays of TEMPO and nitronyl nitroxide radicals with designed arrangements on DNA. Chem. Eur. J. **18**, 178–183 (2012)
44. Y. Morita, Y. Yakiyama, S. Nakazawa, T. Murata, T. Ise, D. Hashizume, D. Shiomi, K. Sato, M. Kitagawa, K. Nakasuji, T. Takui, Triple-stranded metallo-helicates addressable as Lloyd's electron spin qubits. J. Am. Chem. Soc. **132**, 6944–6946 (2010)
45. C.R. Timmel, J.R. Harmer (eds.), *Structural Information from Spin-Labels and Intrinsic Paramagnetic Centers in the Biosciences.* Structure and Bonding, vol. 152 (Springer, Berlin, 2014), pp. 1–332
46. S. Nakazawa, S. Nishida, T. Ise, T. Yoshino, N. Mori, R.D. Rahimi, K. Sato, Y. Morita, K. Toyota, D. Shiomi, M. Kitagawa, H. Hara, P. Carl, P. Höfer, T. Takui, A synthetic

two-spin quantum bit: g-engineered exchange-coupled biradical designed for controlled-NOT gate operations. Angew. Chem. Int. Ed. **51**, 9860–9864 (2012)

47. K. Sato, S. Nakazawa, R. Rahimi, T. Ise, S. Nishida, T. Yoshino, N. Mori, K. Toyota, D. Shiomi, Y. Yakiyama, Y. Morita, M. Kitagawa, K. Nakasuji, M. Nakahara, H. Hara, P. Carl, P. Höfer, T. Takui, Molecular electron-spin quantum computers and quantum information processing: pulse-based electron magnetic resonance spin technology applied to matter spin-qubits. J. Mater. Chem. **19**, 3739–3754 (2009)

48. P. Jordan, P. Fromme, H.T. Witt, O. Klukas, W. Saenger, N. Krauss, Three-dimensional structure of cyanobacterial photosystem I at 2.5 A resolution. Nature **411**, 909–917 (2001)

49. M.V. Fedin, E.G. Bagryanskaya, H. Matsuoka, S. Yamauchi, S.L. Veber, K.Y. Maryunina, E.V. Tretyakov, V.I. Ovcharenko, R.Z. Sagdeev, W-band time-resolved electron paramagnetic resonance study of light-induced spin dynamics in copper-nitroxide-based switchable molecular magnets. J. Am. Chem. Soc. **134**, 16319–16326 (2012)

50. M. Tanabe, H. Matsuoka, Y. Ohba, S. Yamauchi, K. Sugisaki, K. Toyota, K. Sato, T. Takui, I. Goldberg, I. Saltsman, Z. Gross, Time-resolved electron paramagnetic resonance and phosphorescence studies of the lowest excited triplet states of Rh(III) corrole complexes. J. Phys. Chem. A **116**, 9662–9673 (2012)

51. J. Fujisawa, Y. Ohba, S. Yamauchi, A time-resolved electron paramagnetic resonance study of excited triplet porphyrins in fluid solution. J. Am. Chem. Soc. **119**, 8736–8737 (1997)

52. H. Matsuoka, L. Utschig, O. Poluektov, E. Ohmes, Y. Ohba, M.C. Thurnauer, G. Kothe, S. Yamauchi, W-band cw and pulse EPR studies of photosystem I reaction center, in *7th Asia-Pacific EPR/ESR Symposium 2010*, p. 110

53. Y. Umena, K. Kawakami, J.R. Shen, N. Kamiya, Crystal structure of oxygen-evolving photosystem II at a resolution of 1.9 Å. Nature **473**, 55–61 (2011)

54. N. Kamiya, J.R. Shen, Crystal structure of oxygen-evolving photosystem II from Thermosynechococcus vulcanus at 3.7 Å resolution. Proc. Natl. Acad. Sci. U. S. A. **100**, 98–103 (2003)

55. H. Matsuoka, J.R. Shen, A. Kawamori, K. Nishiyama, Y. Ohba, S. Yamauchi, Proton-coupled electron-transfer processes in photosystem II probed by highly resolved g-anisotropy of redox-active tyrosine Yz. J. Am. Chem. Soc. **133**, 4655–4660 (2011)

56. H. Matsuoka, K. Furukawa, T. Kato, H. Mino, J.R. Shen, A. Kawamori, g-Anisotropy of the S_2-state manganese cluster in single crystals of cyanobacterial photosystem II studied by w-band electron paramagnetic resonance spectroscopy. J. Phys. Chem. B **110**, 13242–13247 (2006)

57. A. Kawamori, J.R. Shen, H. Mino, K. Furukawa, H. Matsuoka, T. Kato, in *Photosynthesis: Fundamental Aspects to Global Perspectives*, ed. by A. van der Est, D. Bruce (Allen Press, Lawrence, 2005), pp. 406–408

58. D. Leupold, B. Voigt, W. Beenken, H. Stiel, Pigment-protein architecture in the light-harvesting antenna complexes of purple bacteria: does the crystal structure reflect the native pigment-protein arrangement? FEBS Lett. **480**, 73–78 (2000)

59. P. Atkins, J. de Paula, *Atkins' Physical Chemistry*, 8th edn. (Oxford University Press, Oxford, 2006), p. 856

60. T. Ritz, P. Thalau, J.B. Phillips, R. Wiltschko, W. Wiltschko, Resonance effects indicate a radical-pair mechanism for avian magnetic compass. Nature **429**, 177–180 (2004)

61. K. Maeda, K.B. Henbest, F. Cintolesi, I. Kuprov, C.T. Rodgers, P.A. Liddell, D. Gust, C.R. Timmel, P.J. Hore, Chemical compass model of avian magnetoreception. Nature **453**, 387–390 (2008)

62. G. Link, T. Berthold, M. Bechtold, J.U. Weidner, E. Ohmes, J. Tang, O. Poluektov, L. Utschig, S.L. Schlesselman, M.C. Thurnauer, G. Kothe, Structure of the $P_{700}{}^+A_1{}^-$ radical pair intermediate in photosystem I by high time resolution multifrequency electron paramagnetic resonance: analysis of quantum beat oscillations. J. Am. Chem. Soc. **123**, 4211–4222 (2001)

63. T. Takui, S. Nakazawa, H. Matsuoka, K. Furukawa, K. Sato, D. Shiomi, Molecule-based exchange-coupled high-spin clusters: conventional high-field/high-frequency and pulse-based electron spin resonance of molecule-based magnetically coupled systems, in *EPR of Free Radicals in Solids II: Trends in Method and Applications*, ed. by A. Lund, M. Shiotani, 2nd edn. (Springer, Dordrecht, 2012), pp. 71–162

64. H. Matsuoka, K. Sato, D. Shiomi, T. Takui, 2D electron spin transient nutation spectroscopy of lanthanoid ion $Eu^{2+}(^{8}S_{7/2})$ in a CaF_2 single crystal on the basis of FT-pulsed electron spin resonance spectroscopy: transition moment spectroscopy. Appl. Magn. Reson. **23**, 517–538 (2003)

65. A. Furusawa, P. van Loock, *Quantum Teleportation and Entanglement: A Hybrid Approach to Optical Quantum Information Processing* (Wiley-VCH, Weinheim, 2011)

66. H. Matsuoka, Toward Manipulation of Quantum Spin Information in Biomolecules, Quantum Cybernetics Newsletter, vol. 12, pp. 15, (2014)

67. C. Altenbach, T. Marti, H.G. Khorana, W.L. Hubbell, Transmembrane protein structure: spin labeling of bacteriorhodopsin mutants. Science **248**, 1088–1092 (1990)

68. O.H. Griffith, H.M. McConnell, A nitroxide-maleimide spin label. Proc. Natl. Acad. Sci. U. S. A. **55**, 8–11 (1966)

69. S. Ogawa, H.M. McConnell, Spin label study of hemoglobin conformations in solution. Proc. Natl. Acad. Sci. U. S. A. **58**, 19–26 (1967)

70. L.J. Berliner, J. Grundwald, H.O. Hankovszky, K. Hideg, A novel reversible thiol-specific spin label: papain active site labeling and inhibition. Anal. Biochem. **119**, 450–455 (1982)

71. M.R. Fleissner, E.M. Brustad, T. Kálái, C. Altenbach, D. Cascio, F.B. Peters, K. Hideg, S. Peuker, P.G. Schultz, W.L. Hubbell, Site-directed spin labeling of a genetically encoded unnatural amino acid. Proc. Natl. Acad. Sci. U. S. A. **106**, 21637–21642 (2009)

72. M.J. Schmidt, J. Borbas, M. Drescher, D. Summerer, A genetically encoded spin label for electron paramagnetic resonance distance measurements. J. Am. Chem. Soc. **136**, 1238–1241 (2014)

73. G. Hagelueken, F.G. Duthie, N. Florin, E. Schubert, O. Schiemann, Expression, purification and spin labelling of the ferrous iron transporter FeoB from *Escherichia coli* BL21 for EPR studies. Protein Expr. Purif. **114**, 30–36 (2015)

74. A.J. Fielding, M.G. Concilio, G. Heaven, M.A. Hollas, New developments in spin labels for pulsed dipolar EPR. Molecules **19**, 16998–17025 (2014)

75. T. Kalai, W. Hubbell, K. Hideg, Click reactions with nitroxides. Synthesis **2009**, 1336–1340 (2009)

76. I. Krstic, R. Hänsel, O. Romainczyk, J.W. Engels, V. Dötsch, T.F. Prisner, Long-range distance measurements on nucleic acids in cells by pulsed EPR spectroscopy. Angew. Chem. Int. Ed. **50**, 5070–5074 (2011)

77. A.P. Jagtap, I. Krstic, N.C. Kunjir, R. Hänsel, T.F. Prisner, S.T. Sigurdsson, Sterically shielded spin labels for in-cell EPR spectroscopy: analsis of stability in reducing environments. Free Radic. Res. **49**, 78–85 (2015)

78. I.A. Kirilyuk, A.A. Bobko, I.A. Grigorev, V.V. Khramtsov, Synthesis of the tetraethyl substituted pH-sensitive nitroxides of imidazole series with enhanced stability towards reduction. Org. Biomol. Chem. **2**, 1025–1030 (2004)

79. S. Schreier, J.C. Bozelli, N. Marin, R.F.F. Vieira, C.R. Nakaie, The spin label amino acid TOAC and its use in studies of peptides: chemical, physicochemical, spectroscopic, and conformational aspects. Biophys. Rev. **4**, 45–66 (2012)

80. N. Florin, O. Schiemann, G. Hagelueken, High-resolution crystal structure of spin labelled (T21R1) azurin from Pseudomonas aeruginosa: a challenging structural benchmark for in silico spin labelling algorithms. BMC Struct. Biol. **14**(16), 1–10 (2014)

81. L. Urban, H.J. Steinhoff, Hydrogen bonding to the nitroxide of protein bound spin labels. Mol. Phys. **111**, 2873–2881 (2013)

82. M.R. Fleissner, M.D. Bridges, E.K. Brooks, D. Cascio, T. Kalai, K. Hideg, W.L. Hubbell, Structure and dynamics of a conformationally constrained nitroxide side chain and applications in EPR spectroscopy. Proc. Natl. Acad. Sci. U. S. A. **108**, 16241–16246 (2011)

83. G.W. Reginsson, N.C. Kunjir, S.T. Sigurdsson, O. Schiemann, Trityl radicals: spin labels for nanometer distance measurements. Chem. Eur. J. **18**, 13580–13584 (2012)

84. N.C. Kunjir, G.W. Reginsson, O. Schiemann, S.T. Sigurdsson, Measurements of short distances between trityl spin labels with CW EPR, DQC and PELDOR. Phys. Chem. Chem. Phys. **15**, 19673–19685 (2013)

85. Z. Yang, Y. Liu, P. Borbat, J.L. Zweier, J.H. Freed, W.L. Hubbell, Pulsed ESR dipolar spectroscopy for distance measurements in immobilized spin labeled proteins in liquid solution. J. Am. Chem. Soc. **134**, 9950–9952 (2012)

86. D. Goldfarb, Gd^{3+} spin labeling for distance measurements by pulse EPR spectroscopy. Phys. Chem. Chem. Phys. **16**, 9685–9699 (2014)

87. M. Qi, A. Gross, G. Jeschke, A. Godt, M. Drescher, Gd(III)-PyMTA label is suitable for in-cell EPR. J. Am. Chem. Soc. **136**, 15366–15378 (2014)

88. E. Matalon, T. Huber, G. Hagelueken, B. Graham, A. Feintuch, V. Frydman, G. Otting, D. Goldfarb, Angew. Chem. Int. Ed. **52**, 11831–11834 (2013)

89. H. Yagi, D. Banerjee, B. Graham, T. Huber, D. Goldfarb, O. Gottfried, J. Am. Chem. Soc. **133**, 10418–10421 (2011)

90. H.Y. Ching, P. Demay-Drouhard, H.C. Bertrand, C. Policar, L.C. Tabares, S. Un, Nanometric distance measurements between Mn(II)DOTA centers. Phys. Chem. Chem. Phys. **17**(36), 23368–23377 (2015). doi:10.1039/c5cp03487f

91. T.F. Cunningham, M.R. Putterman, A. Desai, W.S. Horne, S. Saxena, The double histidine Cu(II)-binding motif: a highly rigid, site-specific spin probe for ESR distance measurements. Angew. Chem. Int. Ed. **54**, 6330–6334 (2015)

92. A.V. Astashkin, H. Hara, A. Kawamori, The pulsed electro-electron double-resonance and 2-spin echo study of the oriented oxygen-evolving and mn-depleted preparations of photosystem-II. J. Chem. Phys. **108**, 3805–3812 (1998)

93. C. Elsässer, M. Brecht, R. Bittl, Pulsed electron-electron double resonance on multinuclear metal clusters: assignment of spin projection factors based on the dipolar interaction. J. Am. Chem. Soc. **124**, 12606–12611 (2002)

94. Z. Yang, M. Kurpiewski, M. Ji, J.E. Townsend, P. Mehta, L. Jen-Jacobson, S. Saxena, ESR spectroscopy identifies inhibitory Cu(II) sites in a DNA modifying enzyme to reveal determinants of catalytic specificity. Proc. Natl. Acad. Sci. U. S. A. **109**, E993–E1000 (2012)

95. D. Abdullin, N. Florin, G. Hagelueken, O. Schiemann, EPR-based approach for the localization of paramagnetic metal ions in biomolecules. Angew. Chem. Int. Ed. **54**, 1827–1831 (2015)

96. S. Milikisyants, F. Scarpelli, M.G. Finiguerra, M. Ubbink, M.A. Huber, Pulsed EPR method to determine distances between paramagnetic centers with strong spectral anisotropy and radicals: the dead-time free RIDME sequence. J. Magn. Reson. **201**, 48–56 (2009)

97. D. Abdullin, F. Duthie, A. Meyer, E.S. Müller, G. Hagelueken, O. Schiemann, Comparison of PELDOR and RIDME for distance measurements between nitroxides and low spin Fe(III) ions. J. Phys. Chem. B **119**(43), 13534–13542 (2015). doi:10.1021/acs.jpcb.5b02118

98. A.V. Astashkin, Mapping the structure of metalloproteins with RIDME. Methods Enzymol. **563**, 251–284 (2015). doi:10.1016/bs.mie.2015.06.031

99. R. Ward, O. Schiemann, Structural information from oligonucleotides. Struct. Bond. **152**, 249–282 (2014)

100. P.Z. Quin, I.S. Haworth, Q. Cai, A.K. Kusnetzow, G.P. Grant, E.A. Price, G.Z. Sowa, A. Popova, B. Herreos, H. He, Measuring nanometer distances in nucleic acids using a sequence-independent nitroxide probe. Nat. Protoc. **2**, 2354–2365 (2007)

101. O. Schiemann, A. Weber, T.E. Edwards, T.F. Prisner, S.T. Sigurdsson, Nanometer distance measurements on RNA using PELDOR. J. Am. Chem. Soc. **125**, 3434–3435 (2003)

102. N. Piton, Y. Mu, G. Stock, T.F. Prisner, O. Schiemann, J.W. Engels, Base-specific spin labeling of RNA for structure determination. Nucleic Acids Res. **35**, 3128–3143 (2007)

103. C. Giordano, F. Fratini, D. Attanasio, L. Cellai, Preparation of spin-labeled 2-amino-dA, dA, dC and 5-methyl-dC phosphoramidites for the automatic synthesis of EPR active oligonucleotides. Synthesis **4**, 565–572 (2001)

104. P. Ding, D. Wunnicke, H.J. Steinhoff, F. Seela, Site-directed spin-labeling of DNA by the azide-alkyne 'click' reaction: nanometer distance measurements on 7-deaza-2-'-deoxyadenosin and 2'-deoxyuridine nitroxide conjugates spatially separated or linked to a 'dA-dT' base pair. Chem. Eur. J. **16**, 14385–14396 (2010)

105. O. Schiemann, P. Cekan, D. Margraf, T.F. Prisner, S.T. Sigurdsson, Relative orientation of rigid nitroxides by PELDOR: beyond distance measurements in nucleic acids. Angew. Chem. Int. Ed. **48**, 3292–3295 (2009)

106. G.W. Reginsson, S. Shelke, C. Rouillon, M.F. White, S.T. Sigurdsson, O. Schiemann, Protein-induced changes in DNA structure and dynamics observed with non-covalent site-directed spin-labelling and PELDOR. Nucleic Acids Res. **41**(1), e11 (2013). doi:10.1093/nar/gks817

107. S.A. Shelke, S.T. Sigurdsson, Site-directed nitroxide spin labeling of biopolymers. Struct. Bond. **152**, 121–162 (2014)

108. G.J. Shevlev, O.A. Krumkacheva, A.A. Lomzov, A.A. Kuzhelev, O.Y. Rogozhnikova, D.V. Trukhin, T.I. Troitskaya, V.M. Tormyshev, M.V. Fedin, D.V. Pyshnyi, E.G. Bagryanskaya, Physiological-temperature distance measurements in nucleic acids using triarylmethyl-based spin labels and pulsed dipolar EPR spectroscopy. J. Am. Chem. Soc. **136**, 9874–9877 (2014)

109. X. Zhang, P. Cekan, S.T. Sigurdsson, P.Z. Qin, Studying RNA using site-directed spin-labeling and continuous-wave electron paramagnetic resonance spectroscopy. Methods Enzymol. **469**, 303–328 (2009)

110. O. Schiemann, T.F. Prisner, Long-range distance determinations in biomacromolecules by EPR spectroscopy. Q. Rev. Biophys. **40**, 1–53 (2007)

111. P. Schöps, P.E. Spindler, A. Marko, T.F. Prisner, Broadband spin echoes and broadband SIFTER in EPR. J. Magn. Reson. **250**, 55–62 (2015)

112. A.D. Milov, K.M. Salikhov, M.D. Shirov, Application of ENDOR in electron-spin echo for paramagnetic center space distribution in solids. Fiz. Tverd. Tela **23**, 975–982 (1981)

113. G. Jeschke, DEER distance measurements on proteins. Annu. Rev. Phys. Chem. **63**, 419–446 (2012)

114. G.W. Reginsson, O. Schiemann, Pulsed electron-electron double resonance on biomacromolecules: beyond nanometer distance measurements. Biochem. J. **434**, 353–363 (2011)

115. D. Margraf, P. Cekan, T. Prisner, S. Sigurdsson, O. Schiemann, Ferro- and antiferromagnetic exchange coupling constants in PELDOR spectra. Phys. Chem. Chem. Phys. **11**, 6708–6714 (2009)

116. K. Ayabe, K. Sato, S. Nakazawa, S. Nishida, K. Sugisaki, T. Ise, Y. Morita, K. Toyota, D. Shiomi, M. Kitagawa, S. Suzuki, K. Okada, T. Takui, Pulsed electron spin nutation spectroscopy for weakly exchange-coupled multi-spin molecular systems with nuclear hyperfine couplings: a general approach to bi- and triradicals and determination of their spin dipolar and exchange interactions. Mol. Phys. **111**, 2767–2787 (2013)

Adiabatic Quantum Computing on Molecular Spin Quantum Computers

Satoru Yamamoto, Shigeaki Nakazawa, Kenji Sugisaki, Kazunobu Sato, Kazuo Toyota, Daisuke Shiomi, and Takui Takeji

Abstract A molecular spin quantum computer (MSQC) is a model of QCs, in which we manipulate bus electron spins with client nuclear spins by pulse-based electron spin/magnetic resonance (ESR/MR) techniques applied to well-defined open-shell molecular entities. The spin manipulation executes quantum computation ranging over all Hilbert space, which is achieved by sets of quantum gate operations, called universal gates. The bus electron spin quantum bits (qubits) interact extensively with other electron spins and relatively localized nuclear spins as client qubits. Since the electron spins play the central role in MSQCs, MSQCs can simply be regarded as ESR-QCs. Generally compared with NMR-QC, ESR-QCs have advantages in fast gate operations, global control in client qubits, and initialization process. On the other hand, apparent disadvantages are fast decoherence and technical difficulties in current spin manipulation technology.

In this chapter, we introduce the implementation of an adiabatic quantum computation from the theoretical point of view. The main issue is quantum operations in realistic Adiabatic Quantum Computers (AQCs) based on molecular spin systems, suggesting that the established experimental schemes and protocols render MSQCs realistic. For this purpose, an algorithm is selected for an adiabatic factorization problem of 21, as we compare with the comparable algorithm of NMR experiments with three nuclear qubits. Toward adiabatic quantum computation on MSQCs, two molecular spin systems are selected: One is a molecular spin composed of three exchange/dipole-coupled electrons as electron-only spin qubits and the other an electron-bus qubit with two client nuclear spin qubits. Their electronic spin structures are well characterized particularly in terms of quantum mechanical behavior as interpreted by their spin Hamiltonians. The implementation of AQC has been achieved by establishing ESR/MR pulse sequences applied to the spin Hamiltonians in a fully controlled manner of spin manipulation. The conquered pulse sequences have been compared with the NMR-QC experiments and

S. Yamamoto • S. Nakazawa • K. Sugisaki • K. Sato • K. Toyota • D. Shiomi • T. Takeji (✉)
Department of Chemistry and Molecular Materials Science, Graduate School of Science,
Osaka City University, 3-3-138, Sugimoto, Sumiyoshi, Osaka 558-8585, Japan
e-mail: takui@sci.osaka-cu.ac.jp

© Springer New York 2016   79
T. Takui et al. (eds.), *Electron Spin Resonance (ESR) Based Quantum Computing*,
Biological Magnetic Resonance 31, DOI 10.1007/978-1-4939-3658-8_4

standard QCs. A significant result is that MSQCs can perform adiabatic quantum computations efficiently as same as standard QCs, and the computations can be performed in ESR timescale even if the client nuclear spin qubits participate in the computation processes.

Keywords Molecular spin qubits • Adiabatic quantum computing • Pulse sequences

1   Introduction

In the current era, chemists or materials scientists in emerging fields discuss the quantum states of electrons and nuclei in materials, and they have attempted to implement molecular quantum devices at various levels in microscopic scales. Their attempts are categorized as bottom-up approaches. On the computer technology, down-sizing approaches have been facing physical limits of classical computers (CCs) manufactured on current technology [1, 2], in which further device miniaturization gives rise to quantum interference. Quantum behavior of molecules, especially spin-bearing entities, underlain by molecular optimization for quantum functioning, has attracted considerable attention [3–10], and the relevant interests from the viewpoint of spin science range widely. One major issue is the observations for functionalized spin properties and the other one is the manipulation or control of spin qubits at a desired manner in molecular systems. Quantum computers (QCs) can afford to contribute to range over these problems, which execute calculations beyond the limits of CCs and will require us to establish further molecular optimizations for scalable and practical molecular spin quantum computers (MSQCs). This is an important aspect of implementing QCs as well as a current target in spin science.

According to enormous computational capability, nowadays CC is an essential source for any analyses in pure and applied sciences, but it is known that the total computational capability is intrinsically restricted by its physical "classical" reality [2, 11, 12] and most quantum problems belonging to NP (Non-deterministic Polynomial time) class are not possible to solve efficiently [13–15]. QC is a new paradigm in that bits relevant to quantum states (qubits) are capable of processing quantum problems much faster since QC utilizes the superpositions of the states and/or their entanglement to speed up the processing [13, 14]. In fact, QC has expanded computational ability from CCs and solves BQP (Bounded-error Quantum Polynomial time) class containing some part of the NP class in polynomial time [16–18], e.g., Shor's factorization algorithm [19–23].

Since Shor's algorithm appeared, many experimental attempts have been performed [24] and the first experiment was carried out by highly sophisticated pulsed NMR techniques [25]. The first experiment was made by manipulating C, H, and F nuclear qubits of dimethyl fluoromalonate molecule in solution. It has been claimed that quantum entanglement as the heart of QC was not been established in any NMR experiments in solution. Another factorization experiment was proposed by Peng et al., which factorizes 21 by an Adiabatic Quantum Computer (AQC) with only three qubits. This is the quantum algorithm which we will discuss below as a relevant version of electron spin qubits.

We describe in this chapter how to perform adiabatic quantum computation by implementing AQCs by using MSQCs. As discussed below, AQC is a computation model of the ground state manipulation by the Hamiltonian of the system under study [26]. Then the algorithm of AQC, i.e., adiabatic quantum algorithm (AQUA) is defined by the time-dependent Hamiltonian path. The first quest is how to make performable formula of AQUA for spin resonance techniques. This answer has already been proven in NMR-QCs, and it is based on a replacement approach of the time-dependent Hamiltonian to the time evolution operator. The second quest is the focus of our recent research into how to simulate the time evolution operators by MSQCs. This issue contains AQC and quantum simulation also by using advanced microwave (MW)-based ESR spin technology. In this context, MSQC belongs to the class of ESR-QC, which allows us to manipulate client nuclear spins via bus electron spin qubits. This is not just the simple scaling of NMR to ESR because some physical parameters are different in order of magnitude from each other. In this chapter, we show that qubits generated by open-shell molecules, whose spin properties are optimized, can perform AQC in ESR timescale.

Referred to truly realistic QCs, it is worth noting the recently established MSQC techniques. The MSQC implements that nuclear spin spins as client qubits in molecular spins, while electron spins play the role of bus qubits, then the system can be controlled by both pulsed radiofrequency and pulsed MW techniques [27]. This approach requires particular molecular optimization which renders electron or nuclear spins of molecular spins functioning as addressable spin qubits. The optimization includes g- or A-tensor engineering to distinguish between the qubits [28–33]. It is worth noting that the implementation of CNOT (Controlled-NOT) gates as two-qubit quantum gates has been for the first time achieved for synthetic molecular electron spins [30], and chemistry emerges in the field of quantum computing and quantum information processing (QIP). Furthermore, recently arbitrary wave-form generator (AWG) techniques have been developing to satisfy the manipulation for more than a few molecular electron spins by generating sophisticated sequences of radiation pulses. By virtue of the AWG-based technical development, molecular spin quantum technology has been coming to engineer a large number of the pulses now.

2 Adiabatic Quantum Computer

Algorithms of AQC, AQUAs, are based on the adiabatic theorem (Fig. 1). Let us assume time evolution of a quantum system under following conditions: (1) One prepares a ground state of Hamiltonian as an initial state, (2) the Hamiltonian of the quantum system is varied slowly from the initial state to the final one, and (3) there

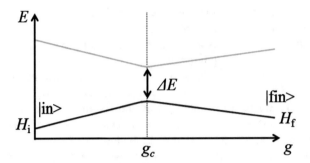

Fig. 1 Schematic view of AQC. The *top* and *bottom* lines indicate the ground and first excited states of a quantum system, respectively. The Hamiltonian of the system moves from the initial Hamiltonian (H_i) to the final one (H_f). g denotes a variable changing from 0 to 1 and corresponding to the initial state ($g = 0$) and final one ($g = 1$). The minimum energy gap is ΔE at $g = g_c$

is no intersection between the ground state and exited states during the evolution period. Under these assumptions, the adiabatic theorem indicates that the quantum system stays in the ground state of the time-dependent Hamiltonian [26].

From the viewpoint of the quantum computation, there is a possibility to find a ground state of the Hamiltonian by the adiabatic theorem. This is because if one develops the quantum system to the known final Hamiltonian, then one can conquer its unknown final state. This is Adiabatic Quantum Computing. Note that the required time of AQC depends on the energy gap (ΔE) between the ground and exited states, which corresponds to the change of speed for the Hamiltonian in a precise manner. Therefore, the computational time is defined as polynomials of the energy gap against the size of problems (N). In general, the computational time of AQC is unknown because of the computational complexity for the energy surface of the quantum systems, even though there are proven cases executing calculations faster than CCs, e.g., adiabatic searching algorithms ($\sqrt{N}$) [34] as the same order of Grover's algorithm in standard QCs. Except for this problem, AQC has the same properties of QCs: (1) AQCs are equivalent to standard QCs [35], and (2) AQCs have error correcting codes [36].

Throughout this chapter, we name a time-dependent Hamiltonian of AQUA as an ideal Hamiltonian or algorithm Hamiltonian, since ESR-QC does not operate the Hamiltonian in any direct manner.

2.1 Adiabatic Factorization Algorithm of 21

Here, we introduce an adiabatic factorization algorithm of 21. This algorithm is proposed by Peng et al. [25]. The ideal/final Hamiltonian (or say the problem Hamiltonian: $\hat{H}_f$), is Eq. (1),

$$\hat{H}_f/\hbar = \left(\hat{N} - \hat{x}\hat{y}\right)^2 \tag{1}$$

where, $\hat{N} = 21\hat{I}$ and $(\hat{x}, \hat{y})$ is the binary representation of natural numbers by qubits. It is obvious to find that the ground state is given by Eq. (2).

$$\langle \hat{H}_f \rangle = 0 \Leftrightarrow (\langle \hat{x} \rangle, \langle \hat{y} \rangle) = (7, 3) \quad \text{or} \quad (3, 7) \tag{2}$$

This is because the final Hamiltonian of Eq. (1) is a positive operator. In the case of factorizing 21, this algorithm is performed by only three qubits. Without loss of generality, one can write down $\hat{x}$ and $\hat{y}$ as Eqs. (3) and (4) assuming $\langle \hat{x} \rangle \leq \langle \hat{y} \rangle$ and both are odd numbers. This indicates $\langle \hat{x} \rangle^2 \leq \hat{N}$ and $\langle \hat{y} \rangle^2 \geq \hat{N}$ because of the relation of $\langle \hat{x} \rangle \times \langle \hat{y} \rangle \approx \hat{N}$.

$$3 \leq \langle \hat{x} \rangle \leq \sqrt{21} \Rightarrow \hat{x} = \left(\hat{I} - \hat{\sigma}_z^1 \right) + \hat{I} \tag{3}$$

$$\sqrt{21} \leq \langle \hat{y} \rangle \leq 21/3 \Rightarrow \hat{y} = 2\left(\hat{I} - \hat{\sigma}_z^2 \right) + \left(\hat{I} - \hat{\sigma}_z^3 \right) + \hat{I} \tag{4}$$

where $\hat{\sigma}_z^i$ is the $\hat{\sigma}_z$ value of the ith spin. In Eqs. (3) and (4), 3 indicates the minimum prime number which gives the restriction to the minimum value of $\langle \hat{x} \rangle$ and the maximum value of $\langle \hat{y} \rangle$. The ground state of $\hat{H}_f$ is $|\downarrow\downarrow\downarrow\rangle$ which allows one to calculate the values of $(\langle \hat{x} \rangle, \langle \hat{y} \rangle) = (3, 7)$ from Eqs. (3) and (4). This adiabatic algorithm is not efficient in a certain case when the solutions of $\hat{x}$ and need the same bit length, that gives two solutions of $(\langle \hat{x} \rangle, \langle \hat{y} \rangle)$ and $(\langle \hat{y} \rangle, \langle \hat{x} \rangle)$ with $\Delta E_{min} = 0$. However, there are some possibilities to calculate other $\hat{N}$ problems fast, and this algorithm allows us to carry out AQC experiments with operations by a small number of qubits. Expanding Eq. (1), we obtain the following expression:

$$\hat{H}_f/\hbar \sim 84\hat{\sigma}_z^1 + 88\hat{\sigma}_z^2 + 44\hat{\sigma}_z^3 - 20\hat{\sigma}_z^1\hat{\sigma}_z^2 - 10\hat{\sigma}_z^1\hat{\sigma}_z^3 + 20\hat{\sigma}_z^2\hat{\sigma}_z^3 - 16\hat{\sigma}_z^1\hat{\sigma}_z^2\hat{\sigma}_z^3 \tag{5}$$

which is utilized for implementing pulse sequences of radiofrequency or MW frequency irradiation in magnetic resonance QC experiments. In this transformation, an identity operator $\hat{I}$ is neglected.

2.2 Time Evolution Formula of AQC for Spin-Resonance Molecular Systems

To perform AQC, we need to define an adiabatic path of a time-dependent ideal Hamiltonian. A typical method defines two ideal Hamiltonians, which are named an initial Hamiltonian ($\hat{H}_i$) and a final Hamiltonian ($\hat{H}_f$) presented above. They connect the path in a linear manner. In order to compare with NMR-QC experiments, the following parameters and initial Hamiltonian are adopted (Eqs. (6), (8), and (9)) [25].

$$\hat{H}_{i}/\hbar = 30\sum_{i=1}^{3}\sigma_{x}^{i} \tag{6}$$

The coefficients of Eq. (6) are selected and the Hamiltonian has the same order of the norm with the final one. If not, the algorithm must need more time required. As mentioned above, it is hard to manipulate spin Hamiltonians of the real systems including its coupling constants between spins in ESR/NMR-QC. However, we can simulate behavior of the quantum system with the time-dependent ideal Hamiltonian by affecting the time evolution operator (Eq. (7)) to the initial state.

$$\hat{U} = \hat{T}\int_{t_{i}}^{t_{f}} \exp\left(-i\hat{H}\left(t\right)/\hbar\right)dt \tag{7}$$

where $\hat{T}$ denotes time-ordered products, $\hat{H}\left(t_{f}\right) = \hat{H}_{f}$, $\hat{H}\left(t_{i}\right) = \hat{H}_{i}$, and $t_{i} < t_{f}$. Approximating to the finite time step for pulse calculations,

$$\hat{U} = \prod_{m=1}^{5} \exp\left(-0.028 \times i\hat{H}_{m}/\hbar\right) \tag{8}$$

$$\hat{H}_{m} = (m/5)^{2}\hat{H}_{f} + \left\{1 - (m/5)^{2}\right\}\hat{H}_{i} \tag{9}$$

are obtained. Note that $\hat{H}_{i}$ (Eq. (6)) is needed not to commute with $\hat{H}_{f}$ (Eq. (5)) because of avoiding crossing of energy levels between the ground state and exited states, and the restriction is satisfied in Eqs. (8) and (9). A simple example is that if $\hat{H}_{m}$ is composed of only $\hat{\sigma}_{z}^{i}$ operators, the operator $\hat{U}$ will never change the $\hat{\sigma}_{z}^{i}$ values, thus never give rise to spin flipping. Therefore, $\hat{U}$ must contain the noncommutative operators in $\hat{H}_{m}$ terms, and simulating the time evolution by ESR/NMR experiments needs Trotter expansion into the commutative operators (Eqs. (10)–(12)).

$$\hat{U} = \prod_{m=1}^{5} \hat{U}_{mi} \times \hat{U}_{mf} \times \hat{U}_{mi} \tag{10}$$

$$\hat{U}_{mi} = \exp\left(-i0.028\left\{1 - (m/5)^{2}\right\}\hat{H}_{i}/2\hbar\right) \tag{11}$$

$$\hat{U}_{mf} = \exp\left(-i0.028(m/5)^{2}\hat{H}_{f}/\hbar\right) \tag{12}$$

In this approach, the theoretical fidelity is known to be 0.91 [25], and the implementation procedure is shown in Sect. 3. The explicit formula of Eqs. (10)–(12) and (10)–(12) is

$$\hat{U}_{mi} = \prod_{i=1}^{3} \exp\left(-i0.42\{1 - s_m\}\hat{\sigma}_x^i\right) \tag{13}$$

$$\begin{aligned}
\hat{U}_{mf} &= \exp\left(-i2.352 s_m \hat{\sigma}_x^1\right) \times \exp\left(-i2.464 s_m \hat{\sigma}_x^2\right) \times \exp\left(-i1.232 s_m \hat{\sigma}_x^3\right) \\
&\times \exp\left(-i0.56 s_m \hat{\sigma}_x^1 \hat{\sigma}_x^2\right) \times \exp\left(+i0.56 s_m \hat{\sigma}_x^2 \hat{\sigma}_x^3\right) \times \exp\left(-i0.28 s_m \hat{\sigma}_x^3 \hat{\sigma}_x^1\right) \\
&\times \exp\left(-i0.448 s_m \hat{\sigma}_x^1 \hat{\sigma}_x^2 \hat{\sigma}_x^3\right)
\end{aligned} \tag{14}$$

$$s_m = (m/5)^2 \tag{15}$$

and thus, the adiabatic factorization is performed by operations given in Eqs. (13)–(15). Note that the elements of $\hat{U}_{mi}$ ($\hat{U}_{mf}$) are commutable with itself, which means one can choose the order of operations in the unitary operator.

3 Spin Hamiltonian in Pulsed ESR Techniques

The spin Hamiltonian of open-shell molecules is written by Eq. (16) in Schrödinger picture. From the viewpoint of QCs, we term Eq. (16) the spin Hamiltonian of molecular spin QCs (MSQCs).

$$\begin{aligned}
\hat{H}_{MSQC} &= \sum_{i=1}^{N} \mathbf{S}^i g_e^i \beta_e \mathbf{B} - \sum_{i=1}^{M} \mathbf{I}^i g_n^i \beta_n^i \mathbf{B} + \sum_{i<j}^{N,N} \mathbf{S}^i (j+D)_e^{ij} \mathbf{S}^j \\
&+ \sum_{i=j=1}^{N,M} \mathbf{S}^i A^{ij} \mathbf{I}^j + \sum_{i<j}^{M,M} \mathbf{I}^i (j+D)_n^{ij} \mathbf{I}^j
\end{aligned} \tag{16}$$

where, N and M denote the number of electrons and nuclei, respectively. This Hamiltonian contains effects of both the static magnetic field and the irradiation fields from micro/radio waves in $\mathbf{B}$ term. The first and second terms denote Zeeman interactions and g^i is a second rank tensor which is related to the Larmor frequency ω_0 of an ith spin ($\omega_{0,e}^i = g_{zz}^i \beta_e B_z / \hbar$ and $\omega_{0,n}^i = -g_{zz}^i \beta_n^i B_z / \hbar$ where B_z denotes the static magnetic field which is parallel to the z-axis). The interactions between spins are described also by second rank tensors of J, D, and A, which denote exchange, spin-dipolar, and hyperfine interactions, respectively. MSQC is assumed to satisfy three conditions for the following pulse sequence study: (1) small anisotropy of the g-tensor for electrons and nuclei, (2) strong magnetic field limit for electrons, which the Zeeman term is much larger than others and (3) hyperfine co-axial system for solid-state ESR studies. The condition (3) is not always needed but this restriction leads the theoretical approach more easily or accurately. Note that there is the case that Eq. (16) can be regarded as an exact Hamiltonian in ensemble systems.

Especially, the molecules hosting spins embedded in the lattices of single crystals are the case. Therefore, these systems have been employed in most of QC experiments on open-shell molecules, e.g., in establishing qubit initialization and entanglement conditions [27, 37, 38], and we also focus on similar systems in this chapter.

3.1 Effective Hamiltonian: Approach for Spin Qubits

For an analytical pulse sequence study, the spin Hamiltonian of MSQCs, Eq. (16) is needed to transform to an effective spin Hamiltonian. The effective spin Hamiltonian is an approximated Hamiltonian for the time evolution of the spin systems. There are some analytical techniques for the approximation of the effective spin Hamiltonian, e.g., Floquet Approach (FA) [39, 40], variations of perturbation theory [41–43] and Secular Averaging Approach (SAA) [41]. In this chapter, we deal with SAA as the most basic approach in order to manipulate molecular spins as spin qubits. The simple form of the effective spin Hamiltonian is due to an interaction picture using rotational frames and all spin manipulations composed of the spin rotation period and time evolution period. The perturbed Hamiltonian in the rotating frame is regarded as an effective spin Hamiltonian of the qubit system.

Alternatively, one can choose other approaches for AQC. The core or heart of the AQUA is the quantum simulation of time evolution which is composed of selective single qubit operations and time evolution of Ising type interactions ($S_z^i S_z^j$), two-spin operations around the z-axis between spin qubits. Therefore, replacement of the generation part for the Ising type interaction allows us to perform AQC in another theoretical model, e.g., perturbation theory (see [43]). In principle, more accurate theory needs a larger number of pulses.

3.2 Effective Hamiltonian: Three Electron System in SAA

Equation (16) for the three electron system can be written by Eq. (17) in Schrödinger picture.

$$\hat{H}_{3e} = \sum_{i=1}^{3} \hat{\mathbf{S}}^i g^i \beta_e \mathbf{B} + \sum_{i<j}^{3,3} \hat{\mathbf{S}}^i (J+D)^{ij} \hat{\mathbf{S}}^j \tag{17}$$

Since there are no MW irradiation during the time evolution period, $\mathbf{B}$ term only contains the static magnetic field in the z-direction ($\mathbf{B} = (0, 0, B_z)$). Then, the spin Hamiltonian is described by Eq. (18).

$$\hat{H}_{3e} = \sum_{i=1}^{3} \left(\sum_{k=x,y,z} \hat{S}_k^i g_{kz}^i \beta_e B_z \right) + \sum_{i<j}^{3,3} \hat{\mathbf{S}}^i (J + D)^{ij} \hat{\mathbf{S}}^j \tag{18}$$

There are two methods to transform to the rotational frame: an individual rotating frame and common rotating frame. Here, we introduce the individual rotating frame first. The non-perturbed Hamiltonian and the perturbed Hamiltonian are given by Eqs. (19) and (20), respectively. Where time-dependent spin operators are given by Eqs. (21)–(23).

$$\hat{H}_{3e}^0 = \sum_{i=1}^{3} \hbar\omega_{0,e}^i \hat{S}_z^i \tag{19}$$

$$\hat{H}_{3e}^{int} = \sum_{i=1}^{3} \left(\sum_{k=x,y} \hat{S}_k^i(t) g_{kz}^i \beta_e B_z \right) + \sum_{i<j}^{3,3} \left(\sum_{k,l=x,y,z} \hat{S}_k^i(t)(J+D)_{kl}^{ij} \hat{S}_l^j(t) \right) \tag{20}$$

$$\hat{S}_x^i(t) = \cos\left(\omega_{0,e}^i t\right) \hat{S}_x^i - \sin\left(\omega_{0,e}^i t\right) \hat{S}_y^i \tag{21}$$

$$\hat{S}_y^i(t) = \sin\left(\omega_{0,e}^i t\right) \hat{S}_x^i + \cos\left(\omega_{0,e}^i t\right) \hat{S}_y^i \tag{22}$$

$$\hat{S}_z^i(t) = \hat{S}_z^i \tag{23}$$

There is no approximation in Eqs. (19) and (20). Secular approximation assumes time averaging of the Hamiltonian under the condition of fast Larmor rotations. In the zeroth order approximation, this approach gives rotating terms related to Larmor frequency as zero in the case of the small anisotropy of g-tensors [41] and smaller interactions between spins than Larmor terms. Therefore, the perturbed Hamiltonian of the three electron system in the time evolution can be written by Eq. (24) in the individual rotating frames.

$$\hat{H}_{3e}^{int} = \sum_{i<j}^{3,3} \hat{S}_z^i (J + D)_{zz}^{ij} \hat{S}_z^j \tag{24}$$

The perturbed Hamiltonian of Eq. (24) is adopted for following pulse sequence study (Sect. 4) as an effective spin Hamiltonian of the qubit system. On the other hand, in solution ESR experiments the same procedure can be executed by only annihilating the anisotropic tensor parameters (Eq. (25)).

$$\hat{H}_{3e,\ sol}^{int} = \sum_{i<j}^{3,3} \hat{S}_z^i J \hat{S}_z^j \tag{25}$$

The formula of the common rotating frame is slightly different from Eqs. (19), (20), and (21)–(23) and the interaction picture is represented in Eqs. (26), (27), and (28)–(30), respectively.

$$\hat{H}^0_{3e} = \sum_{i=1}^{3} \hbar\omega^1_{0,e}\hat{S}^i_z \tag{26}$$

$$\hat{H}^{int}_{3e} = \sum_{i=1}^{3}\left(\sum_{k=x,y}\hat{S}^i_k(t)g^i_{kz}\beta_e B_z\right) + \sum_{i<j}^{3,3}\left(\sum_{k,l=x,y,z}\hat{S}^i_k(t)(J+D)^{ij}_{kl}\hat{S}^j_l(t)\right)$$
$$+\sum_{i=2}^{3}\hat{S}^i_z(g^i_{zz}-g^1_{zz})\beta_e B_z \tag{27}$$

$$\hat{S}^i_x(t) = \cos\left(\omega^1_{0,e}t\right)\hat{S}^i_x - \sin\left(\omega^1_{0,e}t\right)\hat{S}^i_y \tag{28}$$

$$\hat{S}^i_y(t) = \sin\left(\omega^1_{0,e}t\right)\hat{S}^i_x + \cos\left(\omega^1_{0,e}t\right)\hat{S}^i_y \tag{29}$$

$$\hat{S}^i_z(t) = \hat{S}^i_z \tag{30}$$

This picture indicates that all spins are rotating in a common Larmor frequency frame of the first spin and the deviation of the rotational speed for the second and the third spins makes a difference in Eq. (27). The secular approximation can also be applied to this picture,

$$\hat{H}^{int}_{3e} = \sum_{i<j}^{3,3}\hat{S}^i_z(J+D)^{ij}_{zz}\hat{S}^j_z + \sum_{i=2}^{3}\hat{S}^i_z(g^i_{zz}-g^1_{zz})\beta_e B_z \tag{31}$$

$$\hat{H}^{int}_{3e,\,sol} = \sum_{i<j}^{3,3}\hat{S}^i_z J\hat{S}^j_z + \sum_{i=2}^{3}\hat{S}^i_z(g^i_{iso}-g^1_{iso})\beta_e B_z \tag{32}$$

Equation (31) for a diluted single-crystal ESR case and Eq. (32) for a solution ESR case are obtained. The extra terms can be eliminated by spin manipulations as shown in Sect. 4.4.

3.3 Effective Hamiltonian: One Electron System with Two Nuclear Spins in SAA

The same secular approach for the three electron system is applicable to one electron system with two nuclear client qubits. The spin Hamiltonian of this system can be written by Eq. (33) in Schrödinger picture.

$$\hat{H}_{1e+2n} = \hat{S}^1 g^1 \beta_e \mathbf{B} - \sum_{i=2}^{3} \hat{I}^i g^i \beta_n^i \mathbf{B} + \sum_{j=2}^{3} \hat{S}^1 A^{1j} \hat{I}^j + \hat{I}^2 (J+D)^{23} \hat{I}^3 \qquad (33)$$

Applying the static magnetic field $\mathbf{B} = (0, 0, B_z)$,

$$\hat{H}_{1e+2n} = \sum_{k=x,y,z} \hat{S}_k^1 g_{kz}^1 \beta_e B_z - \sum_{i=2}^{3} \left(\sum_{k=x,y,z} \hat{I}_k^i g_{kz}^i \beta_n B_z \right) + \sum_{j=2}^{3} \hat{S}^1 A^{1j} \hat{I}^j$$

$$+ \hat{I}^2 (J+D)^{23} \hat{I}^3 \qquad (34)$$

is obtained. In the case of transforming the individual rotating frame, the Larmor frequency is selected under the condition of $\omega_{0,e}^1 = g_{zz}^1 \beta_e B_z / \hbar$ and $\omega_{0,n}^i = -g_{zz}^i \beta_n^i B_z / \hbar$. Then, the Hamiltonian in interaction picture is represented by Eqs. (35) and (36),

$$\hat{H}_{1e+2n}^0 = \hbar \omega_{0,e}^1 \hat{S}_z^1 + \sum_{i=2}^{3} \hbar \omega_{0,n}^i \hat{I}_z^i \qquad (35)$$

$$\hat{H}_{1e+2n}^{int} = \sum_{k=x,y} \hat{S}_k^1(t) g_{kz}^1 \beta_e B_z - \sum_{i=2}^{3} \left(\sum_{k=x,y} \hat{I}_k^i(t) g_{kz}^i \beta_n B_z \right)$$

$$+ \sum_{j=2}^{3} \left(\sum_{k,l=x,y,z} \hat{S}_k^1(t) A_{kl}^{1j} \hat{I}_l^j(t) \right) + \sum_{k,l=x,y,z} \hat{I}_k^2(t)(J+D)_{kl}^{23} \hat{I}_l^3(t) \qquad (36)$$

where the same definition is applied for nuclear spin operators, i.e., Eqs. (21)–(23) and (37)–(39).

$$\hat{I}_x^i(t) = \cos\left(\omega_{0,n}^i t\right) \hat{I}_x^i - \sin\left(\omega_{0,n}^i t\right) \hat{I}_y^i \qquad (37)$$

$$\hat{I}_y^i(t) = \sin\left(\omega_{0,n}^i t\right) \hat{I}_x^i + \cos\left(\omega_{0,n}^i t\right) \hat{I}_y^i \qquad (38)$$

$$\hat{I}_z^i(t) = \hat{I}_z^i \qquad (39)$$

Then, we discuss the secular approximation in the rotating frame. As well as the three electron system, the time-dependent electron spin operators in Eq. (36) are averaged out and vanishing in terms of this approximation on the basis of the fast electron Larmor rotations. The problem is with nuclear spin operators. The interactions between the nuclei spins are possible and the approximation only applies to their secular terms. This is because the nuclear Larmor terms are much larger than those interactions. On the other hand, hyperfine tensors, interactions between electron and nucleus, do not allow the same secular approach since these are not small enough than the Larmor terms of the nuclear spins. Then the spin Hamiltonian of the system in the time evolution can be written by Eq. (40).

$$\hat{H}_{1e+2n}^{int} = \sum_{j=2}^{3} \left(\sum_{l=x,y,z} \hat{S}_z^1 A_{zl}^{1j} \hat{I}_l^j(t) \right) + \hat{I}_z^2 (J+D)_{zz}^{23} \hat{I}_z^3 \tag{40}$$

Equation (40) is a time-dependent perturbed Hamiltonian in interaction picture. The trigonometric part of $\hat{I}_{x,y}^i(t)$ makes it hard to calculate pulse sequences by using analytical techniques. Therefore, we assume a co-axial system for hyperfine tensors in order to apply the static magnetic field (B_0) parallel to both the principal axes. Then, the Hamiltonian in the representation of time evolution operators is time-independent and can be written by Eq. (41).

$$\hat{H}_{1e+2n}^{int} = \sum_{j=2}^{3} \hat{S}_z^1 A_{zz}^{1j} \hat{I}_z^j + \hat{I}_z^2 (J+D)_{zz}^{23} \hat{I}_z^3 \tag{41}$$

Equation (41) is also adopted as an effective spin Hamiltonian of spin qubits composed of one electron system with the two nuclear spins in the following pulse sequence study of a diluted single crystal (see Sect. 4). On the other hand, in the solution ESR study, the same procedure can be executed only by changing the parameters of the tensor into the isotropic term. Since there is no anisotropic term in a solution case, the restrictions between the static magnetic field and the hyperfine axis are not needed. The secular formula is written by Eq. (42).

$$\hat{H}_{1e+2n,\,sol}^{int} = \sum_{j=2}^{3} \hat{S}_z^1 A_{iso}^{1j} \hat{I}_z^j + \hat{I}_z^2 J^{23} \hat{I}_z^3 \tag{42}$$

The common rotating frame formula for nuclear spins is written in Eqs. (43) and (44), whose formula also has the individual frame between electron and nuclei spins, of necessity. The notation of the electron and nuclear spin part is given by Eqs. (28)–(30) and (45)–(47), respectively.

$$\hat{H}_{1e+2n}^{0} = \hbar\omega_{0,e}^1 \hat{S}_z^i + \sum_{i=2}^{3} \hbar\omega_{0,n}^2 \hat{I}_z^i \tag{43}$$

$$\hat{H}_{1e+2n}^{int} = \sum_{k=x,y} \hat{S}_k^1(t) g_{kz}^1 \beta_e B_z - \sum_{i=2}^{3} \left(\sum_{k=x,y} \hat{I}_k^i(t) g_{kz}^i \beta_n B_z \right) + \sum_{j=2}^{3} \left(\sum_{k,l=x,y,z} \hat{S}_k^1(t) A_{kl}^{1j} \hat{I}_l^j(t) \right)$$
$$+ \sum_{k,l=x,y,z} \hat{I}_k^2(t)(J+D)_{kl}^{23} \hat{I}_l^3(t) + I_z^3 (g_{zz}^3 - g_{zz}^2) \beta_n^3 B_z \tag{44}$$

$$\hat{I}_x^2(t) = \cos\left(\omega_{0,n}^2 t\right)\hat{I}_x^i + \sin\left(\omega_{0,n}^2 t\right)\hat{I}_y^i \tag{45}$$

$$\hat{I}_y^2(t) = \sin\left(\omega_{0,n}^2 t\right)\hat{I}_x^i + \cos\left(\omega_{0,n}^2 t\right)\hat{I}_y^i \tag{46}$$

$$\hat{I}_z^i(t) = \hat{I}_z^i \tag{47}$$

This difference between Eqs. (36) and (44) only appears in a third spin term and this gives rise to a g-shift during the time evolution. By using the same procedure as the individual rotating frame of this system, we obtain Eqs. (48) and (49) for a diluted single crystal study and solution study, respectively. This extra term can be also eliminated by spin manipulations (see Sect. 4.4).

$$\hat{H}_{1e+2n}^{int} = \sum_{j=2}^{3} \hat{S}_z^1 A_{zz}^{1j} \hat{I}_z^j + \hat{I}_z^2 (J+D)_{zz}^{23} \hat{I}_z^3 + I_z^3 \left(g_{zz}^3 - g_{zz}^2\right)\beta_n^3 B_z \tag{48}$$

$$\hat{H}_{1e+2n,\ sol}^{int} = \sum_{j=2}^{3} \hat{S}_z^1 A_{iso}^{1j} \hat{I}_z^j + \hat{I}_z^2 J^{23} \hat{I}_z^3 + I_z^3 \left(g_{iso}^3 - g_{iso}^2\right)\beta_n^3 B_z \tag{49}$$

4 Pulse Operations in AQC

An operation set of ESR-QC experiments is assumed to manipulate arbitrary spin rotations (x- and y-axis directions) for each spin and to perform the time evolution with the effective spin Hamiltonian given in Sects. 3.2 and 3.3 ($\hat{H}_{3e}^{int}$ and $\hat{H}_{1e+2n}^{int}$, respectively). These systems allow us to implement Universal Quantum Gates (UQG), where UQG is a gate set which can perform any quantum operations [14]. This is on the basis of a theory that arbitrary single spin rotation of one qubit and CNOT gates between any qubits can perform UQG. When all the spin qubits of the system can be operable individually, CNOT gates are equivalent to Ising type operations ($S_z^i S_z^j$) between arbitrary two qubits (i and j). Therefore, two problems arise: (1) How to operate Ising type interaction between arbitrary two qubits and (2) How to simulate time evolution of AQUA by UQG.

The operation set, we assumed in this section, can be written by operator sets of (50) and (51).

$$\left\{\sigma_x^i, \sigma_y^i, \hat{H}_{3e}^{int}\right\} \quad \text{for the three electron system} \tag{50}$$

$$\left\{\sigma_x^i, \sigma_y^i, \hat{H}_{1e+2n}^{int}\right\} \quad \text{for the one electron and two nuclear system} \tag{51}$$

In terms of AQUA, the problem is how to operate adiabatic time evolution of the factorization algorithm of 21 by pulsed ESR operations. From a discussion on Sect. 2, the time evolution operator is written by Eqs. (10) and (13)–(15) where $\hat{U}$ is a total adiabatic path of the ground state. Then, we implement operators Eqs. (13) and (50) in order to perform the time evolution of Eqs. (10) and (13)–(15).

$$\hat{U}_{mi} = \prod_{i=1}^{3} \exp\left(-i0.42\{1 - s_m\}\hat{\sigma}_x^i\right) \tag{52}$$

$$s_m = (m/5)^2 \tag{53}$$

$$\hat{U}_z = \exp\left(-i2.352s_m\hat{\sigma}_x^1\right) \times \exp\left(-i2.464s_m\hat{\sigma}_x^2\right) \times \exp\left(-i1.232s_m\hat{\sigma}_x^3\right) \tag{54}$$

$$\hat{U}_{zz} = \exp\left(-i0.56s_m\hat{\sigma}_x^1\hat{\sigma}_x^2\right) \times \exp\left(+i0.56s_m\hat{\sigma}_x^2\hat{\sigma}_x^3\right) \times \exp\left(-i0.28s_m\hat{\sigma}_x^3\hat{\sigma}_x^1\right) \tag{55}$$

$$\hat{U}_{zzz} = \exp\left(-i0.448s_m\hat{\sigma}_x^1\hat{\sigma}_x^2\hat{\sigma}_x^3\right) \tag{56}$$

$$\hat{U}_{zzz} = \exp\left(+i0.56s_m\hat{\sigma}_x^2\hat{\sigma}_x^3\right) \tag{57}$$

The contents of Sect. 4 are:

(1) Arbitrary rotations of spin qubits around the x-/y-/z- axis.

    1. Arbitrary rotations of spin qubits (x-/y-axis): Eq. (13).
    2. Arbitrary rotations of spin qubits (z-axis): Eq. (54).

(2) Two-qubit operations of Eq. (55) depending on interaction picture.

    1. Two-qubit operation in the individual rotating frame.
    2. Two-qubit operation in the common rotating frame.

(3) Three qubit operation and higher order qubit operations.

    1. Three qubit operation: Eq. (56).
    2. Higher order (>3) qubit operations.

(4) Fast two-qubit operation between nuclei spins.

    1. Fast two-qubit operation between nuclei spins: Eq. (57).

(5) Pulse sequences for AQC.

    1. AQC pulse sequence in a three electron system.
    2. AQC pulse sequence in a one electron system with two nuclear spins.

From the viewpoint of UQG, (1) and (2) are the generation of UQG. On the other hand, (3) and (4) are computational methods applying UQG. For the understanding of figures for the pulse sequence during this section, the pulse operations are depicted as given in Fig. 2. The time of the pulse interval and the direction of the irradiation are also given with the pulses.

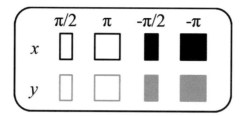

Fig. 2 Notation of pulse operations. *Black (gray)* blocks indicate the rotation around the *x*-(*y*-) axis. Square (oblong) blocks indicate the rotational angles of $\pi(\pi/2)$. The filled block means a minus angle operation. Other pulse operations around the *x*- and *y*-axes are circled by dotted lines with a number/word

4.1 Arbitrary Rotations of Spin Qubits (x-/y-Axis)

The most basal qubit operation is a single spin rotation, which can be performed by irradiating a MW pulse in ESR-QC experiments. There are two types of pulses, selective pulses, and nonselective pulses. The former one rotates a single spin in a system and the latter one rotates some species of spins in a system. Most qubit manipulations in QC need selective operations but the operation of Eq. (52) can be performed by nonselective ones. Although the exact formula of the pulse operation is calculated by the effective spin Hamiltonian with MW irradiations, which contain correctable artifacts in the MW irradiation e.g., Bloch-Siegert shift [41] etc., here we discussed only the simple formulae of pulses as operation sets of (58) and (62).

2α radian rotation to i^{th} spin by a selective pulse (*x-/y*-axis):

$$\exp\left(-i\alpha\sigma_x^k\right), \exp\left(-i\alpha\sigma_y^k\right) \tag{58}$$

2α radian rotation by a nonselective pulse (*x-/y*-axis):

$$\prod_{k=1}^{3}\exp\left(-i\alpha\sigma_x^k\right), \prod_{k=1}^{3}\exp\left(-i\alpha\sigma_y^k\right) \tag{59}$$

The nonselective *x*-pulse in Eq. (62) can obviously perform Eq. (52) and parameter α should be taken as Eq. (60).

$$\alpha = 0.84\{1 - s_m\} \tag{60}$$

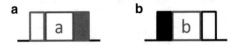

Fig. 3 The pulse sequence of single spin operations. (**a**) Corresponds to the Eq. (58). (**b**) Corresponds to Eq. (62). Dotted blocks of a and b are the $\theta = 2\alpha$ rotation around the x- and y-axes, respectively

4.2 Arbitrary Rotations of Spin Qubits (z-axis)

The single qubit operations around the z-direction can be performed by single spin rotations around the x- and y-axes. With selective pulses, the arbitrary rotation (2α radian) around the z-axis can be written by Eqs. (61) and (62). Figure 3 shows the pulse sequence for Eqs. (61) and (62).

$$\exp\left(-i\alpha\sigma_z^k\right) = \exp\left(i\frac{\pi}{4}\sigma_y^k\right) \cdot \exp\left(-i\alpha\sigma_x^k\right) \cdot \exp\left(-i\frac{\pi}{4}\sigma_y^k\right) \tag{61}$$

$$\exp\left(-i\alpha\sigma_z^k\right) = \exp\left(-i\frac{\pi}{4}\sigma_x^k\right) \cdot \exp\left(-i\alpha\sigma_y^k\right) \cdot \exp\left(i\frac{\pi}{4}\sigma_x^k\right) \tag{62}$$

Then Eq. (54) is operated by the selective pulses with the parameter set of Eq. (63). The sequence of Eq. (61) or (62) is utilized in the calculations for the first, second and third qubits.

$$\alpha_1 = 4.704 s_m, \alpha_2 = 4.928 s_m \quad \text{and} \quad \alpha_3 = 2.464 s_m \tag{63}$$

4.3 Two-Qubit Operations in Individual Rotating Frames

The interaction between qubits needs the time evolution of the effective spin Hamiltonian in general cases. The two-qubit interactions are the essential part of quantum algorithms to speed up. Here, we introduce the method to create two spin interactions between two arbitral spins, σ_z^i and $\sigma_z^j (i \neq j)$, in the secular approximation of the individual rotating frame. The target effective Hamiltonians at Eqs. (24), (25), (41), and (42) are composed of two spin interactions only.

$$\hat{H}_{3e}^{int} = \sum_{i<j}^{3,3} \hat{S}_z^i (J+D)_{zz}^{ij} \hat{S}_z^j \tag{64}$$

$$\hat{H}_{3e, sol}^{int} = \sum_{i<j}^{3,3} \hat{S}_z^i J \hat{S}_z^j \tag{65}$$

$$\hat{H}_{1e+2n}^{int} = \sum_{j=2}^{3} \hat{S}_z^1 A_{zz}^{1j} \hat{I}_z^j + \hat{I}_z^2 (J+D)_{zz}^{23} \hat{I}_z^3 \tag{66}$$

$$\hat{H}_{1e+2n,\,sol}^{int} = \sum_{j=2}^{3} \hat{S}_z^1 A_{iso}^{1j} \hat{I}_z^j + \hat{I}_z^2 J^{23} \hat{I}_z^3 \tag{67}$$

In the three spin system, the operator $\exp(-i\alpha^{ij}\sigma_z^i\sigma_z^j t/\hbar)$ can be written by Eqs. (68) and (69),

$$\exp(-i\alpha^{ij}\sigma_z^i\sigma_z^j t/\hbar)|_{i\neq k\neq l} = \exp(-iHt/2\hbar) \cdot \exp(-iH^{-k}t/2\hbar) \tag{68}$$

$$= \exp(-iH^{-k}t/2\hbar) \cdot \exp(-iHt/2\hbar) \tag{69}$$

where, $H = \sum_{i<j}^{3} \alpha^{ij}\sigma_z^i\sigma_z^j$ and $H^{-k} = \sum_{i<j}^{3} \alpha^{ij}\sigma_z^i\sigma_z^j|_{i\neq k\neq j} - \sum_{i\neq k}^{3} \alpha^{ik}\sigma_z^i\sigma_z^k$. The operator $\exp(-iH^{-k}t/\hbar)$ can be achieved via Eqs. (70)–(73).

$$\exp(-iH^{-k}t/2\hbar) = \exp\left(-i\frac{\pi}{2}\sigma_x^k\right) \cdot \exp(-iHt/\hbar) \cdot \exp\left(i\frac{\pi}{2}\sigma_x^k\right) \tag{70}$$

$$= \exp\left(i\frac{\pi}{2}\sigma_x^k\right) \cdot \exp(-iHt/\hbar) \cdot \exp\left(-i\frac{\pi}{2}\sigma_x^k\right) \tag{71}$$

$$= \exp\left(-i\frac{\pi}{2}\sigma_y^k\right) \cdot \exp(-iHt/\hbar) \cdot \exp\left(i\frac{\pi}{2}\sigma_y^k\right) \tag{72}$$

$$= \exp\left(i\frac{\pi}{2}\sigma_y^k\right) \cdot \exp(-iHt/\hbar) \cdot \exp\left(-i\frac{\pi}{2}\sigma_y^k\right) \tag{73}$$

Any decomposed operation sets can be chosen for the pulse sequence in Eqs. (68), (69), and (70)–(73). The calculated pulse sequence corresponding to Eq. (68) with (70) is shown in Fig. 4.

If we do not need to consider the global phase, any pattern of π pulses with the same direction is permitted as given by Eqs. (74)–(77). This phase does not affect the quantum computation results.

$$-\exp(-iH^{-k}t/2\hbar) = \exp\left(-i\frac{\pi}{2}\sigma_x^k\right) \cdot \exp(-iHt/\hbar) \cdot \exp\left(-i\frac{\pi}{2}\sigma_x^k\right) \tag{74}$$

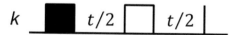

Fig. 4 An example of the pulse sequence of a two spin interaction. The operation $\exp(-i\alpha^{ij}\sigma_z^i\sigma_z^j t/\hbar)$ $(i\neq k, k\neq j, j\neq i)$ is composed of Eqs. (68) and (70). The vertical line indicates the end of the pulse sequence

$$= \exp\left(i\frac{\pi}{2}\sigma_x^k\right) \cdot \exp(-iHt/\hbar) \cdot \exp\left(i\frac{\pi}{2}\sigma_x^k\right) \tag{75}$$

$$= \exp\left(-i\frac{\pi}{2}\sigma_y^k\right) \cdot \exp(-iHt/\hbar) \cdot \exp\left(-i\frac{\pi}{2}\sigma_y^k\right) \tag{76}$$

$$= \exp\left(i\frac{\pi}{2}\sigma_y^k\right) \cdot \exp(-iHt/\hbar) \cdot \exp\left(i\frac{\pi}{2}\sigma_y^k\right) \tag{77}$$

In the case of the opposite sign operator $(\exp(i\alpha^{ij}\sigma_z^i\sigma_z^j t/\hbar))$, the operation can be written by Eqs. (78)–(81), utilizing an $\exp\left(-i\alpha^{ij}\sigma_z^i\sigma_z^j t/\hbar\right)$ operation.

$$\exp\left(i\alpha^{ij}\sigma_z^i\sigma_z^j t/\hbar\right) = \exp\left(-i\frac{\pi}{2}\sigma_x^i\right) \cdot \exp\left(-i\alpha^{ij}\sigma_z^i\sigma_z^j t/\hbar\right) \cdot \exp\left(i\frac{\pi}{2}\sigma_x^i\right) \tag{78}$$

$$= \exp\left(i\frac{\pi}{2}\sigma_x^i\right) \cdot \exp\left(-i\alpha^{ij}\sigma_z^i\sigma_z^j t/\hbar\right) \cdot \exp\left(-i\frac{\pi}{2}\sigma_x^i\right) \tag{79}$$

$$= \exp\left(-i\frac{\pi}{2}\sigma_y^i\right) \cdot \exp\left(-i\alpha^{ij}\sigma_z^i\sigma_z^j t/\hbar\right) \cdot \exp\left(i\frac{\pi}{2}\sigma_y^i\right) \tag{80}$$

$$= \exp\left(i\frac{\pi}{2}\sigma_y^i\right) \cdot \exp\left(-i\alpha^{ij}\sigma_z^i\sigma_z^j t/\hbar\right) \cdot \exp\left(-i\frac{\pi}{2}\sigma_y^i\right) \tag{81}$$

Any decomposed operation sets can be chosen for the pulse sequence in Eqs. (78)–(81). If we do not care about the global phase, any pattern of π pulses with the same direction is permitted as given by Eqs. (82)–(85).

$$-\exp\left(i\alpha^{ij}\sigma_z^i\sigma_z^j t/\hbar\right) = \exp\left(-i\frac{\pi}{2}\sigma_x^i\right) \cdot \exp\left(-i\alpha^{ij}\sigma_z^i\sigma_z^j t/\hbar\right) \cdot \exp\left(-i\frac{\pi}{2}\sigma_x^i\right) \tag{82}$$

$$= \exp\left(i\frac{\pi}{2}\sigma_x^i\right) \cdot \exp\left(-i\alpha^{ij}\sigma_z^i\sigma_z^j t/\hbar\right) \cdot \exp\left(i\frac{\pi}{2}\sigma_x^i\right) \tag{83}$$

$$= \exp\left(-i\frac{\pi}{2}\sigma_y^i\right) \cdot \exp\left(-i\alpha^{ij}\sigma_z^i\sigma_z^j t/\hbar\right) \cdot \exp\left(-i\frac{\pi}{2}\sigma_y^i\right) \tag{84}$$

$$= \exp\left(i\frac{\pi}{2}\sigma_y^i\right) \cdot \exp\left(-i\alpha^{ij}\sigma_z^i\sigma_z^j t/\hbar\right) \cdot \exp\left(i\frac{\pi}{2}\sigma_y^i\right) \tag{85}$$

An example of the pulse sequence is shown in Fig. 5, being composed of Eqs. (83), (71), and (80). And these operations are utilized for Eq. (55).

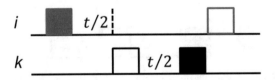

Fig. 5 An example of the pulse sequence of a two-spin interaction. The operation $\exp\left(-i\alpha^{ij}\sigma_z^i\sigma_z^j t/\hbar\right)$ $(i \neq k,\ k \neq j,\ j \neq i)$ is composed of Eqs. (83), (71), and (80). The time is delimited by a dotted line

4.4 Two-Qubit Operations in the Common Rotating Frame

In some cases, experimental restrictions force us to manipulate spins in the common rotating frame, Eqs. (86), (87), (88), and (89). The difference between the individual and common rotating frame originates from the single spin rotating terms around the z-axis in the secular approximation. Here, we show two methods to annihilate these extra terms to develop the same formulas as Eqs. (24), (25), (41), and (42) in the common rotating frame.

$$\hat{H}_{3e}^{int} = \sum_{i<j}^{3,3} \hat{S}_z^i (J + D)_{zz}^{ij} \hat{S}_z^j + \sum_{i=2}^{3} \hat{S}_z^i (g_{zz}^i - g_{zz}^1)\beta_e B_z \tag{86}$$

$$\hat{H}_{3e,\ sol}^{int} = \sum_{i<j}^{3,3} \hat{S}_z^i J \hat{S}_z^j + \sum_{i=2}^{3} \hat{S}_z^i (g_{iso}^i - g_{iso}^1)\beta_e B_z \tag{87}$$

$$\hat{H}_{1e+2n}^{int} = \sum_{j=2}^{3} \hat{S}_z^1 A_{zz}^{1j} \hat{I}_z^j + \hat{I}_z^2 (J + D)_{zz}^{23} \hat{I}_z^3 + I_z^3 (g_{zz}^3 - g_{zz}^2)\beta_n^3 B_z \tag{88}$$

$$\hat{H}_{1e+2n,\ sol}^{int} = \sum_{j=2}^{3} \hat{S}_z^1 A_{iso}^{1j} \hat{I}_z^j + \hat{I}_z^2 J^{23} \hat{I}_z^3 + I_z^3 (g_{iso}^3 - g_{iso}^2)\beta_n^3 B_z \tag{89}$$

The first method is based on the effect of selective inverse pulses for single spin-rotating terms. During the time evolution period, $\exp\left(-i\hat{H}^{int}\Delta t/\hbar\right)$ corresponding its Hamiltonian of Eqs. (86), (87), (88), and (89), the pulses are applied as the single spin rotation of the z-direction, Eqs. (61) and (62). The resulting time evolution $\exp\left(-i\hat{H}^{zz}\Delta t/\hbar\right)$ is given in Eqs. (90) and (91), where the rotation angle ($2\alpha^k$ pulses) for kth spin is given in Table 1. The example is given as Eq. (92) and in Fig. 6 under the condition of Eqs. (86) and (58). Then, the Hamiltonian in the time evolution of the common rotating frame, $\exp\left(-i\hat{H}^{zz}\Delta t/\hbar\right)$, gives the same operator of the case for the individual rotating frame (Eq. (24)).

Table 1 Rotation angle of the spins during the time evolution of $\exp\left(-i\hat{H}^{int}\Delta t/\hbar\right)$

	Rotation angles ($\theta^2 = 2\alpha^2$)	Rotation angles ($\theta^3 = 2\alpha^3$)
Equation (31)	$(g_{zz}^2 - g_{zz}^1)\beta_e B_z \Delta t/\hbar$	$(g_{zz}^3 - g_{zz}^1)\beta_e B_z \Delta t/\hbar$
Equation (32)	$(g_{iso}^2 - g_{iso}^1)\beta_e B_z \Delta t/\hbar$	$(g_{iso}^3 - g_{iso}^1)\beta_e B_z \Delta t/\hbar$
Equation (48)	0	$-(g_{zz}^3 - g_{zz}^1)\beta_n^3 B_z \Delta t/\hbar$
Equation (49)	0	$-(g_{iso}^3 - g_{iso}^1)\beta_n^3 B_z \Delta t/\hbar$

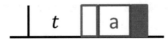

Fig. 6 Generation of $\exp\left(-i\hat{H}^{zz}\Delta t/\hbar\right)$ by the spin rotation around z-axis in the case of Eqs. (86) and (61). The dotted block a is the spin rotation around x-axis which spin number and angles (θ^k) are shown in Table 1

$$\exp\left(-i\hat{H}^{zz}\Delta t/\hbar\right) = \exp\left(-i\hat{H}^{int}\Delta t/\hbar\right) \cdot \exp\left(-i\sum_{k=2}^{3}\alpha^k\sigma_z^k\right) \tag{90}$$

$$= \exp\left(-i\sum_{k=2}^{3}\alpha^k\sigma_z^k\right) \cdot \exp\left(-i\hat{H}^{int}\Delta t/\hbar\right) \tag{91}$$

$$\exp\left(-i\hat{H}^{zz}\Delta t/\hbar\right) = \exp\left(-i\sum_{i<j}^{3,3}\hat{S}_z^i(J+D)_{zz}^{ij}\hat{S}_z^j\Delta t/\hbar\right) \tag{92}$$

The second method is the annihilation approach to the odd order effects. This operation can be performed by two nonselective pulses and does not depend on the evolution time $\exp\left(-i\hat{H}^{int}\Delta t/\hbar\right)$. Then, we define the operator $\hat{H}^{int,-s}$ as a spin flipped Hamiltonian of all spins (Eq. (93)) and this operation can be achieved via Eqs. (94)–(97).

$$\hat{H}^{int,-s}\left(\sigma_z^i\right) = \hat{H}^{int}\left(-\sigma_z^i\right) \tag{93}$$

$$\exp\left(-i\hat{H}^{int,-s}\Delta t/\hbar\right)$$

$$= \exp\left(-i\frac{\pi}{2}\sum_{k=1}^{3}\sigma_x^k\right) \cdot \exp\left(-i\hat{H}^{int}\Delta t/\hbar\right) \cdot \exp\left(i\frac{\pi}{2}\sum_{k=1}^{3}\sigma_x^k\right) \tag{94}$$

$$= \exp\left(i\frac{\pi}{2}\sum_{k=1}^{3}\sigma_x^k\right) \cdot \exp\left(-i\hat{H}^{int}\Delta t/\hbar\right) \cdot \exp\left(-i\frac{\pi}{2}\sum_{k=1}^{3}\sigma_x^k\right) \tag{95}$$

$$= \exp\left(-i\frac{\pi}{2}\sum_{k=1}^{3}\sigma_y^k\right) \cdot \exp\left(-i\hat{H}^{int}\Delta t/\hbar\right) \cdot \exp\left(i\frac{\pi}{2}\sum_{k=1}^{3}\sigma_y^k\right) \tag{96}$$

$$= \exp\left(i\frac{\pi}{2}\sum_{k=1}^{3}\sigma_y^k\right) \cdot \exp\left(-i\hat{H}^{int}\Delta t/\hbar\right) \cdot \exp\left(-i\frac{\pi}{2}\sum_{k=1}^{3}\sigma_y^k\right) \tag{97}$$

If we do not need to consider the global phase, any pattern of π pulses with the same direction is permitted as given by Eqs. (98)–(101).

$$- \exp\left(-i\hat{H}^{\text{int},-s}\Delta t/\hbar\right)$$

$$= \exp\left(-i\frac{\pi}{2}\sum_{k=1}^{3}\sigma_x^k\right)\cdot\exp\left(-i\hat{H}^{\text{int}}\Delta t/\hbar\right)\cdot\exp\left(-i\frac{\pi}{2}\sum_{k=1}^{3}\sigma_x^k\right) \qquad (98)$$

$$= \exp\left(i\frac{\pi}{2}\sum_{k=1}^{3}\sigma_x^k\right)\cdot\exp\left(-i\hat{H}^{\text{int}}\Delta t/\hbar\right)\cdot\exp\left(i\frac{\pi}{2}\sum_{k=1}^{3}\sigma_x^k\right) \qquad (99)$$

$$= \exp\left(-i\frac{\pi}{2}\sum_{k=1}^{3}\sigma_y^k\right)\cdot\exp\left(-i\hat{H}^{\text{int}}\Delta t/\hbar\right)\cdot\exp\left(-i\frac{\pi}{2}\sum_{k=1}^{3}\sigma_y^k\right) \qquad (100)$$

$$= \exp\left(i\frac{\pi}{2}\sum_{k=1}^{3}\sigma_y^k\right)\cdot\exp\left(-i\hat{H}^{\text{int}}\Delta t/\hbar\right)\cdot\exp\left(i\frac{\pi}{2}\sum_{k=1}^{3}\sigma_y^k\right) \qquad (101)$$

Then, the time evolution which is the same evolution in the individual rotating frame is given by Eqs. (102) and (103). The example pulse sequence calculated by Eqs. (94) and (103) is shown in Fig. 7.

$$\exp\left(-i\hat{H}^{zz}\Delta t/\hbar\right) = \exp\left(-i\hat{H}^{\text{int},-s}\Delta t/2\hbar\right)\cdot\exp\left(-i\hat{H}^{\text{int}}\Delta t/2\hbar\right) \qquad (102)$$

$$= \exp\left(-i\hat{H}^{\text{int}}\Delta t/2\hbar\right)\cdot\exp\left(-i\hat{H}^{\text{int},-s}\Delta t/2\hbar\right) \qquad (103)$$

From these methods, the effective spin Hamiltonian in the common rotating frame can be manipulated similarly as in the case of the individual rotating frame; therefore, we will discuss only the effective spin Hamiltonian in the individual rotating frame in the following sections.

Fig. 7 Generation of Eqs. (94) and (103) by the spin rotation around the z-axis for three spin systems

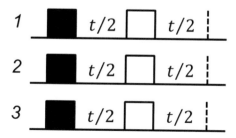

4.5   Three Qubit Operations

In general, UQG can simulate n qubit interactions as n qubit operations. Here, we show a three qubit interaction case which method can expand into the n qubit interactions [44]. At first, the three qubit interaction is decomposed as given by Eqs. (104)–106.

$$\exp\left(-i\alpha^{12}\sigma_z^1\sigma_z^2\sigma_z^3 t/\hbar\right) = \exp\left(-i\frac{\pi}{4}\sigma_x^1\right) \cdot \exp\left(-i\alpha^{12}\sigma_y^1\sigma_z^2\sigma_z^3 t/\hbar\right) \cdot \exp\left(i\frac{\pi}{4}\sigma_x^1\right) \tag{104}$$

$$= \exp\left(-i\frac{\pi}{4}\sigma_x^1\right) \cdot \exp\left(i\frac{\pi}{4}\sigma_x^1\sigma_z^3\right) \cdot \exp\left(-i\alpha^{12}\sigma_z^1\sigma_z^2 t/\hbar\right) \cdot \exp\left(-i\frac{\pi}{4}\sigma_x^1\sigma_z^3\right) \cdot \exp\left(i\frac{\pi}{4}\sigma_x^1\right) \tag{105}$$

$$= \exp\left(-i\frac{\pi}{4}\sigma_x^1\right) \cdot \exp\left(-i\frac{\pi}{4}\sigma_y^1\right) \cdot \exp\left(i\frac{\pi}{4}\sigma_z^1\sigma_z^3\right) \cdot \exp\left(i\frac{\pi}{4}\sigma_y^1\right) \cdot \exp\left(-i\alpha^{12}\sigma_z^1\sigma_z^2 t/\hbar\right)$$

$$\cdot\exp\left(-i\frac{\pi}{4}\sigma_y^1\right) \cdot \exp\left(-i\frac{\pi}{4}\sigma_z^1\sigma_z^3\right) \cdot \exp\left(i\frac{\pi}{4}\sigma_y^1\right) \cdot \exp\left(i\frac{\pi}{4}\sigma_x^1\right) \tag{106}$$

The two-qubit operation terms depend on the method of effective spin Hamiltonian, where we have assumed with secular approximation in the individual rotating frame. The Eq. (106) is utilized to perform the three qubit interaction part (Eq. (56)) of the pulse sequence study. In order to prepare the following section, we denote other two expressions (Eqs. (107) to (110)) calculated from the permutation of Eq. (106).

$$= \exp\left(-i\frac{\pi}{4}\sigma_x^2\right) \cdot \exp\left(-i\frac{\pi}{4}\sigma_y^2\right) \cdot \exp\left(i\frac{\pi}{4}\sigma_z^1\sigma_z^2\right) \cdot \exp\left(i\frac{\pi}{4}\sigma_y^2\right) \cdot \exp\left(-i\alpha^{12}\sigma_z^2\sigma_z^3 t/\hbar\right)$$

$$\cdot\exp\left(-i\frac{\pi}{4}\sigma_y^2\right) \cdot \exp\left(-i\frac{\pi}{4}\sigma_z^1\sigma_z^2\right) \cdot \exp\left(i\frac{\pi}{4}\sigma_y^2\right) \cdot \exp\left(i\frac{\pi}{4}\sigma_x^2\right) \tag{107}$$

$$t = \alpha^{23}t'/\alpha^{12} \tag{108}$$

$$= \exp\left(-i\frac{\pi}{4}\sigma_x^3\right) \cdot \exp\left(-i\frac{\pi}{4}\sigma_y^3\right) \cdot \exp\left(i\frac{\pi}{4}\sigma_z^2\sigma_z^3\right) \cdot \exp\left(i\frac{\pi}{4}\sigma_y^3\right) \cdot \exp\left(-i\alpha^{12}\sigma_z^1\sigma_z^3 t/\hbar\right)$$

$$\cdot\exp\left(-i\frac{\pi}{4}\sigma_y^3\right) \cdot \exp\left(-i\frac{\pi}{4}\sigma_z^2\sigma_z^3\right) \cdot \exp\left(i\frac{\pi}{4}\sigma_y^3\right) \cdot \exp\left(i\frac{\pi}{4}\sigma_x^3\right) \tag{109}$$

$$t = \alpha^{13}t'/\alpha^{12} \tag{110}$$

Note that t' and t'' whose absolute value indicates the evolution time which can range to negative values. In the negative case, adopt Eqs. (78)–(81) or (82)–(85) in

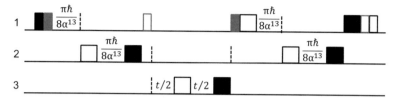

Fig. 8 The pulse sequence of a three spin interaction. The operation $\exp\left(-i\alpha^{12}\sigma_z^1\sigma_z^2\sigma_z^3 t/\hbar\right)$ is composed of Eqs. (69), (71), (79), and (106). $\alpha^{13} > 0$ is assumed in this pulse sequence scheme. The time is delimited by a *dotted line* in 2 and 3

order to transform the positive time evolution. For the operation of $\exp(i\alpha^{12}\sigma_z^1\sigma_z^2\sigma_z^3 t/\hbar)$, one can use the same procedure as given by Eqs. (78)–(81) or (82)–(85). The example pulse sequence of Eq. (106) with Eqs. (69), (71), and (79) is shown in Fig. 8. In this pulse sequence, the sign of α^{13} is assumed to be positive.

4.6 Higher Order (>3) Qubit Operations

The higher qubit interaction ($n > 3$) can be simulated as a same method as a three qubit operation [44]. Only the repetition is needed to simulate four qubit interaction from three qubit interaction. Eq. (111) is obtained as an example utilized by Eq. (106). This is because the first four terms and the last four terms play the role to create an interaction between the controlled first spin and newer fourth spin in Eq. (111).

$$
\begin{aligned}
&\exp\left(-i\alpha^{12}\sigma_z^1\sigma_z^2\sigma_z^3\sigma_z^4 t/\hbar\right) \\
&= \exp\left(-i\frac{\pi}{4}\sigma_x^1\right) \cdot \exp\left(-i\frac{\pi}{4}\sigma_y^1\right) \cdot \exp\left(i\frac{\pi}{4}\sigma_z^1\sigma_z^4\right) \cdot \exp\left(i\frac{\pi}{4}\sigma_y^1\right) \cdot \exp\left(-i\alpha^{12}\sigma_z^1\sigma_z^2\sigma_z^3 t/\hbar\right) \\
&\quad \cdot \exp\left(-i\frac{\pi}{4}\sigma_y^1\right) \cdot \exp\left(-i\frac{\pi}{4}\sigma_z^1\sigma_z^4\right) \cdot \exp\left(i\frac{\pi}{4}\sigma_y^1\right) \cdot \exp\left(i\frac{\pi}{4}\sigma_x^1\right)
\end{aligned}
$$

$$(111)$$

These equations shown in Sect. 4.5 and 4.6 indicate that the spin QCs have the ability for simulating n qubit interactions analytically, and the computational costs of AQC are estimated $2n + 1$ as the number of two-qubit operation parts in order to create a n qubit interaction.

4.7   Fast Two-Qubit Operation Between Nuclear Spins

In general, two spin interactions between nuclei are too weak to manipulate due to the small gyromagnetic ratio of nuclei in comparison with electron one. Here, we introduce a fast operation method by manipulating hyperfine interactions. One electron and two nuclear system (e_1, n_2, and n_3) are assumed as described above. Focusing on the three qubit operations, Eqs. (106) and (107), there is only one two-qubit operation between the second and third spin. Transforming these equations,

$$\exp\left(-i\alpha^{12}\sigma_z^2\sigma_z^3 t/\hbar\right) = \exp\left(-i\frac{\pi}{4}\sigma_y^2\right) \cdot \exp\left(-i\frac{\pi}{4}\sigma_z^1\sigma_z^2\right) \cdot \exp\left(i\frac{\pi}{4}\sigma_y^2\right) \cdot \exp\left(i\frac{\pi}{4}\sigma_x^2\right)$$
$$\cdot \exp\left(-i\frac{\pi}{4}\sigma_x^1\right) \cdot \exp\left(-i\frac{\pi}{4}\sigma_y^1\right) \cdot \exp\left(i\frac{\pi}{4}\sigma_z^1\sigma_z^3\right) \cdot \exp\left(-i\alpha^{12}\sigma_z^1\sigma_z^2 t/\hbar\right)$$
$$\cdot \exp\left(-i\frac{\pi}{4}\sigma_y^1\right) \cdot \exp\left(-i\frac{\pi}{4}\sigma_z^1\sigma_z^3\right) \cdot \exp\left(i\frac{\pi}{4}\sigma_y^1\right)$$
$$\cdot \exp\left(i\frac{\pi}{4}\sigma_x^1\right) \cdot \exp\left(-i\frac{\pi}{4}\sigma_x^2\right) \cdot \exp\left(-i\frac{\pi}{4}\sigma_y^2\right) \cdot \exp\left(i\frac{\pi}{4}\sigma_z^1\sigma_z^2\right) \cdot \exp\left(i\frac{\pi}{4}\sigma_y^2\right)$$

$$(112)$$

is obtained. This transformation is always possible to hyperfine coupled nuclei and the computational cost of AQC is 5 as same as a four qubit interaction for the case of two nuclear spins coupled to the same electron. This cost increases in which two nuclei couple only to other electrons. The pulse sequence is shown in Fig. 9 when the sign of α^{12} and α^{13} is positive and adopting Eqs. (69), (71), and (79).

4.8   AQC Pulse Calculations in a Three Electron System

The pulse operations toward the adiabatic factorization problem of 21 are calculated by the method described above, and the pulse sequence for a three electron system is calculated by connecting these pulse operations. Here, we show the connected pulse sequence when all spin interactions are negative (Fig. 10). As mention later, this pulse sequence can be applied for a phthalocyanine derivative molecule.

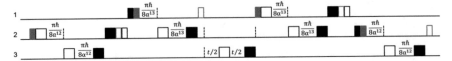

Fig. 9 The pulse sequence of a three spin interaction. The operation $e^{-\alpha^{12}\sigma_z^2\sigma_z^3 t/\hbar}$ is composed of Eqs. (69), (71), (79), and (112) assumed in this pulse sequence scheme. The time is delimited by a dotted line in 2 and 3

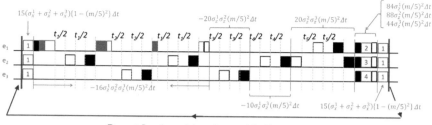

Repeat five times (changing m=1 to 5)

Fig. 10 The pulse sequence for a three electron system which coupling constants are $\alpha^{12}, \alpha^{23}, \alpha^{31} < 0$. This sequence needs to repeat five times with changing the value of $m = 1$ to 5 (see Eqs. (10) and (13)–(15)), where $\Delta t = 0.028/\hbar$. The detail information on the pulse interval (t_1 to t_5) and the dotted blocks are shown in Tables 2 and 3

Table 2 The analytical pulse interval (t_1 to t_5) in the three electron system

t_1/s	t_2/s	t_3/s	t_4/s	t_5/s
$-\pi\hbar/(D_{zz}+J)^{13}$	$-64a_m/(D_{zz}+J)^{12}$	$-80a_m/(D_{zz}+J)^{12}$	$-40a_m/(D_{zz}+J)^{13}$	$-80a_m/(D_{zz}+J)^{23}$

Here, $a_m = 0.028\hbar(m/5)^2$

Table 3 The analytical operation angles and the directions (Block 1–5) in the three electron system

1	2	3	4	5
$30b_m$	$168c_m$	$176c_m$	$88c_m$	$30b_m + \pi/2$
x	y	y	y	x

Here, $b_m = 0.028\left\{1 - (m/5)^2\right\}$ and $c_m = 0.028(m/5)^2$

4.9 AQC Pulse Calculations in a One Electron and Two Nuclear System

The pulse sequence for a one electron and two nuclear system is calculated by connecting these pulse operations. Here, we shows the connected pulse sequence when spin interaction signs are $\alpha^{12} > 0, \alpha^{31} < 0$ (Fig. 11). As mentioned later, this pulse sequence can be applied for a glutaconic acid radical molecule.

5 MSQCs for AQC

This section introduces realistic molecular spin systems for AQC. As discussed before, towering the experiments of the adiabatic factorization algorithm of 21 requires some particular conditions. Here, we summarize the computational conditions as discussed in Sects. 2–4.

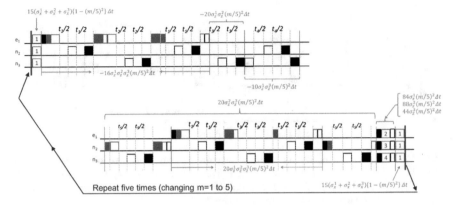

Fig. 11 The pulse sequence for a one electron and two nuclear system which coupling constants are $\alpha^{12} > 0, \alpha^{31} < 0$. This sequence needs to repeat five times with changing the value of $m = 1–5$ (see Eq. (1-6a)), where $\Delta t = 0.028/\hbar$. The detail information on the pulse interval (t_1 to t_5) and the dotted blocks is shown in Tables 4 and 5

Table 4 The analytical pulse interval ($t_1–t_5$) in a one electron and two nuclear system

t_1/s	t_2/s	t_3/s	t_4/s	t_5/s
$-\pi\hbar/A_{zz}^{13}$	$64a_m/A_{zz}^{12}$	$80a_m/A_{zz}^{12}$	$-40a_m/A_{zz}^{13}$	$\pi\hbar/A_{zz}^{12}$

Here, $a_m = 0.028\hbar(m/5)^2$

Table 5 The analytical operation angles and the directions (Block 1–5) in a one electron and two nuclear system

1	2	3	4	5
$30b_m$	$168c_m$	$176c_m$	$88c_m$	$30b_m + \pi/2$
x	y	y	y	x

Here, $b_m = 0.028\left\{1 - (m/5)^2\right\}$ and $c_m = 0.028(m/5)^2$

(1) This AQUA needs 3 qubits to perform AQC.
(2) The spin system is assumed as a fully controlled/coupled manner.
(3) The principle axes of hyperfine tensors should be parallel to the static magnetic field.
(4) The coupling constants between nuclear spins are not important.

(1) was discussed on Sect. 2 in terms of the algorithm, (2) and (3) are assumed to make universal gates easy to implement and discussed in Sects. 3 and 4, and (4) was proven in Sect. 4. The effective spin Hamiltonian (Eqs. (64) and (66)) in the diluted single crystal was chosen in this section since most of QC experiments on MSQCs have been carried out in solid states and such ensemble experiments enable us to establish both qubit initialization and entanglement conditions [27, 37].

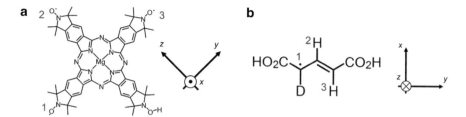

Fig. 12 Molecular systems for AQC. (**a**) A phthalocyanine system for three electron spin qubits. One radical site is reduced by a hydrogen atom. Three electron spins are mostly localized on each NO radical site, which is numbered. (**b**) A trans-glutaconic acid radical molecule for one electron spin bus qubit and two nuclear client qubits. One hydrogen atom is deuterated and the number 1 denotes an unpaired electron spin and the numbers 2 and 3 denote the client qubits. It should be noted that the unpaired electron is delocalized to some extent over the π-conjugation

A phthalocyanine derivative [45] and a 2-deuterated glutaconic acid radical [46–49] are adopted for MSQCs as three electron qubit (3e) system and one electron and three nuclear client qubit (1e + 2n) system, respectively (Fig. 12). These systems are selected to concern above conditions (1)–(4), especially glutaconic acid radical has approximate collinearity between the hyperfine tensors, which is essential for the restriction (3) [46, 48]. We assumed its deuterated derivative and the spin qubits (e_1, H_2, and H_3) is depicted in Fig. 12. On the other hand, a phthalocyanine system with four electron spins has been reported [45]. In this study, we assumed that one of the four nitroxide radical (N − O·) sites is reduced to form the closed shell of N − O − H. Other chemical structures at the NO site are possible. The unpaired electrons (e_1, e_2, and e_3) are numbered in Fig. 2.

5.1 Parameter Sets of the Three Electron Spin Qubit System (D-tensor)

The spin parameters of the phthalocyanine system (Eq. (113)) were calculated by quantum chemical calculations.

$$\hat{H}_{3e}^{int} = S_z^1 (j + D)_{zz}^{12} S_z^2 + S_z^2 (j + D)_{zz}^{23} S_z^3 + S_z^3 (j + D)_{zz}^{31} S_z^1 \qquad (113)$$

The geometry optimization of this Mg-centered phthalocyanine system was carried out at the UB3LYP/6-31G* level of theory using Gaussian 03 software [50–52]. The molecule belongs to a C_s point group with a mirror plane parallel to the HON…Mg…NO• axis. The structure do not have imaginary vibrational frequency at the optimized geometry (Fig. 13).

Since the phthalocyanine derivative has localized electrons with the spin distance larger than 10 Å, the zero field splitting (D-) tensor was calculated by the point dipole approximation with (Eq. (114)) the optimized structure. An angle θ is

Fig. 13 The optimized
structure of the
phthalocyanine triradical
molecule

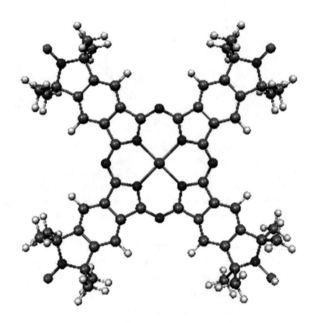

Table 6 The spin distances
and D-values of the zero field
splitting tensor

	1–2	2–3	3–1
Distance /Å	13.31	13.31	18.82
D/h /MHz	−33.11	−33.11	−11.71

defined an angle between the static magnetic field (the z-direction) and the line
connecting two radical sites. The distance was assumed for the mean distance
between N–N and O–O in the nitroxide radical moieties. Table 6 shows the spin
distance and D tensors between the spin sites.

$$D/h = -\frac{3}{2}\frac{\mu_0(g\beta)^2}{4\pi r^3 h}, \quad D_{zz} = D(3\cos^2\theta - 1) \tag{114}$$

5.2 Parameter Sets of the Three Electron Spin Qubit System (J-Coupling)

Exchange coupling constants J in the phthalocyanine triradical system are calculated by means of the broken-symmetry DFT method [52]. It is not trivial to expand
the broken-symmetry DFT method [53], then we assumed a following expansion.
The exchange coupling constants are derived by a Heisenberg Hamiltonian acting
on the unpaired electrons localized onto the NO sites, as Eq. (115).

$$H = -2J_{12}\mathbf{S}_1 \cdot \mathbf{S}_2 - 2J_{23}\mathbf{S}_2 \cdot \mathbf{S}_3 - 2J_{31}\mathbf{S}_3 \cdot \mathbf{S}_1 \tag{115}$$

The numbering of the spin site is given in Fig. 12. The Heisenberg Hamiltonian matrix in the spin function (Slater determinant) basis ($|\alpha\alpha\beta\rangle$, $|\alpha\beta\alpha\rangle$, and $|\beta\alpha\alpha\rangle$) is written by Eq. (116).

$$H \doteq \begin{pmatrix} (-J_{12} + J_{23} + J_{31})/2 & -J_{23} & -J_{31} \\ -J_{23} & (J_{12} + J_{23} - J_{31})/2 & -J_{12} \\ -J_{31} & -J_{12} & (J_{12} - J_{23} + J_{31})/2 \end{pmatrix}$$

$$(116)$$

The C_s symmetry of the phthalocyanine molecule indicates $J_{12} = J_{23}$. In this case, the secular equation is analytically solved, and the following eigenfunctions and eigenvalues of one spin-quartet and two spin-doublet states (Eqs. (117) to (119)) are obtained.

$$\Psi\left(S = \frac{3}{2}, M_S = \frac{1}{2}\right) = \frac{1}{\sqrt{3}}(|\alpha\alpha\beta\rangle + |\alpha\beta\alpha\rangle + |\beta\alpha\alpha\rangle),$$

$$E\left(S = \frac{3}{2}, M_S = \frac{1}{2}\right) = -(J_{12} + J_{23} + J_{31})/2 \qquad (117)$$

$$\Psi\left(S = \frac{1}{2}, M_S = \frac{1}{2}; 1\right) = \frac{1}{\sqrt{6}}(2|\alpha\beta\alpha\rangle - |\alpha\alpha\beta\rangle - |\beta\alpha\alpha\rangle),$$

$$E\left(S = \frac{1}{2}, M_S = \frac{1}{2}; 1\right) = J_{12} + J_{23} - J_{31}/2 \qquad (118)$$

$$\Psi\left(S = \frac{1}{2}, M_S = \frac{1}{2}; 2\right) = \frac{1}{\sqrt{2}}(|\alpha\alpha\beta\rangle - |\beta\alpha\alpha\rangle)$$

$$E\left(S = \frac{3}{2}, M_S = \frac{1}{2}; 2\right) = 3J_{31}/2 \qquad (119)$$

Here, $\Psi(S, M_S; X)$ represents an eigenfunction of the Heisenberg Hamiltonian of the spin quantum number S and magnetic quantum number M_S. X is the difference between the two spin-doublet wave functions. The Eqs. (117)–(119) hold regardless of the absolute signs and magnitudes (ratios) of the J values. (The off-diagonal term of the Heisenberg Hamiltonian between the two spin-doublet eigenfunctions is calculated as $\sqrt{3}(J_{12} - J_{23})/2$, but this is vanished by $J_{12} = J_{23}$.) Since the spin-doublet eigenfunctions in Eqs. (118) and (119) have multideterminantal characters, they cannot be represented from DFT calculation directly. In this case, the structure of the spin eigenfunctions is well defined, then one can derive energy differences between the spin states as well as the exchange coupling constants J from the diagonal terms of the Heisenberg Hamiltonian (Eq. (116)). It should be emphasized that the calculations of the off-diagonal terms in the Heisenberg Hamiltonian are not straightforward in DFT because Kohn–Sham orbitals are not identical between two determinants such as $|\alpha\alpha\beta\rangle$ and $|\alpha\beta\alpha\rangle$.

In the phthalocyanine-based triradical, energy separations among three states (one spin-quartet (**HS**, $M_S = 3/2$) and two broken-symmetry (**BS1** and **BS2**) states with $M_S = 1/2$) are quite small ($<10^{-7}$ Hartree). The tough conditions are adopted that an ultrafine grid for the computations of two-electron integrals and very tight SCF convergence criteria (requested convergence on RMS density matrix is 1.0×10^{-12}, max density matrix is 1.0×10^{-10}, energy is 1.0×10^{-10} Hartree). The calculated DFT energies and $<S^2>$ values, and expected value of the Heisenberg Hamiltonian are summarized in Table 7. The exchange coupling constants J were calculated by utilizing the following equations.

$$J_{12} = J_{23} = \{E(\mathbf{BS1}) - E(\mathbf{HS})\}/2 \tag{120}$$

$$J_{31} = E(\mathbf{BS2}) - E(\mathbf{HS}) - J_{12} \tag{121}$$

The calculated **HS**, **BS1**, and **BS2** are illustrated in Fig. 14. It should be noted that the reliable calculation of exchange coupling constants J in terms of BS-DFT is very difficult because the level of accuracy strongly depends on the nature of the species under study, exchange–correlation functionals, and basis sets. In the present study, we used the UB3LYP/6-31G* level of theory for the calculations because qualitative J values can usually be obtained at this level.

Table 7 The UB3LYP single point energies and $< S^2 >$ values, and expectation value of the Heisenberg Hamiltonian

State	E(UB3LYP/6-31G*)/Hartree	$<S^2>$	$<H(\text{Heisenberg})>$
HS	-3326.33031852657	3.7614	$(-J_{12} - J_{23} - J_{31})/2$
BS1	-3326.33031853021	1.7614	$(J_{12} + J_{23} - J_{31})/2$
BS2	-3326.33031853843	1.7614	$(J_{12} - J_{23} + J_{31})/2$

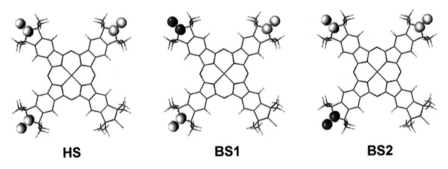

HS   **BS1**   **BS2**

Fig. 14 Contour plot of the spin density of a spin-quartet (**HS**) and two broken-symmetry (**BS1** and **BS2**) states. The isosurface value of the contour plot is set to 0.005

Table 8 The exchange–correlation functional and basis set dependences of the exchange coupling constants J

Functional	Basis set	J_{12}/MHz	J_{23}/MHz	J_{31}/MHz
B3LYP	6-31G*	−12.01	−12.01	−66.03
O3LYP	6-31G*	−8.03	−8.03	−54.02
B3PW91	6-31G*	−14.21	−14.21	−47.83
BMK	6-31G*	−24.18	−24.18	−59.98
B3LYP	6-311G*	−17.30	−17.30	−51.65

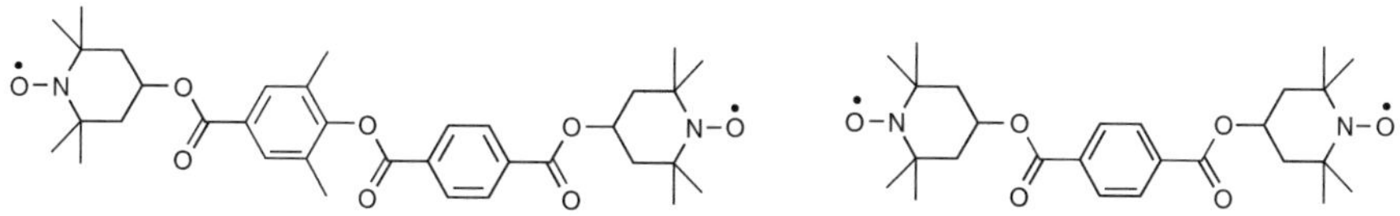

Fig. 15 Weakly exchange-coupled TEMPO biradicals **BIR-1** (*left*) and **BIR-2** (*right*)

Table 8 shows the exchange–correlation functional dependences by using O3LYP, B3PW91, and BMK functionals, and the basis set dependence from 6-31G* to 6-311G*, which indicates that no significant differences in the trend of J values. Another computational examples of exchange coupling constants, biradical molecules (**BIR-1** and **BIR-2**) [30, 54], are calculated by the present computations. Both are also weakly exchange-coupled systems using known TEMPO (2,2,6,6-tetramethylpiperidine 1-oxyl) as shown in Fig. 15. Those experiments were carried out using isotope-labelled samples for **BIR-1** and **BIR-2**, aiming to make ESR lines narrower and to make two TEMPO radicals distinguishable. Experimentally determined exchange coupling constants J in the TEMPO biradicals are +0.07 MHz and less than 0.5 MHz (in absolute value) for **BIR-1** and **BIR-2**, respectively. Note that the Heisenberg exchange coupling Hamiltonian is defined as $H = J_{12}\mathbf{S}_1 \cdot \mathbf{S}_2$ in [30, 54], not as $H = -2J_{12}\mathbf{S}_1 \cdot \mathbf{S}_2$. Therefore, we divided the J value given in Refs. [30] and [54] by a factor of −2 for the purpose of direct comparison. At the UB3LYP/6-31G* level, the J value is calculated to be less than 0.07 MHz for **BIR-1**, and +2.50 MHz for **BIR-2**.

5.3 Total Spin Interactions Between the Spins in the Three Electron Spin Qubit System

A static magnetic field direction is selected for the pulse sequence analysis. In order to have strong interactions between the spin sites, the static magnetic field is assumed to be along the z-direction as given in Fig. 16. The orientation is selected to give suitable interaction strengths. The calculated value of UB3LYP/6-31G* is adopted for J coupling constants. Table 9 shows the D_{zz}-values and the total coupling values $(D_{zz} + J)$. These values are utilized to the coupling constants of

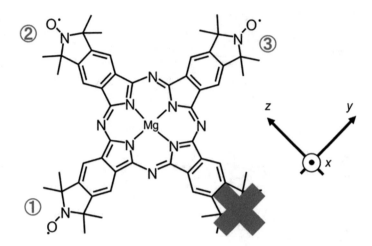

Fig. 16 The molecular structure of the phthalocyanine system. The radical sites are designated by the numbers

Table 9 The interaction strength between the spin sites by theoretical calculation

	1–2	2–3	3–1
θ	$5\pi/4$	$-5\pi/4$	$\pi/2$
$D_{zz}/h/\text{MHz}$	-16.55	-16.55	11.71
$(D_{zz}+J)/h/\text{MHz}$	-28.56	-28.56	-54.32

the effective spin Hamiltonian, which govern pulse intervals (required time) and pulse sequence.

5.4　Parameter Sets of the One Electron and Two Nuclear Spin Qubit System

The spin Hamiltonian parameters of the glutaconic acid derivative were obtained from the X-ray irradiation study [46, 48]. The magnetic field direction is oriented along the z-axis depicted in Fig. 17 because the orientation gives the anisotropic terms of the hyperfine tensors for the deuterated glutaconic acid system, respectively. The adopted hyperfine coupling constants of the glutaconic acid system are $A_{zz}^{12} = +7.0$ MHz and $A_{zz}^{31} = -37.9$ MHz [46, 48]. These values are utilized as the coupling constants of the effective spin Hamiltonian, which govern pulse intervals (required time) and pulse sequence. In this electron spin bus qubit, the exchange interaction between the nuclei was estimated to be much smaller than the hyperfine interactions; therefore, any operation relevant to this interaction is not included in the present pulse sequences.

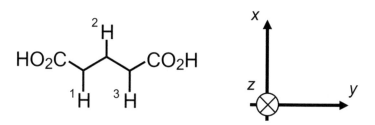

Fig. 17 The molecular structure of the glutaconic acid radical. The hydrogen 1 is deuterated and the direction of the static magnetic field is along the z-direction. The experimental principal values in z,z-direction of hyperfine tensors between the electron and second and third hydrogen nuclei are +7.0 MHz and −36.0 MHz, respectively

6 Pulse Sequence Results: Operation Time of the Sequences

The pulse sequences for the adiabatic factorization of 21 are calculated analytically as shown in Sect. 4.8. A phthalocyanine derivative and a glutaconic acid radical as discussed in Sect. 5 satisfy the signs of the spin coupling constants for the sequences as shown in Table 10.

The simplified pulse sequences are shown in Fig. 18 by reducing the obvious operations from the sequences of Sect. 4.8, and the detailed parameters for the pulse intervals and the rotational angles are given in Table 11. To claim any practical scheme of quantum computation, the spin qubit manipulation based on the pulse sequence must be executed in polynomial time. The sequence generation method for AQC, which is also useful for quantum simulation by using molecular spins, gives the simplest procedure and fulfills the requirement for the computation time.

The required time of MSQC in the context of ESR-QC was estimated as the total time of the pulse intervals, the summation of the time evolution period, shown in Table 12. The phthalocyanine and glutaconic acid systems need 0.176 and 1.31 µs to complete the factorization, respectively. The required time for those systems reflects the spin interaction strength and the sequence generation technique especially for the two nuclear spin manipulation. In the previous NMR-QC experiment on the closed shell molecule, the corresponding required time was approximately 50 ms [25]. The time length is proportional to the strength of two spin interactions generating for the multi-qubit operations. At the NMR-QC case, there are only exchange couplings between the nuclei ranging from 50 to 200 Hz on the basis of the solution NMR experiments. On the other hand, the ESR-QC molecular spins, both the 3e and (1e + 2n) systems, have about 7 up to 55 MHz spin interaction for the qubit manipulations, and thus the 3e and (1e + 2n) systems can speed up performing AQC-base factorization about 2.8×10^5 and 3.8×10^4 times faster than the NMR-QC case, respectively. Besides initialization issues of spin qubits in ensemble, in this context molecular electron spins have a big advantage over NMR-QC cases. As expected for ESR-QC experiments based on the circuit model [30], the present AQC approach demonstrates that hyperfine interactions with reasonable strength ensure marked speedup in performing QC processes.

Table 10 Coupling constants obtained by quantum chemical calculations for the phthalocyanine system

	e_1–e_2	e_2–e_3	e_1–e_3
(a) Coupling constants of the J tensors			
J/h/MHz	−12.01	−12.01	−66.03
(b) Spin distances and coupling constants of the D tensors			
r/Å	13.31	13.31	18.82
D/h/MHz	−33.11	−33.11	−11.71
D_{zz}/h/MHz	−16.55	−16.55	11.71

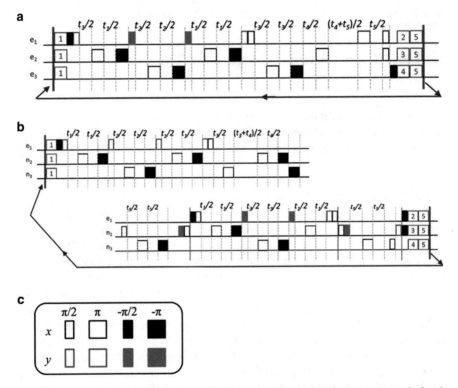

Fig. 18 Conquered pulse sequences for AQC. Time intervals are given in the upper panel of each pulse sequence. Numbered pulse operations in dotted blocks denote rotations around the x- or y-axis direction. (**a**) A pulse sequence in the phthalocyanine derivative for the factorization of 21. The sequence indicates one cycle for m (ranging from 1 to 5); therefore, this sequence is needed to loop at five times along the *arrows*. (**b**) A pulse sequence in the glutaconic acid system for the factorization of 21. The sequence indicates one cycle for m (ranging from 1 to 5); therefore, this sequence is needed to loop at five times along the *arrows*. (**c**) Schematic picture for the operations appearing in the pulse sequences. Narrow and wide pulses denote the $\pi/2$ and π angle rotations, respectively. Black and gray blocks denote the operations for the x- and y-axis direction, respectively

Table 11 Detail parameters of the pulse sequences

	t_1/ns	t_2/ns	t_3/ns	t_4/ns	t_5/ns
(a) Analytical time intervals of the pulse intervals for the phthalocyanine system and the glutaconic acid radical					
Phthalocyanine	$-\pi\hbar/(D_{zz}+J)^{13}$	$-64a_m/(D_{zz}+J)^{12}$	$-80a_m/(D_{zz}+J)^{12}$	$-40a_m/(D_{zz}+J)^{13}$	$-80a_m/(D_{zz}+J)^{23}$
Glutaconic acid	$-\pi\hbar/A_{zz}^{13}$	$64a_m/A_{zz}^{12}$	$80a_m/A_{zz}^{12}$	$-40a_m/A_{zz}^{13}$	$\pi\hbar/A_{zz}^{12}$
(b) Numerical time intervals ($m=1$) of the pulse intervals for the phthalocyanine system and the glutaconic acid radical					
Phthalocyanine	9.158	0.4017	0.5021	0.1306	0.5021
Glutaconic acid	13.89	1.630	2.037	0.1981	71.43

(c) Analytical operation angles and direction of the dotted blocks (see Fig. 3) in the pulse sequences. Here, $b_m = 0.028\left\{1 - (m/5)^2\right\}$ and $c_m = 0.028(m/5)^2$

	θ_1	θ_2	θ_3	θ_4	θ_5
Operation angles	$30b_m$	$168c_m$	$176c_m$	$88c_m$	$30b_m + \pi/2$
Direction	x	y	y	y	x

Table 12 Required times and total operation angles in units of radian

	e_1	e_2	e_1
(a) Required time and total operation angles for the phthalocyanine derivative			
Operation angles	29.8π	35.0π	28.2π
Required time	0.176 μs		
	e_1	n_2	n_3
(b) Those for the glutaconic acid radical			
Operation angles	39.8π	70.0π	53.2π
Required time	1.31 μs		

6.1 Pulse Sequence Results: Operation Angles of the Sequences

Referred to the spin manipulation appearing in the pulse sequences, a larger total number of pulses have to be executed, 140 pulses for the 3e system and 240 pulses for the (1e + 2n) system, than the NMR-QC case with 95 pulses [25], and accordingly the operation angles increased (Table 12). The operation angles relevant to the three spin qubits are 29.8π, 34.9π, 28.2π in units of radian for the 3e system, and 39.8π, 70.0π, 53.2π for the (1e + 2n) system, while 21.5π, 24.0π, 11.5π for the NMR-QC case with three nuclear spin qubits. This is on the basis that our pulse generation method is a fully straight forward method which is ensured to calculate in polynomial time; therefore, there is the space to reduce pulses in terms of single spin rotations. It is worth to mention that although the optimization of the pulse sequence must make the experiments easier to carry out, the optimization problem is harder than what we expect to solve in general. This is the reason why we calculated the pulse sequence analytically.

The straightforward method for the sequence generation in the 3e system takes approximately 1.5 times larger time of the pulse operation/spin rotation angles than the NMR-QC case. For comparison of the two ESR-QC systems, the operation angles in the (1e + 2n) system result from approximately twice a larger number of the pulse operations than the 3e-system. This is due to the replacement techniques of the spin interaction between the nuclear spins (discussed in Sect. 4.7). This operation needs 5 two-qubit manipulations in order to generate the qubit interaction between the nuclei; this term strongly affects the operation time and angles. This operation achieves the (1e + 2n) system to operate fast as the same order as the 3e system, otherwise the (1e + 2n) system needs its required time as the same as NMR-QC experiments.

6.2 Pulse Sequence Results: Discussion

From the experimental viewpoint, we found important difference in the pulse intervals between the spin qubits under study. The pulse intervals between two spins are found to be much smaller in the ESR-QC systems (shorter than 1 ns: about

0.2 ns). This is because AQUA defines the time evolution in which an ideal Hamiltonian contains small interaction terms. Since these terms are optimized for the interaction strength of NMR cases (Table 11b), the adiabatic ESR-QCs can cause much shorter time operation than standard ESR-QCs. Under this condition, we can execute operations of the pulse sequence with somewhat reduced fidelity or perform AQC with scaling up the pulse intervals (resulting in the longer required time). Another paradigm is to implement correct and short time operations (below 0.1 ns) suitable for ESR-QC systems. In this work, we assumed that the ESR-QC experiments were carried out under the conditions of conventional MW frequencies at X-band. In principle, it is possible to set up ESR-QC experiments with the strong static magnetic field, which erase the anisotropic terms of the spin Hamiltonian in the SAA.

The issue above appears particularly in AQC, but not in gate model QC approaches. Simulating the adiabatic path demands larger numbers of operators than the standard QC, whose processes are composed of only single spin rotations and CNOT-gate (two-qubit gate) operations. On the other hand, the basic operations, selective single spin rotations, and two-qubit operations around the z-axis, which we discussed above (Sects. 4.1 and 4.4) is the same as standard QCs. The difference is the following procedures for CNOT-gate and n-qubit operation in standard QC and AQC, respectively. This ensures that if we can perform the standard QC with some molecules then AQC can be performed with them as well.

Elaborate qubit operations are needed not only for the time interval but also for the single spin rotations operated for the ESR-QC systems. We did not treat pulse generating techniques in this chapter; nevertheless, this is also an essential technical element for achieving the spin ensemble QCs. For example, Rabi operations about spin flips take sub-nanosecond for electrons and few µs for nuclei (e.g., π pulses) [30, 37, 38]. The spin rotation time is at least the same order as a typical short period of qubit manipulations, then the generation of the pulse forms can be a significantly tough task in current pulse-MW technology. The theoretical approach shown in Sect. 4 is also known to help pulse designing, and numerical calculations will help more elaborate spin rotations by pulses. It is worth to mention that recent AWG techniques must help us perform numerically calculated pulses for specific cases.

The formidable task is the Rabi operation of nuclei for the complex system composed of electron and nuclei spins. This operation takes much time, therefore one needs to eliminate the spin interactions between electrons and nuclei during the operating period, and it needs additional pulses for the electrons. Based on the estimation from the numbers of the pulses and the Rabi frequencies of nuclear spins, the required time for executing the AQC algorithm depends on the operation time of the spins in both the present ESR-QC systems, resulting in a marked difference from the NMR-QC experimental scheme. As described above, the spin rotation time of nuclear spins (few µs) is estimated to be much larger than electron spins, therefore the true required time seems to strongly depend on the spin rotations in the $(1e + 2n)$ system. This is the total costs for AQC with the complex system. Nevertheless, clearing this hindrance promises us fast quantum computations in ESR timescale with nuclear spins.

7 Conclusions

In this chapter, we have described the adiabatic factorization of 21 by MSQCs. Implementation of spin qubit operations as the pulse sequences has proved how fast the factorization is processed on real molecular ESR-QCs in the solid state, compared with the previously documented NMR-QC experiments. The pulse sequences implemented assume the experimental conditions of ESR. The theoretical approach to AQCs here contains the treatment of both three electron spins as qubits (3e system) and a one electron-bus spin with two nuclear client spins coupled to the electron spin, (1e + 2n) system. We applied the secular approach under the restriction between the principal axes of hyperfine tensors and the static magnetic field, and the approach can also help utilize other molecules as spin qubits by pulse ESR techniques (e.g., average Hamiltonian method [39–41] etc.). The CPU time of AQCs indicates the same behavior as standard QCs. The spin interaction strength of the z-direction plays the central role and this suggests that molecular spin qubits with spin properties optimized can afford to perform adiabatic quantum computing with much faster than NMR-QC cases. On the other hand, the static magnetic field (assumed as X-band) does not affect the required time directly but the secular approximation and the pulse shape can be influential.

The numbers of pulses at the 3e and (1e + 2n) systems increase from the NMR-QC experiments. This difference between the 3e system and NMR one is on the basis of the pulse sequence calculation approach, therefore the spin rotation of the 3e system is expected to be decreased down to the NMR pulse sequence. Another important aspect is the difference between the 3e and (1e + 2n) systems. The basis of the theoretical treatment of different kinds of spins as qubits demands proper spin operations.

The pulse intervals in the present AQC algorithm are found to be much small in ESR-QC cases. This is a particular issue intrinsic to AQC, contrasting with standard gate model approaches to QC. In this context, improved MW spin technology is encouraged to develop from the experimental side.

Finally, we emphasize that the present approach to perform AQC on MSQCs requires only three spin qubits and such a small number of qubits are not enough to solve intractable problems with CCs. We note that AQC is another approach to QC but equivalent to the standard quantum gate model. All physically realized qubits face their scalability in extending the QC capability [3, 28–33]. ESR-QC suggests that the scalability is materials challenge and chemistry can reach an important milestone if more than ten addressable synthetic spin qubits are prepared in optimized molecular frames. Based on the possible scenario, we have illustrated how chemistry contributes to the development of QC/QIP in spite of the fact that quantum chemistry or quantum chemical calculations performed on QCs is still a challenge for current QC/QIP technology underlain by quantum gate/circuit models. It is worth mentioning that in this work we have achieved adiabatic quantum computing (AQC) on MSQCs composed of a few addressable qubits and demonstrated that molecular spins can afford to execute realistic quantum computing.

Acknowledgments This work has been supported by Grants-in-Aid for Scientific Research on Innovative Areas "Quantum Cybernetics" and Scientific Research (B) from MEXT, Japan. The support for the present work by the FIRST project on "Quantum Information Processing" from JSPS, Japan and by the AOARD project on "Quantum Properties of Molecular Nanomagnets" (Award No. FA2386-13-1-4030) is also acknowledged.

References

1. R.W. Keyes, Rep. Prog. Phys. **68**, 2701–2746 (2005)
2. S. Lloyd, Nature **406**, 1047–1054 (2000)
3. M. Galbiati, S. Tatay, C. Barraud, A.V. Dediu, F. Petroff, R. Mattana, P. Seneor, MRS. Bull. **39**, 602–607 (2014)
4. E. Coronado, A.J. Epstein, eds. Molecular spintronics and quantum computing. *J. Mater. Chem.*, *2009*, *19*, 1661–1768.
5. S.D. Jiang, K. Goss, C. Cervetti, L. Bogani, Sci. China Chem. **55**, 867–882 (2012)
6. Y. Li, H.J. Yang, Chem. Lett. **39**, 796–802 (2010)
7. C.T. Rodgers, Pure Appl. Chem. **81**, 19–43 (2009)
8. Z.G. Zhou, L.X. Liu, Curr. Org. Chem. **18**, 459–474 (2014)
9. I. Ratera, J. Veciana, Chem. Soc. Rev. **41**, 303–349 (2012)
10. A.V. Golovin, D.A. Ponomarev, V.V. Takhistov, J. Theor. Comput. Chem. **9**, 125–153 (2010)
11. C. Bennett, E. Bernstein, G. Brassard, U. Vazirani, J. SIAM Comput. **26**, 1510–1523 (1997)
12. S. Aaronson, ACM SIGACT News **36**, 30–52 (2005)
13. R.P. Feynman, Int. J. Theor. Phys. **21**, 467–488 (1982)
14. M.A. Nielsen, I.L. Chuang, *Quantum Computation and Quantum Information* (Cambridge University Press, Cambridge, 2000)
15. Y. Wang, Statist. Sci. **27**, 373 (2012)
16. D. Bacon, W. van Dam, Commun. Acm. **53**, 84–93 (2010)
17. P.W. Shor, J. SIAM, Sci. Statist. Comput. **26**, 1484–1509 (1997)
18. A. Gepp, P. Stocks, Genet. Program. Evol. M **10**, 181–228 (2009)
19. C.-Y. Lu, D.E. Browne, T. Yang, J.-W. Pan, Phys. Rev. Lett. **99**, 250504 (2007)
20. B.P. Lanyon, T.J. Weinhold, N.K. Langford, M. Barbieri, D.F.V. James, A. Gilchrist, A.G. White, Phys. Rev. Lett. **99**, 250505 (2007)
21. A. Politi, J.C.F. Matthews, J.L. O'Brien, Science **325**, 1221 (2009)
22. E.L.A. Martine-Lopez, T. Lawson, X.Q. Zhou, J.L. O'Brien, Nature Photon. **6**, 773–776 (2012)
23. E. Lucero, Nat. Phys. **8**, 719–723 (2012)
24. L.M.K. Vandersypen, M. Steffen, G. Breyta, C.S. Yannoni, M.H. Sherwood, I.L. Chung, Nature **414**, 883–887 (2001)
25. X.-H. Peng, Z. Liao, N. Xu, G. Qin, X. Zhou, D. Suter, J. Du, Phys. Rev. Lett. **101**, 220405 (2008)
26. E. Farhi, J. Goldstone, S. Gutman, M. Sipser, arXiv:quant-ph/0001106
27. M. Mehring, J. Mende, Phys. Rev. A **73**, 052303 (2006)
28. G.A. Timco, S. Carretta, F. Troiani, F. Tuna, R.J. Pritchard, C.A. Muryn, E.J.L. McInnes, A. Ghirri, A. Candini, P. Santini, G. Amoretti, M. Affronte, R.E.P. Winpenny, Nat. Nanotechnol. **4**, 173–178 (2009)
29. K. Sato, S. Nakazawa, R. Rahimi, T. Ise, S. Nishida, T. Yoshino, N. Mori, K. Toyota, D. Shiomi, Y. Yakiyama, Y. Morita, M. Kitagawa, K. Nakasuji, M. Nakahara, H. Hara, P. Carl, P. Höfer, T. Takui, J. Mater. Chem. **19**, 3739–3754 (2009)

30. S. Nakazawa, S. Nishida, T. Ise, T. Yoshino, N. Mori, R. Rahimi, K. Sato, Y. Morita, K. Toyota, D. Shiomi, M. Kitagawa, H. Hara, P. Carl, P. Höfer, T. Takui, Angew. Chem. Int. Ed. **51**, 9860–9864 (2012)
31. Y. Morita, Y. Yakiyama, S. Nakazawa, T. Murata, T. Ise, D. Hashizume, D. Shiomi, K. Sato, M. Kitagawa, K. Nakasuji, T.J. Takui, Am. Chem. Soc. **132**, 6944–6946 (2010)
32. H. Atsumi, K. Maekawa, S. Nakazawa, D. Shiomi, K. Sato, M. Kitagawa, T. Takui, K. Nakatani, Chem. Eur. J. **18**, 178–183 (2012)
33. H. Atsumi, S. Nakazawa, C. Dohno, K. Sato, T. Takui, K. Nakatani, Chem. Commun. **49**, 6370–6372 (2013)
34. J. Roland, N. Cerf, J. Phys. Rev. A **65**, 042308 (2002)
35. D. Aharonov, W. van Dam, J. Kempe, Z. Landau, S. Lloyd, O. Regev, SIAM J. Comput. **37**, 166–194 (2007)
36. S.P. Jordan, E. Farhi, P.W. Shor, Phys. Rev. A. **74**, 052322 (2006)
37. T. Yoshino, S. Nishida, K. Sato, S. Nakazawa, R.D. Rahimi, K. Toyota, D. Shiomi, Y. Morita, M. Kitagawa, T. Takui, J. Phys. Chem. Lett. **2**, 449–453 (2011)
38. M. Mehring, J. Mende, W. Scherer, Phys. Rev. Lett. **90**, 153001 (2003)
39. M.M. Maricq, Phys. Rev. B **25**, 6622 (1982)
40. A. Llor, Chem. Phys. Lett. **204**, 217 (1993)
41. M. Mehring, V.A. Weberruss, (eds.), *Object-Oriented Magnetic Resonance; Classes and Objects, Calculations and Computations* (Academic Press, San Diego, 2001)
42. P.P. Borbat, J.H. Freed, *Structural Information from Spin-Labels and Intrinsic Paramagnetic Centres in the Biosciences Structure and Bonding*, vol. 152 (Springer, Berlin, 2013), pp. 1–82
43. M.Y. Volkov, K.M. Salikhov, Appl. Magn. Reson. **41**, 145–154 (2011)
44. C.H. Tseng, S. Somaroo, Y. Sharf, E. Knill, R. Laflamme, T.F. Havel, D.G. Cory, Phys. Rev. A **61**, 012302 (1993)
45. A.G.M. Barrett, G.R. Hanson, A.J.P. White, D.J. Williams, A.S. Micallef, Tetrahedron **63**, 5244–5250 (2007)
46. H.R. Falle, M.A. Whitehea, Can. J. Chem. **50**, 139–151 (1972)
47. L. Thomas, T.J. Srikrishan, Chem. Crystallogr. **33**, 689–693 (2003)
48. C. Heller, T.J. Cole, Chem. Phys. **37**, 243–250 (1962)
49. Y. Atalay, D. Avci, A.J. Basoglu, Mol. Struct. **787**, 90–95 (2006)
50. M.J. Frisch, G.W. Trucks, H.B. Schlegel, G.E. Scuseria, M.A. Robb, J.R. Cheeseman, G. Scalmani, V. Barone, B. Mennucci, G.A. Petersson, H. Nakatsuji, M. Caricato, X. Li, H.P. Hratchian, A.F. Izmaylov, J. Bloino, G. Zheng, J.L. Sonnenberg, M. Hada, M. Ehara, K. Toyota, R. Fukuda, J. Hasegawa, M. Ishida, T. Nakajima, Y. Honda, O. Kitao, H. Nakai, T. Vreven, J.A. Montgomery Jr., J.E. Peralta, F. Ogliaro, M. Bearpark, J.J. Heyd, E. Brothers, K.N. Kudin, V.N. Staroverov, R. Kobayashi, J. Normand, K. Raghavachari, A. Rendell, J.C. Burant, S.S. Iyengar, J. Tomasi, M. Cossi, N. Rega, M.J. Millam, M. Klene, J.E. Knox, J.B. Cross, V. Bakken, C. Adamo, J. Jaramillo, R. Gomperts, R.E. Stratmann, O. Yazyev, A.J. Austin, R. Cammi, C. Pomelli, J.W. Ochterski, R.L. Martin, K. Morokuma, V.G. Zakrzewski, G.A. Voth, P. Salvador, J.J. Dannenberg, S. Dapprich, A.D. Daniels, Ö. Farkas, J.B. Foresman, J.V. Ortiz, J. Cioslowski, D.J. Fox, *GAUSSIAN 03 (Revision D.01)* (Gaussian, Inc., Wallingford, CT, 2004)
51. M. Shoji, K. Koizumi, Y. Kitagawa, T. Kawakami, S. Yamanaka, M. Okumura, K. Yamaguchi, Chem. Phys. Lett. **432**, 343–347 (2006)
52. K. Yamaguchi, Chem. Phys. Lett. **33**, 330–335 (1975)
53. M. Shoji, K. Koizumi, T. Hamamoto, T. Taniguchi, R. Takeda, Y. Kitagawa, T. Kawakami, M. Okumura, S. Yamanaka, K. Yamaguchi, Polyhedron **24**, 2708–2715 (2005)
54. K. Ayabe, K. Sato, S. Nishida, T. Ise, S. Nakazawa, K. Sugisaki, Y. Morita, K. Toyota, D. Shiomi, M. Kitagawa, T. Takui, Phys. Chem. Chem. Phys. **14**, 9137–9148 (2012)

Free-Time and Fixed End-Point Multitarget Optimal Control Theory Applied to Quantum Computing

K. Mishima and K. Yamashita

Abstract Quantum computing and quantum information science are expected to be one of the newest technologies in the next generation. In this article, we focus on theoretical and numerical studies on quantum computing and entanglement generation using molecular internal degrees of freedom (electronic, vibrational, and rotational). We have proposed one method of creating the Bell states and arbitrary linear superposition states in molecular vibrational–rotational modes by using sequential chirped laser pulses. In addition, the numerical simulations of Deutsch–Jozsa algorithm using several combinations of the molecular internal states are reported and compared them from the viewpoint of fidelity of the measurement results of the sender. It turned out that rotational modes of polar molecules coupled by dipole–dipole interaction are the most promising candidates for molecular quantum computing. In connection with quantum computing and entanglement manipulation by external laser fields, we have constructed free-time and fixed end-point optimal control theories (FRFP-OCTs) for the quantum systems without and with dissipation. Using the theories, we have performed simulations of entanglement generation and maintenance. From the numerical results, we have found that FRFP-OCT is more efficient than the conventional fixed-time and fixed end-point optimal control theory (FIFP-OCT) because the optimal time duration of the external laser fields can also be determined exactly using FRFP-OCT.

Keywords Quantum computing • Free-time and fixed end-point multitarget optimal control theory • Molecular internal degrees of freedom • Entanglement • Deutsch-Jozsa algorithm

K. Mishima (✉) • K. Yamashita
Department of Chemical System Engineering, Graduate School of Engineering,
The University of Tokyo, Tokyo 113-8656, Japan
e-mail: erdao@tcl.t.u-tokyo.ac.jp

© Springer New York 2016   119
T. Takui et al. (eds.), *Electron Spin Resonance (ESR) Based Quantum Computing*,
Biological Magnetic Resonance 31, DOI 10.1007/978-1-4939-3658-8_5

1 Introduction

In recent years, quantum computing and quantum information science have become one of the most important and attractive research topics in a variety of disciplines, e.g., mathematics, information science, physics, etc. [1]. These new kinds of technologies are predicted to be much more advantageous compared with the classical computers and classical information science and the benefit obtained by these technologies is assumed to be beyond measure in our everyday life. For instance, quantum computers are predicted to be able to solve mathematical problems that today's fastest computers could not solve in years. In particular, entanglement or entangled state plays a key role for quantum computing and quantum information processing. For example, arbitrary quantum states of two-level system can be teleported through classical communication with the help of maximally entangled Bell state from one place to other macroscopic distant places (quantum teleportation) [2], which has no counterpart in classical mechanics. As opposed to the quantum teleportation, classical information can be teleported by using the maximally entangled Bell state (superdense coding) [3]. Needless to say, entanglement is also an essential ingredient in quantum computing.

At present, theoretical investigations of the mechanism of quantum computing and quantum information science have become mature although some of the important theoretical problems, e.g., definition of entanglement degree of multi-partite systems, have not yet been solved and are still controversial. Yet, one can say that we are now reaching a stage of experimental realizations of quantum computing and quantum information processing proposed and investigated theoretically and numerically. To apply quantum computing and quantum information processing to realistic quantum systems, a number of microscopic quantum systems have been proposed. Just to mention a few, cavity quantum electrodynamics (cavity QED) [4], trapped ions [5–7], neutral atoms trapped in optical lattices [8], nuclear magnetic resonance (NMR) [9, 10], superconducting circuits [11], silicon-based nuclear spin [12], diamond-based quantum computer [13, 14] are some of the promising candidates of quantum computing devices.

However, investigation of utilization of molecular internal degrees of freedom for quantum computing and quantum information science, in particular, electronic, vibrational, and rotational degrees of freedom, is still in its infancy. Although molecules are also quantum systems, very few chemists have yet examined how to use molecular internal degrees of freedom for quantum computing and quantum information science from the chemical viewpoint. The pioneering numerical investigation of usage of molecular vibrational states for constructing elementary quantum gates was reported by de Vivie-Riedle and coworkers at the beginning of this century [15]. Later on, they have stick to pursuing "molecular vibrational" quantum computing in a number of papers [16–21]. Soon after their works, some of the other research groups have extended their works and have proposed new ideas of quantum computing and quantum information science [22–30]. The purpose of many of these works is to numerically construct elementary gate pulses using optimal control theory (OCT) [31]. Instead of using tailored laser pulses, Teranishi and coworkers have developed a quantum computation scheme to process arbitrary quantum gate operations by using the free propagation of the wave packet of I_2 molecule [32].

Although the "vibrational" quantum computers are the mainstream for the investigations of molecular quantum computing, two-qubit system consisting of one vibrational and one rotational modes of molecules has also been investigated by several researchers [33, 34]. In [33], single- and two-qubit operations, e.g., NOT and CNOT gates, within rotational and vibrational states of a diatomic molecule using strong-field molecular alignment are proposed. Numerical calculations of IR quantum gate pulses for $^{12}C^{16}O$ molecule using a genetic algorithm instead of employing OCT have been investigated by Momose and coworkers [34].

Another possibility is to use *inter*molecular states instead of the *intra*molecular states mentioned earlier. In [35], one of the methods of realizing quantum phase gate and generation of entanglement rotational modes of two polar molecules coupled by dipole–dipole interaction has been proposed. Unlike their research, we have numerically constructed several universal gates and applied them to the Deutsch–Jozsa algorithm as shown later in detail [36].

On the other hand, attempts of experimental realizations of quantum computers using molecular internal degrees of freedom have also begun to be done in recent years. For example, Vala and coworkers experimentally demonstrated the Deutsch–Jozsa algorithm for three-qubit functions by utilizing pure coherent superposition states of Li_2 rovibrational eigenstates [37]. Rovibrational wave-packet manipulation using phase- and amplitude-modulated midinfrared femtosecond laser pulses for $^{12}C^{16}O$ and $^{14}N^{16}O$ molecules have been investigated experimentally and numerically by Momose and coworkers for the purpose of applying their techniques to quantum computing [38]. Ohmori and coworkers experimentally demonstrated coherent control of wave packet interference, wave packet interferometry, using vibrational wave packets of I_2 molecule with the aim of retrieving quantum information such as amplitudes and phases of eigenfunctions involved in the wave packet [39–43].

This present situation implies that the research of quantum computing using molecular internal degrees of freedom is gradually attracting many physical chemists and chemical physicists in quite recent years.

Interesting aspects of molecules compared with physical systems such as atoms, photons, electron spins, nuclear spins, etc., are that they possess a variety of quantum mechanical internal degrees of freedom. If we restrict ourselves only to two-qubit systems, several kinds of combinations of modes can be considered. The two-qubit combination studied most frequently is vibrational–vibrational qubit combination as mentioned earlier. Since the investigation of molecular quantum computers is still immature, we predict that there will be a number of unsolved problems up to now and recommend chemists to investigate molecular quantum computing in more detail in the future although many of the chemists including us have already contributed to the improvement of the molecular quantum computers.

The present article is organized as follows. In Sect. 2, we present our proposed method of generation of entanglement and arbitrary superposition states using vibrational and rotational modes of molecules. In addition, we shall show numerical results based on the scheme. In Sect. 3, we first introduce some of the basic concepts of quantum computers for chemists' convenience who are not familiar with quantum computers. Then, for this article to be self-contained, OCT will briefly be reviewed because molecular quantum computing strongly relies on OCT as mentioned earlier. Our calculation results or some improvement of the present OCT will also be presented. In Sect. 4, our development of free-time and fixed end-point optimal control theories (FRFP-OCTs) without and with dissipation is presented and the theory and the algorithm are applied to entanglement generation and maintenance. One will find that FRFP-OCT is more convenient and advantageous than fixed end-point optimal control theory (FIFP-OCT). Finally, Sect. 5 is devoted to concluding remarks.

2 Generation of Entanglement and Arbitrary Superposition States Using Vibrational and Rotational Modes of Molecules [44]

2.1 Scheme of Generation of Arbitrary Quantum States in Vibrational and Rotational Modes of Molecules

In Fig. 1, we show the scheme of arbitrary superposition states using the molecular rovibrational modes of closed shell molecules. Here, 0_v denotes no quantum in the vibrational mode and 1_v corresponds to one quantum in the vibrational mode. The same holds for 0_r and 1_r for rotational mode. The initial state is assumed to be a separable state $|0_v0_r\rangle$. By shining a microwave pulse, the following superposition state can be obtained: $a|0_v0_r\rangle + b|0_v1_r\rangle$. When we irradiate an IR laser pulse to this

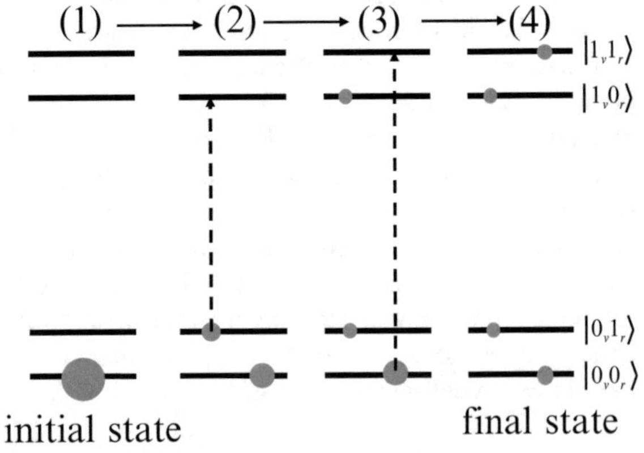

Fig. 1 Scheme of arbitrary state generation using the molecular rovibrational modes

state, we obtain $c|0_v0_r\rangle + d|0_v1_r\rangle + e|1_v0_r\rangle$. Finally, using another IR laser pulse to this state, we have $f|0_v0_r\rangle + g|0_v1_r\rangle + h|1_v0_r\rangle + q|1_v1_r\rangle$ as a final state. Note that steps 2 and 3 are interchangeable. Of course, entangled states such as $u|0_v1_r\rangle + w |1_v0_r\rangle$ and $x|0_v0_r\rangle + y|1_v1_r\rangle$ are the special cases of the arbitrary superposition states. The fact that any arbitrary superposition states of two-mode system can be created at least means that there is a possibility to process two-qubit quantum algorithms with the choice of vibrational and rotational modes of molecules. (This conclusion will be shown numerically in Sect. 3.5.) Therefore, it is very important to numerically show that arbitrary superposition states can be created by external fields.

The mechanism of creating entangled states is explained as follows. The interaction Hamiltonian of molecules with laser pulses is given by

$$W(R,\theta,t) = -E(t)\mathrm{d}(R)\cos\theta, \tag{1}$$

where R is the internuclear distance, θ is the angle between the molecular axis and the laser polarization direction, $\mathrm{d}(R)$ is the transition dipole moment, and $E(t)$ is the external laser field. Because this Hamiltonian contains the product of the vibrational parameter R and the rotational parameter θ, it follows that the entanglement between the vibrational and rotational degrees of freedom can be created when the external laser pulse is on. On the other hand, if the external laser pulse is off, the degree of entanglement cannot be changed. This feature is very particular to molecular systems. As far as we know, this kind of mechanism of entanglement generation is not found in any quantum systems other than the combination of molecular vibrational and rotational modes.

2.2 Numerical Calculation of Generation of Entanglement and Arbitrary Superposition States

The total Hamiltonian for the rovibrational states of diatomic molecules in a given electronic state irradiated by laser fields is given by

$$\hat{H}_{\mathrm{tot}}(R,\theta,t) = \hat{H}_0(R,\theta) + W(R,\theta,t), \tag{2}$$

where

$$\hat{H}_0 = T^N(R) - \frac{1}{2\mu_{\mathrm{red}}R^2}H^{\mathrm{ROT}}(\theta) + V(R), \tag{3}$$

Here, $T^N(R)$ is the vibrational kinetic part with vibrational coordinate R, $H^{\mathrm{ROT}}(\theta)$ is the rotational part of the total Hamiltonian with θ being the angle between the molecular axis and the laser polarization direction, μ_{red} is the reduced mass of the molecule, and $V(R)$ is the potential energy.

The Schrödinger equation for the rovibrational states of diatomic molecules using the total Hamiltonian of Eq. (2) is expressed as

$$\dot{c}_{v,l}(t) = -i\varepsilon_v c_{v,l}(t) - i\frac{l(l+1)}{2\mu_{\text{red}}}\sum_{v'=0}c_{v',l}(t)\int_0^\infty \chi_v^*(R)\chi_{v'}(R)\mathrm{d}R$$

$$+iE(t)\sum_{v'=0}\left[c_{v',l-1}(t)\frac{l}{\sqrt{4l^2-1}}\int_0^\infty \mathrm{d}RR^2\chi_v^*(R)\mathrm{d}(R)\chi_{v'}(R)\right. \tag{4}$$

$$\left.+\sum_{v'=0}c_{v',l+1}(t)\frac{l+1}{\sqrt{(2l+1)(2l+3)}}\int_0^\infty \mathrm{d}RR^2\chi_v^*(R)\mathrm{d}(R)\chi_{v'}(R)\right],$$

where ε_v is the vibrational energy for the vibrational quantum number v, l is the rotational principal quantum number, $\chi_v(R)$ is the vibrational wavefunction for quantum number v, and $c_{v,l}(t)$ represents the amplitude for the rovibrational wavefunction with the quantum numbers v and l. The external successive IR and microwave chirped laser pulses are expressed as

$$E(t) = \sum_{j=1}^{3} E_j(t-T_j)\cos\left\{\omega_j(t-T_j)+\frac{b_j}{2}(t-T_j)^2\right\}, \tag{5}$$

where ω_j is the resonant pulse frequency, b_j is the linear chirp rate, and $E_j(t)$ is given by the following Gaussian line shape,

$$E_j(t) = E_j^0\exp\left(-\frac{4\ln2}{\text{FWHM}_j^2}t^2\right), \tag{6}$$

where FWHM_j is the full-width at half maximum for the jth pulse and E_j^0 is the peak amplitude of the jth pulse. In the following, we assume that the linearly polarized fields are irradiated to the molecule.

To obtain the appropriate external fields, we use the Landau–Zener formula for population transfer that is given by [45–47]

$$p_i = 1 - \exp\left\{-\pi\frac{(\mathrm{d}E_i^0)^2}{2b_i}\right\} \quad \text{if } b_i \neq 0, \tag{7}$$

where d denotes the transition dipole matrix element and b_i is the absolute value of the chirp rate of the ith pulse.

Here, we shall show one of the numerical examples. The numerical result of the transfer $|0_v0_r\rangle \rightarrow (|0_v1_r\rangle + |1_v0_r\rangle)/\sqrt{2}$ based on the scheme shown in Fig. 1 is presented in Fig. 2. In this case, the equations of $p_1=1$ and $p_2=1/2$ have to be satisfied. Then, we have set $b_1=0.0855$ cm^{-1}/ps and $b_2=3.30$ cm^{-1}/ps. From Fig. 2, we can see that by using one IR field and one microwave external field, the Bell state $(|0_v1_r\rangle + |1_v0_r\rangle)/\sqrt{2}$ can be created almost completely. However, there is a detrimental effect that has to be taken into account experimentally. That is, the initial external field has to be long or strong enough to satisfy $p_1=1$. The chirp rate

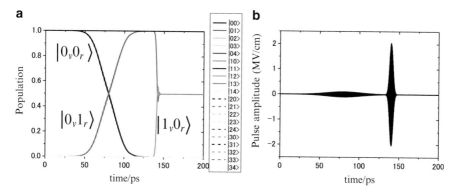

Fig. 2 Generation of the Bell state $(|0_v1_r\rangle + |1_v0_r\rangle)/\sqrt{2}$ in the HF molecule in the electronically ground state. Panel (**a**) shows the time evolution of the populations and panel (**b**) shows the external field amplitudes. The electronic ground state of the HF molecule is assumed

b_2 should be large for large α_{01} and be small for large α_{10}, where the wavefunction is $\alpha_{01}|0_v1_r\rangle + \alpha_{10}|1_v0_r\rangle$. In the former case, the second pulse has to have small pulse amplitude or large chirp rate. On the other hand, in the latter case, the reverse holds. To realize the former case, one should note that the rotational energy gap in most of the molecules is so small that care has to be taken in order not to excite the molecule to unexpected energy levels, e.g., $|0_v2_r\rangle$. In fact, we have confirmed that the virtual transition to $|0_v2_r\rangle$ takes place in the present situation. On the other hand, to realize the latter case, the chirp rate has to be so small that the chirp rate has to be adjusted appropriately in the experiments. The maximally entangled state is achieved at $p_2 = 1/2$. If p_2 shifts from this value, the entanglement degree decreases unilaterally. It is clear that the state $|0_v1_r\rangle$ can be created without the second and third pulses while the second adiabatic chirped pulse is necessary for generating the state $|1_v0_r\rangle$. Since two sequential chirped pulses are necessary for creating the state $|1_v0_r\rangle$, this state is relatively difficult to create from the experimental point of view.

3 Quantum Algorithms

3.1 Quantum Gates

Quantum gates are the counterparts of logic gates of classical computer circuits. The definition of operations of the classical single bit logic gates is given by truth table. For example, the operation of NOT gate is to flip the bits: $0 \rightarrow 1$ and $1 \rightarrow 0$.

In what follows, we list some important quantum gates that are usually used in quantum circuits:

Hadamard gate: $H_{dm} = \frac{1}{\sqrt{2}}\begin{bmatrix} 1 & 1 \\ 1 & -1 \end{bmatrix}$ for single-qubit gate,

NOT gate: $\text{NOT} = \begin{bmatrix} 0 & 1 \\ 1 & 0 \end{bmatrix}$ for single-qubit gate,

CNOT (controlled-not) gate: $\text{CNOT} = \begin{bmatrix} 1 & 0 & 0 & 0 \\ 0 & 1 & 0 & 0 \\ 0 & 0 & 0 & 1 \\ 0 & 0 & 1 & 0 \end{bmatrix}$ for two-qubit gate,

ID gate: $\text{ID} = \begin{bmatrix} 1 & 0 \\ 0 & 1 \end{bmatrix}$ for single-qubit gate,

Z gate: $Z = \begin{bmatrix} 1 & 0 \\ 0 & -1 \end{bmatrix}$ for single-qubit gate,

$\pi/8$ gate: $T = \begin{bmatrix} 1 & 0 \\ 0 & \exp(i\pi/4) \end{bmatrix}$ for single-qubit gate,

Phase gate: $S = \begin{bmatrix} 1 & 0 \\ 0 & i \end{bmatrix}$ for single-qubit gate,

Toffoli gate: $U_T = \begin{bmatrix} 1 & 0 & 0 & 0 & 0 & 0 & 0 & 0 \\ 0 & 1 & 0 & 0 & 0 & 0 & 0 & 0 \\ 0 & 0 & 1 & 0 & 0 & 0 & 0 & 0 \\ 0 & 0 & 0 & 1 & 0 & 0 & 0 & 0 \\ 0 & 0 & 0 & 0 & 1 & 0 & 0 & 0 \\ 0 & 0 & 0 & 0 & 0 & 1 & 0 & 0 \\ 0 & 0 & 0 & 0 & 0 & 0 & 0 & i \\ 0 & 0 & 0 & 0 & 0 & 0 & -i & 0 \end{bmatrix}$ for three-qubit gate.

For processing the quantum computation, the two-level unitary gates such as shown earlier must be universal [48]. Here, the term "universal" means that one can implement an arbitrary two-level unitary transformation on the space of arbitrary numbers of qubits. For example, using the Gray codes, it has been proven that single qubit and CNOT gates are universal [1]. It should be emphasized that the global unitary transformations such as CNOT gate cannot be reduced to the direct product of two single-qubit gates. Therefore, if the total Hamiltonian can be reduced to the product of two single-qubit unitary transformations, it is impossible to perform universal quantum computation and quantum information processing.

3.2 Deutsch–Jozsa Algorithm

So far, several quantum algorithms have been proposed which outperform the corresponding classical algorithms. These include the Grover's algorithm, Shor's algorithm, the quantum Fourier transform, the Deutsch–Jozsa algorithm, etc. [1]. In particular, the Deutsch–Jozsa algorithm of our concern here was found by Deutsch and coworkers [49, 50]. For example, the Shor's algorithm is a quantum algorithm for integer factorization [51]. On a quantum computer, to factor an integer N, Shor's algorithm takes polynomial time in $\log N$, specifically $O((\log N)^3)$, demonstrating

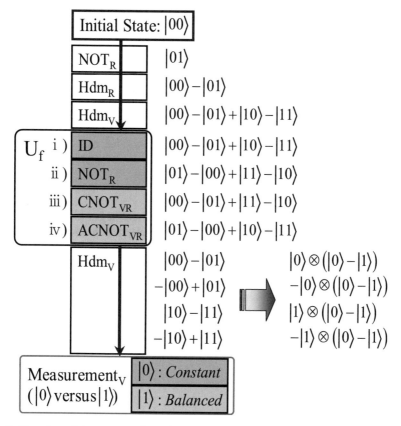

Fig. 3 Flowchart of the two-state Deutsch–Jozsa algorithm

that integer factorization is in the complexity class BQP. This is exponentially faster than the best-known classical factoring algorithm.

The flowchart of the two-state Deutsch–Jozsa algorithm is shown in Fig. 3. In short, the story of the Deutsch–Jozsa algorithm is as follows. Let us assume two persons, Alice and Bob. Alice holds the so-called query register while Bob holds the so-called answer register. First, they come close together and they make some promises before they go far apart from each other. When they are close together, Alice promises to send the number 0 or 1 to Bob and he promises to calculate some function f and to send her the answer 0 or 1. At this time, Bob promises to use two kinds of functions f. That is, he sends her the same number for all the numbers that he obtains from her (constant function) or he sends 0 for half of the numbers that he obtains from her and 1 for the remaining half (balanced function). After that, they go far apart from each other. The purpose of this algorithm is that Alice must clarify whether the function f that Bob applies is constant or balanced, which is contained in the oracle denoted by U_f. It is known that classically the algorithm scales as $O(2^n)$, while quantum mechanically it scales as $O(n)$, where n is the number of qubit registers that Alice holds. This demonstrates the significant speedup of quantum parallelism compared with classical algorithms, in particular, when n is very large. In other words, the advantage of quantum parallelism is obtained when the quantum circuit becomes very large.

In the flowchart of Fig. 3, the initial state of the whole Hilbert space is $|00\rangle$. First, Bob applies the NOT gate and the transition $|00\rangle \rightarrow |01\rangle$ occurs. Bob then applies the Hadamard gate Hdm_R and Alice the Hadamard gate Hdm_V. At this moment, the state of the whole system becomes $|00\rangle - |01\rangle + |10\rangle - |11\rangle$. To this quantum superposition state, the unitary transformation, the so-called oracle,

$$U_f : \quad |x, y\rangle \rightarrow \left| x, y \bigoplus f(x) \right\rangle, \tag{8}$$

is applied. Here, $\bigoplus$ denotes addition modulo 2. The rule of Eq. (8) must be applied for all four possible definitions of f. According to the four definitions, U_f is defined by the four operations (i)–(iv) in Fig. 3. Alice then applies the Hadamard transformation Hdm_V. If she recognizes that she obtains the state $\pm|0\rangle$ by her own measurement, f is constant, while f is balanced if she obtains the state $\pm|1\rangle$. These states can be distinguished by measuring their own qubit as shown in Fig. 3.

In all the presentations later, the subscripts of the first and the second entries for elementary quantum gates refer to control bit and target bit, respectively. In addition, we shall use abbreviations E, V, and R for electronic, vibrational, and rotational states, respectively.

3.3   Optimal Control Theory

As already mentioned in Sect. 1, to process quantum computing, it is necessary to tailor elementary gate laser pulses appropriately. This particularly holds for molecules. This is because unlike spins molecular modes of internal degrees of freedom are essentially "qudits," not "qubits." In this section, we will briefly review conventional OCT and multitarget OCT (MTOCT). For more details, we recommend the readers to refer to [52, 53].

If the purpose is just to drive one specific wave function $\psi_i(t)$ to the desired wave function $\Phi(T)$ at the fixed time $t = T$, the objective functional to be maximized is given by [52]

$$J = |\langle \psi_i(T)|\Phi(T)\rangle|^2 - \alpha_0 \int_0^T [E(t)]^2 dt - 2\text{Re}[\langle \psi_i(T)|\Phi(T)\rangle \\ \times \int_0^T \langle \psi_f(t)| \frac{\partial}{\partial t} + i[H_0 + V - \mu E(t)]|\psi_i(t)\rangle dt], \tag{9}$$

where H_0 is the 0th-order Hamiltonian, V is the potential energy, μ is the transition dipole moment, $E(t)$ is the laser pulse to be optimized, and T is the fixed final time of the laser pulse. The second term restricts the laser intensity, where α_0 is usually called the penalty factor. $|\psi_f(t)\rangle$ is the Lagrange multiplier for $|\psi_i(t)\rangle$.

To incorporate the effect of slow turn-on and turn-off of the laser pulses adequate for practical experimental tailoring, the penalty factor in Eq. (9) is replaced by [53]

$$-\alpha_0 \int_0^T \frac{[E(t)]^2}{s(t)} \, dt, \tag{10}$$

where

$$s(t) = \sin^2(\pi t/T). \tag{11}$$

In this case, the optimized external field is expressed as

$$E(t) = -\frac{s(t)}{\alpha_0} \text{Im}\{\langle \psi_i(t)|\psi_f(t)\rangle\langle \psi_f(t)|\mu|\psi_i(t)\rangle\}. \tag{12}$$

In all the calculations shown later, we have taken this effect into account.

Although the above formalisms may be applicable to tailoring the gate laser pulses, they are not appropriate for tailoring *general-purpose* global gate pulses. In other words, the given gate pulse has to process the given quantum gate for any inputs and the corresponding outputs. In this case, one of the best choices is to resort to multitarget optimal control theory (MTOCT) [54]. For MTOCT, the objective functional to be maximized is given by

$$
\begin{aligned}
J_{\text{MTOCT}} = \sum_{k=1}^z &\Big\{ |\langle \psi_{ik}(T)|\Phi_{fk}(T)\rangle|^2 - \alpha_0 \int_0^T \frac{[E(t)]^2}{s(t)} \, dt - 2\text{Re}\big\{ \langle \psi_{ik}(T)|\Phi_{fk}(T)\rangle \\
&\times \int_0^T \langle \psi_{fk}(t)| \frac{\partial}{\partial t} + i[H_0 + V - \mu E(t)]|\psi_{ik}(t)\rangle dt \big\} \Big\},
\end{aligned}
\tag{13}
$$

where z is the number of control targets, k denotes the number of targets ranging from 1 to z, $|\Phi_{fk}(T)\rangle$ is the kth target at time $t = T$, $|\psi_{ik}(t)\rangle$ is the wavefunction of the system of the kth target, and $|\psi_{fk}(t)\rangle$ is the Lagrange multiplier for $|\psi_{ik}(t)\rangle$. In this case, the optimal external field reads

$$E(t) = -\frac{zs(t)}{\alpha_0} \sum_{k=1}^z \text{Im}\{\langle \psi_{ik}(t)|\psi_{fk}(t)\rangle\langle \psi_{fk}(t)|\mu|\psi_{ik}(t)\rangle\}. \tag{14}$$

The number of the control targets z has to be chosen as follows. Recently, de Vivie-Riedle and coworkers [17] proposed a method for phase-correct and basis-set-independent quantum gates in order to perform the correct universal quantum computing. As far as we know, their work is the first one where the phase correction was taken into account adequately. The requirement of the phase-correct quantum gate is that, for example, the NOT operation for the superposition state,

$$|00\rangle + |01\rangle + |10\rangle + |11\rangle \rightarrow (|01\rangle + |00\rangle + |11\rangle + |10\rangle)e^{i\varphi_5}, \qquad (15)$$

must be optimized in addition to the following four conventional pure basis state optimizations,

$$\begin{aligned} |00\rangle &\rightarrow |01\rangle e^{i\varphi_1}, \\ |01\rangle &\rightarrow |00\rangle e^{i\varphi_2}, \\ |10\rangle &\rightarrow |11\rangle e^{i\varphi_3}, \\ |11\rangle &\rightarrow |10\rangle e^{i\varphi_4}. \end{aligned} \qquad (16)$$

If we do not impose the requirement of Eq. (15), the superposition state will evolve as:

$$|00\rangle + |01\rangle + |10\rangle + |11\rangle \rightarrow |01\rangle e^{i\varphi_1} + |00\rangle e^{i\varphi_2} + |11\rangle e^{i\varphi_3} + |10\rangle e^{i\varphi_4}, \qquad (17)$$

which is not the correct NOT operation, because in general $\varphi_1 \neq \varphi_2 \neq \varphi_3 \neq \varphi_4$. Likewise, we must impose additional constraints for the other quantum gates we have in mind. As de Vivie-Riedle and coworkers pointed out [17], the phase correction of quantum gates is one of the key issues for the implementation of quantum algorithms. Therefore, for two-qubit systems, z has to be more than 4, and according to their suggestion, their proposal will be taken into account in all the following calculations.

There are two methods to measure the gate fidelities: the average transition probability given by

$$\overline{P} = \frac{1}{z} \sum_{k=1}^{z} \left| \langle \psi_{ik}(T) | \Phi_{fk}(T) \rangle \right|^2, \qquad (18)$$

and the fidelity expressed as

$$F = \frac{1}{z^2} \left| \sum_{k=1}^{z} \langle \psi_{ik}(T) | \Phi_{fk}(T) \rangle \right|^2. \qquad (19)$$

The average transition probability cannot take into account the phase relation between $\psi_{ik}(T)$ and $\Phi_{fk}(T)$, while the fidelity can. If one uses the average transition probability, the phase correction cannot be determined, while the fidelity is useful for clarifying the phase correction. Therefore, we define the laser pulses that have the largest fidelity as the optimal gate pulses in the following calculations.

In what follows, we will show our numerical results by using some of the combinations of molecular internal degrees of freedom.

3.4 Combination of Intramolecular Electronic and Vibrational States [55]

When one regards electronic and vibrational states as qubits, special care must be taken. Usually, the eigenstates of control and target qubits are orthonormalized states in each Hilbert space. If we consider electronic and vibrational states as two-qubit system, the electronic eigenstates are usually orthonormalized, while the vibrational eigenstates that the electronic eigenstates involve are usually not orthonormalized for each electronic eigenstate. Unless they are orthonormalized, efficient quantum computing cannot be expected. This is because if the states are not orthogonal among each other, we cannot distinguish them reliably by measurement, as is well known from quantum mechanics. In order to circumvent this difficulty, the vibrational eigenstates of the electronic excited state should be written as a linear combination of the vibrational eigenstates of the electronic ground state:

$$|i'_V\rangle = \sum_{j=0} c_{i,j}|j_V\rangle, \tag{20}$$

where $|i'_V\rangle$ is the ith real vibrational eigenfunction of the electronic excited state, $|j_V\rangle$ is the jth vibrational eigenfunction of the electronic ground state, and $c_{i,j}$ is the coefficient required to perform a unitary transformation among the vibrational eigenfunctions.

The total Hamiltonian for the electronic and vibrational states of diatomic molecules in the ground and excited electronic states irradiated by the laser pulses is given by:

$$\hat{H}_{tot}(R,t) = \begin{bmatrix} T^N(R) + V_g(R) & W(R,t) \\ W(R,t) & T^N(R) + V_e(R) \end{bmatrix}, \tag{21}$$

where

$$W(R,t) = -d(R)E(t). \tag{22}$$

Here, $T^N(R)$ is the vibrational kinetic component with vibrational coordinate R; $V_g(R)$ and $V_e(R)$ are the potential energy curves (PECs) for the electronic ground and excited states, respectively; $d(R)$ is the transition dipole moment dependent on R; and $E(t)$ is the external laser pulse. In the calculations, we have taken the electronic ground and excited states as $X^1\Sigma_g^+$ and $A^1\Sigma_u^+$, respectively, of Li_2 and Na_2 molecules.

Using the total Hamiltonian of Eq. (21), the Schrödinger equation for our system is given by

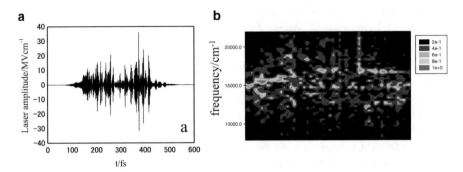

Fig. 4 (**a**) Optimized laser pulse after 1500 iterations of MTOCT, and (**b**) FROG representation for NOT_V gate of the Na_2 molecule

$$
i\frac{\partial}{\partial t}\begin{pmatrix} \psi_g(R,t) \\ \psi_e(R,t) \end{pmatrix} = \hat{H}_{tot}(R,t)\begin{pmatrix} \psi_g(R,t) \\ \psi_e(R,t) \end{pmatrix}, \tag{23}
$$

where $\psi_g(R,t)$ is the wavefunction in the electronic ground state and $\psi_e(R,t)$ is that in the electronic excited state.

In Fig. 4, we show the optimized laser pulse (panel a), frequency resolved optical gating (FROG) representation (panel b) for NOT_V gate of Na_2 molecule. In panel a, we can see that the optimized laser pulse contains very low laser amplitudes from $t = 0$–100 fs to $t = 500$–600 fs, and the laser is virtually on from $t = 100$–500 fs. From panel b, we notice that the laser frequency mainly consists of the value 15,000 cm^{-1} which almost corresponds to the resonant transition frequency between $X^1\Sigma_g^+$ and $A^1\Sigma_u^+$ states of Na_2 molecule: $\hbar\omega_0 = 15,325.4367\,cm^{-1}$. Using the optimized laser pulse, the final population of $|11\rangle$ state reaches 90.03 % at the target time $T = 600$ fs for the transition $|10\rangle \rightarrow |11\rangle$.

From the snapshots of motion of wave packets for the transition $|10\rangle \rightarrow |11\rangle$ of NOT_V gate (not shown here), it is clear that the wave packet oscillates twice on the electronically excited state until the target state is reached. From $t = 0$–100 fs, the laser pulse is negligibly small so that the initial wave packet on the excited electronic state just propagates on the identical PEC. However, from $t = 100$–500 fs, some portion of the wave packet on the electronic excited state transfers from the state to the electronic ground state because the laser pulse is on. During this period, the wave packet on the electronic excited state changes to the one-node shape and at around $t = 500$ fs, the wave packet on the electronic ground state disappears. After around $t = 500$ fs, the wave packet only freely propagates on the electronic excited state because the laser pulse is almost off. The final wave packet at $t = 600$ fs is very similar to the target state $|11\rangle$. Almost all the optimized laser pulses obtained for the combination of the electronic and vibrational qubits contain these kinds of low-amplitude intensities for the initial and final free propagations of the wave packets. This kind of low-amplitude parts of the optimized laser pulses is necessary, e.g., for generating or destructing the nodes to reach the final target states with high

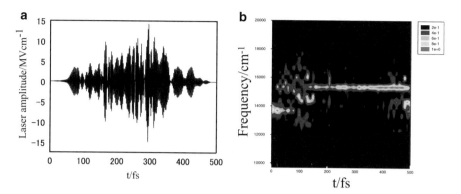

Fig. 5 In panel (**a**), optimized laser pulse after 999 iterations of MTOCT and in panel (**b**), FROG representation for CNOT$_{EV}$ gate of the Na$_2$ molecule are presented

fidelity. This seems to be very different from vibrational–rotational and vibrational–vibrational qubits in which case the laser pulses do not contain these low-amplitude intensities for the initial and final periods of the laser pulses.

In Fig. 5, we show the optimized laser pulse (panel a) and FROG (panel b) of CNOT$_{EV}$ for Na$_2$ molecule. Roughly speaking, NOT$_V$ gate at least performs the transformations $|00\rangle \rightarrow |01\rangle$, $|01\rangle \rightarrow |00\rangle$, $|10\rangle \rightarrow |11\rangle$, and $|11\rangle \rightarrow |10\rangle$. All these transformations include the vibrational transitions with the change of vibrational quantum number being unity. This is reflected in the complicated FROG in panel b of Fig. 4. However, CNOT$_{EV}$ gate performs the transformations $|00\rangle \rightarrow |00\rangle$, $|01\rangle \rightarrow |01\rangle$, $|10\rangle \rightarrow |11\rangle$, and $|11\rangle \rightarrow |10\rangle$. In this case, the two former transitions do not include the vibrational transition so that the FROG has a simpler form for CNOT$_{EV}$ gate than for NOT$_V$ gate as shown in panel b of Fig. 5.

From the snapshots of the wave packet dynamics of the transition $|00\rangle \rightarrow |00\rangle$ for CNOT$_{EV}$ gate (not shown here), the wave packet again oscillates twice until the target state is reached. From $t = 0$–50 fs, the strength of the laser pulse is negligibly small and the initial wave packet is the eigenstate $|00\rangle$ so that the initial wave packet retains the initial shape. However, from $t = 50$–450 fs, some portion of the wave packet on the electronically ground state transfers from the state to the electronically excited state because the laser pulse is on. During this period, using the shapes of PECs and the laser pulse, the wave packets on the electronic ground and excited states change to the one- or two-node shape and at around $t = 450$ fs, the wave packet on the electronic excited state disappears and the wave packet almost reaches the target state $|00\rangle$. After around $t=450$ fs to the target time $T = 500$ fs, the laser pulse is almost off so that the wave packet nearly retains the target eigenstate $|00\rangle$.

As mentioned earlier, almost all the optimized laser pulses contain the low-amplitude intensities for the initial and final periods. In Fig. 4, this fact was used for the free propagation on the electronic excited state since the target state is not the vibrational eigenfunction of the electronic excited state, while in Fig. 5 this

Table 1 Average transition probabilities of the quantum gates for DJ_E of the Na_2 molecule

Gates	Population (%)	f_1	f_2	f_3	f_4
(*Operations*)					
NOT_V	91.76				
Hdm_V	89.74				
Hdm_E	75.84				
U_f		89.66	79.00	85.00	85.84
Hdm_E		80.46	80.46	67.96	67.96
(*Measurements*)					
Correct		72.34	74.90	58.62	62.38
False		27.66	25.10	41.38	37.62

Constant and balanced functions can be distinguished correctly with an accuracy of at least 58.62 %

Table 2 Average transition probabilities of the quantum gates for DJ_V of the Na_2 molecule

Gates	Population (%)	f_1	f_2	f_3	f_4
(*Operations*)					
NOT_E	86.59				
Hdm_E	88.44				
Hdm_V	80.31				
U_f		87.46	76.14	83.64	83.53
Hdm_E		82.23	82.23	82.37	82.37
(*Measurements*)					
Correct		80.42	87.58	66.54	78.72
False		19.58	12.42	33.46	21.28

Constant and balanced functions can be distinguished correctly with an accuracy of at least 66.54 %

is used for the wave packet to be able to remain the target eigenfunction of the electronic ground state until the target time. Therefore, it turns out that the low-amplitude intensities of the laser pulses for the initial and final periods are used for the free propagation as well as for the wave packet to remain to be the vibrational eigenfunction.

By concatenating all the optimized laser pulses and tracking the wave packet motion, the summary of the quality of the Deutsch–Jozsa algorithm for each quantum gate and the fidelity of the measurement results shown in Tables 1, 2, 3, and 4 were obtained. Let us compare this with Table I of [17] (vibrational–vibrational qubits) and Table 5 (vibrational–rotational qubits). The results for vibrational–rotational qubits of $C^{12}O^{16}$ molecule [56] indicate that constant and balanced functions can be distinguished correctly with an accuracy of at least 96.11 % (as shown in the next section). This is slightly larger than that for the vibrational–vibrational qubits of the acetylene molecule, 94.28 % [17]. However, for electronic–vibrational qubits constant and balanced functions can be distinguished correctly with an accuracy of at least 83.12 %. This corresponds to Table 4 (DJ_V of Li_2 molecule). In addition, we notice that DJ_V is better than DJ_E for both the

Table 3 Average transition probabilities of the quantum gates for DJ_E of the Li_2 molecule

Gates	Population (%)	f_1	f_2	f_3	f_4
(*Operations*)					
NOT_V	95.49				
Hdm_V	96.04				
Hdm_E	90.52				
U_f		91.36	87.22	93.82	90.57
Hdm_E		91.14	91.14	84.52	84.52
(*Measurements*)					
Correct		84.03	76.86	85.59	77.83
False		15.97	23.14	14.41	22.17

Constant and balanced functions can be distinguished correctly with an accuracy of at least 76.86 %

Table 4 Average transition probabilities of the quantum gates for DJ_V of the Li_2 molecule

Gates	Population (%)	f_1	f_2	f_3	f_4
(*Operations*)					
NOT_E	92.67				
Hdm_E	85.23				
Hdm_V	90.87				
U_f		91.05	88.18	92.58	91.15
Hdm_E		93.39	93.39	91.11	91.11
(*Measurements*)					
Correct		90.44	83.12	83.63	86.09
False		9.56	16.88	16.37	13.91

Constant and balanced functions can be distinguished correctly with an accuracy of at least 83.12 %

Table 5 Average transition probabilities of the quantum gates

Gates	Population (%)	f_1	f_2	f_3	f_4
(*Operations*)					
NOT_R	98.63				
Hdm_R	97.86				
Hdm_V	94.80				
U_f		88.19	90.28	92.02	93.87
$Hdmv$		89.41	88.99	91.39	88.23
(*Measurements*)					
Correct		96.27	99.29	96.11	97.52
False		3.73	0.71	3.90	2.48

Constant and balanced functions can be distinguished correctly with an accuracy of at least 96.11 %

molecules. Because these values are the maximum possible values that MTOCT produced with our intuitive initial guess, a real maximum reliability will be higher for any two-qubit combination. This also holds for all the following results obtained by MTOCT.

3.5   Combination of Intramolecular Vibrational and Rotational States [56]

Next, let us proceed to the case of the combination of intramolecular vibrational and rotational modes of molecules in the electronically ground state. The molecule of our target is closed-shell $C^{12}O^{16}$ molecule. Among the various gate pulses calculated for this molecule, the most difficult one is the Hdm$_V$ gate (Fig. 6). This gate deserves detailed consideration. The essence of the difficulty is that this gate involves the disallowed transition for rotational modes, e.g., $|00\rangle \rightarrow |00\rangle + |10\rangle$. From the population evolution, we can see that the allowed transitions $|00\rangle \rightarrow |01\rangle$ and $|00\rangle \rightarrow |11\rangle$ occur first. In effect, the FROG shows strong peaks for the frequencies of these transitions within about 20 ps. The pulse shape also shows this tendency, with slowly varying and rapidly varying components. From 20 to 50 ps, very complicated transitions take place, especially among the states $|00\rangle$, $|01\rangle$, $|10\rangle$, and $|11\rangle$. From 50 ps, by using IR and microwave frequencies, the populations of the states $|01\rangle$ and $|11\rangle$ go down and the state $|00\rangle + |10\rangle$ is created. The form of the laser pulse actually consists of a slowly varying sine function (rotational transition) and a rapidly oscillating sine function (vibrational transition). This is actually reflected in the split FROG in panels (b) and (c): the IR frequency components are shown in panel (b) and the microwave frequency components in panel (c). This is the method for counteracting the so-called forbidden transition that OCT has produced. The essential features are the same for other types of transition. From several calculations, it was revealed that these kinds of transitions require longer pulses than other types of gate operations (note that the Hdm$_V$ gate pulse requires more than 60 ps time duration).

The CNOT$_{VR}$ gate is shown in Fig. 7. In panel (d), the transition $|10\rangle \rightarrow |11\rangle$ is demonstrated. We can see that the dominant transition consists of $|10\rangle \rightarrow |11\rangle$ and $|02\rangle \rightarrow |11\rangle$, where the $|02\rangle$ state is transiently populated by vibrational transitions. The transition $|10\rangle \rightarrow |11\rangle$ does not require any vibrational transition, but OCT chooses to include the vibrational transition in order for the gate to be universal. In addition, we have also checked that the population transitions $|00\rangle \rightarrow |00\rangle$, $|01\rangle \rightarrow |01\rangle$, and $|11\rangle \rightarrow |10\rangle$ follow the transitions $|00\rangle \rightarrow |01\rangle \rightarrow |00\rangle$, $|01\rangle \rightarrow |00\rangle \rightarrow |01\rangle$, and $|11\rangle \rightarrow |02\rangle$, $|11\rangle \rightarrow |10\rangle$, respectively (not shown here). In the CNOT$_{VR}$, the transition patterns are a little less complicated than those for the Hdm$_V$ gate, because they satisfy the selection rule of rotational transition compared with those for the latter.

As can be understood from these two examples, for quantum computing using rovibrational qubits, the selection rule for rotational transition plays a key role in determining the optimal laser pulse and the gate fidelity.

The summary of the quality of the Deutsch–Jozsa algorithm for each quantum gate and the fidelity of the measurement results is demonstrated in Table 5. Let us compare this with Table I of [17]. Our results indicate that constant and balanced functions can be distinguished correctly with an accuracy of at least 96.11 %. This is slightly larger than that for the vibrational–vibrational qubits of the acetylene

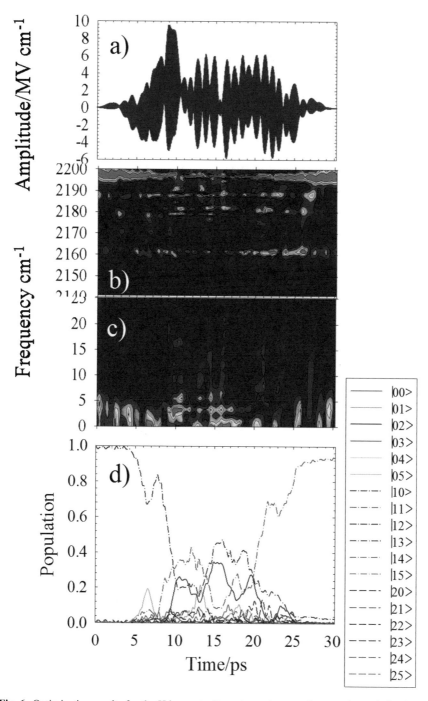

Fig. 6 Optimization results for the Hdm$_V$ gate. From top to bottom, they are the optimized gate pulse (**a**), FROG ((**b**) and (**c**)), and the population transition of $|00\rangle \rightarrow |00\rangle + |10\rangle$ (**d**). Panel (**b**) shows the IR frequency components and panel (**c**) shows the microwave frequency components of the external field

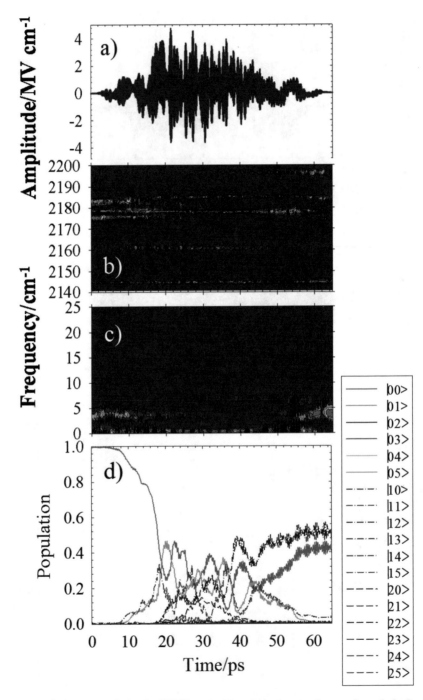

Fig. 7 Optimization results for the CNOT$_{VR}$ gate. From top to bottom, they are the optimized gate pulse (**a**), FROG ((**b**) and (**c**)), and the population transition of $|10\rangle \rightarrow |11\rangle$ (**d**). Panel (**b**) shows the IR frequency components and panel (**c**) shows the microwave frequency components of the external field

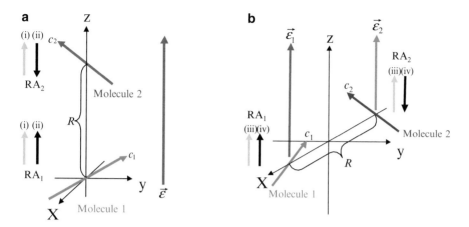

Fig. 8 Four configurations of two polar molecules studied in the present article. In the figure, R is the intermolecular distance, RA_1 and RA_2 represent the rotational axes for molecule 1 and molecule 2, respectively, $\vec{\varepsilon}$'s are the laser polarizations, and c's are molecule-fixed coordinates that are parallel to the dipole moment

molecule: 94.28 % [17]. This means that the combination of vibrational and rotational qubits is a little bit better than the other cases discussed until here, at least from the numerical viewpoint.

3.6 Combination of Intermolecular Rotational States [36]

This type of combination of molecular internal degrees of freedom is quite different from the previous examples. In the present case, a quantum system that carries a qubit is different. In addition, the nonlocal operation such as CNOT gate can be carried out through nonlocal interaction such as dipole–dipole interaction. Furthermore, we have extended the conventional one-laser pulse OCT to multiple-pulse OCT, which is quite similar to the spirit as proposed in [57, 58].

In the present calculations, we assume four cases: four configurations of two polar molecules that are shown in Fig. 8. In panel (a), two different molecules, NaCl and NaBr, are the target molecules whose rotational axes are parallel to z-axis. In this case, one laser pulse addresses two molecules simultaneously. In the case when the rotational axes are numbered as (i), the interaction between the two molecules is attractive, while they are numbered as (ii), the interaction is repulsive. In panel (b), two identical molecules, NaCl or NaBr, are the target molecules whose rotational axes are also parallel to z-axis. In this case, two different laser pulses address each molecule. In the case when the rotational axes are numbered as (iii), the interaction between the two molecules is repulsive, while they are numbered as (iv), the interaction is attractive. In both panels (a) and (b), the linearly polarized laser polarizations are parallel to z-axis.

For notational convenience, we define the case when the rotational axes are numbered as (i) in panel (a) of Fig. 8, where the molecule 1 is NaCl and the molecule 2 is NaBr as NaCl–NaBr (I). On the other hand, we define the case when the rotational axes are numbered as (ii) in panel (a) of Fig. 8 where the molecule 1 is NaCl and the molecule 2 is NaBr as NaCl–NaBr (II). In the similar manner, we define the case when the rotational axes are numbered as (iv) in panel (b) of Fig. 8 where the molecule 1 is NaCl and the molecule 2 is NaCl as NaCl–NaCl (I). On the other hand, we define the case when the rotational axes are numbered as (iii) in panel (b) of Fig. 8 where the molecule 1 is NaCl and the molecule 2 is NaCl as NaCl–NaCl (II). Likewise, we define the cases for the system consisting of two NaBr molecules as NaBr–NaBr (I) and NaBr–NaBr (II), respectively.

For designing *general-purpose* universal gate pulses, we have treated case (a) and case (b) in Fig. 8 separately. For the one-pulse technique in the cases of NaCl–NaBr (I) and NaCl–NaBr (II), the objective functional is expressed as

$$
J = \sum_{k=1}^{z} \left\{ |\langle \psi_{ik}(T)|\Phi_{fk}\rangle|^2 - \alpha_0 \int_0^T \frac{|E(t)|^2}{s(t)} dt \right.
$$
$$
\left. -2\mathrm{Re}\left\{ \langle \psi_{ik}(T)|\Phi_{fk}\rangle \int_0^T \langle \psi_{fk}(t)|i[\hat{H} - \vec{\mu}_1 \cdot \vec{E}(t) - \vec{\mu}_2 \cdot \vec{E}(t)] + \frac{\partial}{\partial t}|\psi_{ik}(t)\rangle dt \right\} \right\},
$$
$$
(24)
$$

The Hamiltonian $\hat{H}$ is given by

$$
\hat{H} = \hat{H}_0 + \hat{V}, \qquad (25)
$$

where $\hat{H}_0$ denotes the diagonal part of the Hamiltonian which satisfies

$$
\hat{H}_0|j_1, m_1, j_2, m_2\rangle = \left\{ \frac{1}{2I_1}j_1(j_1+1) + \frac{1}{2I_2}j_2(j_2+1) \right\} |j_1, m_1, j_2, m_2\rangle, \qquad (26)
$$

where I_1 and I_2 represent the rotational constants for the control bit and target bit molecules, respectively. $\hat{V}$ is the rotational dipole–dipole coupling operator which can be written as

$$
\hat{V} = \frac{\mu_1 \mu_2}{4\pi\varepsilon_0} \frac{1}{R^3} \left\{ \vec{v}_1 \cdot \vec{v}_2 - 3(\vec{v}_1 \cdot \hat{R})(\vec{v}_2 \cdot \hat{R}) \right\}, \qquad (27)
$$

where μ_1 and μ_2 are the dipole moments for the first and second molecules, respectively, $\vec{v}_i$ is the unit vector of the orientation of the ith molecule, R is the distance between the two molecules, and $\hat{R}$ is the unit vector from the center of the first molecule to the second molecule. For case (a), the optimized gate pulse is given by

$$E(t) = -\frac{zs(t)}{\alpha_0} \sum_{k=1}^{z} \text{Im}\{\langle \psi_{ik}(t)|\psi_{fk}(t)\rangle\langle \psi_{fk}(t)|\mu_1 \cos\theta_1 + \mu_2 \cos\theta_2|\psi_{ik}(t)\rangle\}. \quad (28)$$

On the other hand, in case (b) of Fig. 8, we assume that the individual molecules are irradiated by respective optimized laser pulses. The objective functional in this case is given by

$$J = \sum_{k=1}^{z}\left\{|\langle\psi_{ik}(T)|\Phi_{fk}\rangle|^2 - \alpha_1\int_0^T \frac{|E_1(t)|^2}{s_1(t)}dt - \alpha_2\int_0^T \frac{|E_2(t)|^2}{s_2(t)}dt,\right.$$
$$\left.-2\text{Re}\left\{\langle\psi_{ik}(T)|\Phi_{fk}\rangle\int_0^T \langle\psi_{fk}(t)|i[\hat{H} - \vec{\mu}_1 \cdot \vec{E}_1(t) - \vec{\mu}_2 \cdot \vec{E}_2(t)] + \frac{\partial}{\partial t}|\psi_{ik}(t)\rangle dt\right\}\right\},$$
$$(29)$$

where it is assumed that the laser pulse $\vec{E}_1(t)$ addresses the first molecule (control bit) and $\vec{E}_2(t)$ addresses the second molecule (target bit) individually. The second and third terms restrict the laser intensity, where $\alpha_1/s_1(t)$ and $\alpha_2/s_2(t)$ are the penalty factors for the first and second molecules, respectively. Therefore, the optimized control and target gate pulses are expressed as

$$E_1(t) = -\frac{zs_1(t)}{\alpha_1} \sum_{k=1}^{z}\text{Im}\{\langle\psi_{ik}(t)|\psi_{fk}(t)\rangle\langle\psi_{fk}(t)|\mu_1 \cos\theta_1|\psi_{ik}(t)\rangle\},$$
$$(30)$$
$$E_2(t) = -\frac{zs_2(t)}{\alpha_2} \sum_{k=1}^{z}\text{Im}\{\langle\psi_{ik}(t)|\psi_{fk}(t)\rangle\langle\psi_{fk}(t)|\mu_2 \cos\theta_2|\psi_{ik}(t)\rangle\},$$

where the quantities with subscript 1 are related to the control bit and those with subscript 2 are related to the target bit.

In Fig. 9, we show the optimized laser pulse of the first qubit in panel (a), the FROG representation of the pulse in panel (b), the optimized laser pulse of the second qubit in panel (c), and the FROG representation of the pulse in panel (d), respectively. The target population evolution of this figure is $|00\rangle \rightarrow |00\rangle$ for CNOT gate for the case NaCl–NaCl (II) with R being equal to 5.0 nm as shown in panel (e). From panel (e), we can see that the population transfer mainly takes place in the Hilbert space of our interest. However, the transient population transfer to $|2, 0, 0, 0\rangle$ takes place due to the dipole coupling between $|01\rangle$ and $|10\rangle$. From the Fourier transforms of the laser pulses, it is clear that the off-resonant frequency of the laser pulses has the strongest intensity at around 0.9 cm^{-1}. The discussion in Fig. 6 also holds for the role of this off-resonant component. The final population of $|00\rangle$ is 99.31 %.

The eigenenergies of the rotational eigenstates of NaCl molecule are 0.0, 0.4336, 1.301, 2.602 cm^{-1} for the ground state, the first excited state, the second excited state, and the third excited state, respectively. Comparing with these values with the frequency components shown in the FROG, the frequency of the laser pulses is

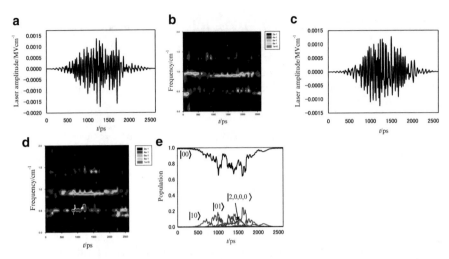

Fig. 9 (**a**) Optimized control gate pulse, (**b**) FROG representation of the optimized control gate pulse, (**c**) optimized target gate pulse, (**d**) FROG representation of the optimized target gate pulse, (**e**) population evolution of $|00\rangle \rightarrow |00\rangle$ for CNOT gate of the case NaCl–NaCl (II) with R being equal to 5.0 nm. The population of $|00\rangle$ state reaches 99.31 % at the target time $T = 2621.42$ ps

almost resonant between the ground and the first excited states. However, we find the laser frequency of around 0.9 cm^{-1} in the FROG, that is, off-resonant component that lies between the first and the second excited states. As explained in [59], in a pair of two-level atoms interacting with each other by the dipole–dipole coupling, a new dipole–dipole interaction-induced resonance takes place at the frequency of the sum of the resonant frequencies of the ground and the first excited states of two atoms. This also holds for the rotational modes of molecules. Actually, the laser frequency of around 0.9 cm^{-1} is almost the same as the sum of the resonant frequencies of the ground and the first excited states of two NaCl molecules (0.8672 cm^{-1}).

Although not shown here, almost all the optimized laser pulses have a similar structure of the FROG for the cases NaCl–NaCl (I), NaCl–NaCl (II), NaBr–NaBr (I), and NaBr–NaBr (II).

In Table 6, we show some examples of the transition probabilities of each quantum gate and the correctness of the measurement. The corresponding flowchart of the two-state Deutsch–Jozsa algorithm is shown in Fig. 10. Comparing the case NaCl–NaBr

(I) with R being equal to 5.0 nm and that with R being equal to 8.5 nm, we can see that the distinguishability is better for the latter than the former. This is due to the fact that the fidelity of Hdm$_2$ gate plays a key role in the two-state Deutsch–Jozsa algorithm because Hdm$_2$ gate is used twice. Therefore, because the fidelity of Hdm$_2$ gate with R being equal to 8.5 nm is larger than that with R being equal to 5.0 nm, the distinguishability is better for the case with R being equal to 8.5 nm. On the other hand, in the case NaCl–NaBr (I) with R being equal to 12.0 nm, we notice

Table 6 Examples of the average transition probabilities of the quantum gates

System	R (nm)	NOT (%)	Hdm_1 (%)	Hdm_2 (%)	f_1 (%)	f_2 (%)	f_3 (%)	f_4 (%)	f_5 (%)	f_6 (%)	f_7 (%)	f_8 (%)	Measurement			
													C_1	C_2	C_3	C_4
NaCl-NaBr (I) (Attractive)																
	5.0	98.32	98.82	94.74	96.33	95.77	95.40	96.15	94.71	94.71	96.63	96.63	98.55	94.96	97.29	98.15
	8.5	98.76	99.38	98.16	99.35	98.08	94.53	96.10	99.18	99.18	99.30	99.30	98.13	99.63	99.05	97.45
	12.0	99.64	99.43	99.88	99.58	99.58	85.12	82.70	99.39	99.39	99.39	99.39	99.51	99.71	83.10	80.62
NaCl-NaBr (II) (Repulsive)																
	5.0	99.05	99.48	95.79	98.82	99.14	97.46	99.55	96.75	96.75	95.25	95.25	97.63	98.06	96.64	97.61
	8.5	99.54	98.64	99.43	98.56	99.01	97.15	97.61	99.03	99.03	98.88	98.88	97.87	98.24	97.32	98.65
	12.0	99.79	99.60	99.65	99.46	99.75	83.16	87.06	99.74	99.74	99.73	99.73	99.65	99.71	82.51	90.25
NaCl-NaCl (I) (Attractive)																
	5.0	96.76	97.92	95.85	96.31	96.87	95.78	96.08	97.77	97.77	91.75	91.75	98.75	97.36	96.63	96.48
	8.5	97.94	98.65	96.86	96.35	97.58	97.52	98.03	97.20	97.20	97.86	97.86	93.71	95.90	95.39	97.41
NaCl-NaCl (II) (Repulsive)																
	5.0	96.97	98.04	95.71	95.28	96.38	97.44	96.80	96.30	96.30	95.54	95.54	98.44	97.62	99.01	98.47
	8.5	98.21	98.14	98.48	96.91	99.11	97.28	96.97	97.61	97.61	98.25	98.25	96.27	98.21	96.71	97.27
	5.0	98.81	98.35	98.97	98.20	97.80	98.43	98.25	98.97	98.97	98.44	98.44	99.53	99.57	98.12	97.95

In this table, C_1, C_2, C_3, and C_4 designate the correctness of the measurement after f_5, f_6, f_7, and f_8, respectively

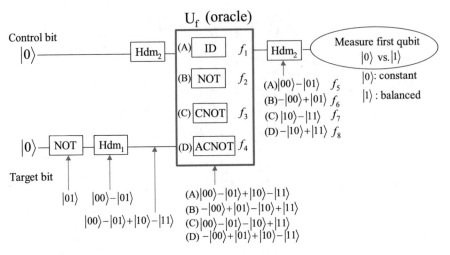

Fig. 10 Flowchart of the two-state Deutsch–Jozsa algorithm

that the correctness of constant function is very good (~99 %). This is because since the quantum circuit for the constant function only contains the local unitary operations, the dipole–dipole interaction is negligibly small so that the local operation can be performed with high fidelity when R is very large. However, the correctness of balanced function is very small (~80 %). This is simply because for the balanced function the quantum circuit contains not only the local unitary operations but also the global unitary operations such as CNOT and ACNOT gates. If the dipole–dipole interaction is very weak, the fidelities of CNOT and ACNOT gates deteriorate significantly. This holds also for other cases shown later.

On the other hand, comparing the cases NaCl–NaBr (I) and NaCl–NaBr (II), it can be seen that the distinguishability is better for the case NaCl–NaBr (II) than that of the case NaCl–NaBr (I) for all the values of R. First, this is because the fidelity of the first gate, NOT gate, which influences significantly the following gates is higher for the repulsive configuration than for the attractive configuration. Second, this is due to the fact that the fidelity of Hdm_2 gate for the repulsive case is larger than that for the attractive case.

Next, we compare the cases NaCl–NaCl (I) and NaCl–NaCl (II). We notice that the repulsive configuration shows better distinguishability than the attractive configuration in the same manner as in the NaCl–NaBr system shown earlier. In general, we can see that the probability of population transfer is better for the repulsive configuration than for the attractive configuration, which leads to the better distinguishability for the repulsive configuration. Although not shown here, when R is equal to 12.0 nm, the distinguishability deteriorates significantly for both the attractive and the repulsive cases in the same manner as in the cases NaCl–NaBr (I) and NaCl–NaBr (II).

Finally, we concentrate on the case NaBr–NaBr (II). This example is the best performance of the two-state Deutsch–Jozsa algorithm in all our calculations. In this case, constant and balanced functions can be distinguished correctly with an accuracy of at least 97.95 %. In this case, the fidelities of each gate are equally very high so that the minimum distinguishability also amounts to a large value.

Summarizing, we predict that the fidelity of the general-purpose quantum gates is very large and the performance of the two-state Deutsch–Jozsa algorithm is very good when using the *inter*molecular rotational–rotational qubits.

Let us compare the present Table 6 with Table I of [17] (*intra*molecular vibrational–vibrational qubits), Table 5 ($^{12}C^{16}O$ molecule) and the results of $^{14}N^{16}O$ [60] (*intra*molecular vibrational–rotational qubits), and Tables 1, 2, 3, and 4 (*intra*molecular electronic–vibrational qubits). As shown earlier, Table 5 indicates that constant and balanced functions can be distinguished correctly with an accuracy of at least 96.11 % in $^{12}C^{16}O$ molecule when the control bit is vibrational and the target bit is rotational. On the other hand, if the molecular system is $^{14}N^{16}O$ molecule, constant and balanced functions can be distinguished correctly with an accuracy of at least 94.76 % when the control bit is rotational and the target bit is vibrational. This is similar to that for the vibrational–vibrational qubits of the acetylene molecule, 94.28 % [17]. However, for the electronic–vibrational qubits of Li_2 molecule, constant and balanced functions can be distinguished correctly with an accuracy of at least 83.12 %. This is the worst distinguishability reported up to now. On the other hand, our present results show that the distinguishability is 97.95 % for the case NaBr–NaBr (II) with the interval $R = 5.0$ nm, which is the best performance of the two-state Deutsch–Jozsa algorithm compared with any of the *intra*molecular vibrational–vibrational, vibrational–rotational, and electronic–vibrational qubits reported so far. Therefore, up to now, the *inter*molecular rotational–rotational qubits are the most promising candidate for quantum computing when using the molecular degrees of freedom as qubits.

Although we do not show the details, the average transition probabilities and the fidelity of CNOT and ACNOT gates can be much more enhanced even if we enlarge R than R investigated earlier (5.0–12.0 nm). The method for enhancing the average transition probabilities and the fidelity of CNOT and ACNOT gates is to elongate T more than that explored in the above examples ($T = 2000$–5000 ps). In fact, in [61, 62], we have analytically predicted that the temporal duration of the incident laser fields for generating the maximally entangled Bell states becomes longer for smaller entangling interaction matrix elements. For example, for the ACNOT gate for the case NaCl–NaBr (I) with R being equal to 12.0 nm, T demonstrated in Table 6 was 5242.72 ps, $\overline{P} = 0.8858$, and $F = 0.8332$. On the other hand, when T is equal to 20,971.4 ps, $\overline{P} = 0.9787$ and $F = 0.9755$. As a second example, for the CNOT gate for the case NaCl–NaBr (I) with R being equal to 12.0 nm, T demonstrated in Table 6 was 5242.72 ps, $\overline{P} = 0.8937$, and $F = 0.7657$. On the other hand, when T is equal to 20,971.4 ps, $\overline{P} = 0.9752$ and $F = 0.9724$.

The consequence that the combination of intermolecular rotational qubits gives the best performance of quantum computing may be attributed to the fact that the eigenenergies between the nearest levels increase with increasing rotational quantum number so that it becomes difficult to occupy higher energy levels for purely rotational modes if the strength of external fields is sufficiently small. Therefore, the purely rotational states of molecules can be regarded as a "qubit" although the rotational states constitute a "qudit" in principle. Furthermore, a large number of rotational states of molecules can be coupled by dipole–dipole interactions and by selecting appropriate positions and directions of molecules, multiqubit quantum computing will become possible with high fidelity. This fact satisfies the criterion of scalability required for realization of quantum computers. However, it seems to be not so easy to do so if the intramolecular states are regarded as qubits.

4 Free-Time and Fixed End-Point Optimal Control Theory (FRFP-OCT)

So far, we have used conventional FIFP-OCT to tailor optimal laser pulses, especially for constructing general-purpose optimal gate pulses for quantum computing. Needless to say, OCT can be used not only for quantum computing but also for control problems of a variety of physical and chemical phenomena [31, 63].

In our previous publications [61, 62], we have found that the entanglement generation in general quantum systems crucially rely on the strength of entangling interactions among distinct quantum systems. We have stressed that if the entangling interactions are strong, the maximally entangled state can be created in short time. This in turn implies that if the strength of the entangling interactions is weak, long laser fields are necessary for creating the maximally entangled states. In the simplest case, the time duration of the laser pulses by which the maximally entangled states can be created is inversely proportional to the strength of the entangling interaction. Although our previous findings have assumed simplified entangling interactions, the tendency we found there has turned out to be quite general in the sense that it also holds for the case when the entangling interactions are complicated as shown in the previous section (Sect. 3.6). Therefore, it can easily be recognized that we need a new OCT that works well even if we do not know the necessary time duration of the laser pulses to create the maximally entangled state efficiently because the actual entangling interactions are usually much more complicated in molecular systems. If this is the case, the necessary OCT will become *free-time* and fixed end-point optimal control theory (FRFP-OCT) since the optimal temporal duration of the laser pulses is not known exactly in advance. Currently, OCT in quantum systems proposed so far has been limited to the *fixed-time* and fixed end-point optimal control theory (FIFP-OCT). Consequently, we have constructed one of the versions of FRFP-OCTs that can optimize the objective functional and the temporal duration of the laser pulses simultaneously [64, 65]. One of the advantages of our theory is that one does not need to try various final fixed times to achieve the best control of quantum dynamics. To demonstrate the utility of our theory it has been applied to the optimization of laser pulses that can create maximally entangled states efficiently, but it may also be applied to various physical and chemical quantum control problems. As a demonstration, we have applied the theory to entanglement generation in the situation sketched in panel a of Fig. 8.

On the other hand, realistic quantum systems that we observe experimentally and calculate theoretically are always interacting with surrounding environment by way of entangling interactions. If the whole quantum system is the sum of the system of our interest and the huge surrounding environment, the quantum state is maintained in pure state (no decoherence). However, the surrounding environment is traced out and our attention is paid only to our small quantum system, our system becomes mixed state (decoherence). This can be easily verified by using, e.g., the von-Neumann entropy used to measure entanglement degree of the pure state of composite systems. In many quantum control problems, the decoherence is unfavorable and should be suppressed.

Quantum computing and quantum information science are also not exceptions. It was pointed out that the decoherence might become one of the crucial obstacles for quantum computers and entanglement generation and manipulation because quantum information processing must be performed in pure states in most cases [66, 67]. Therefore, to achieve accurate quantum computing and quantum information processing in the quantum system in contact with the surrounding environment, it is crucial to maintain the coherence by external active manipulation of the target quantum system. It should be noted that the decoherence was completely neglected in the earlier calculations.

At present, there are two methods to suppress decoherence that are proposed theoretically. One of these is to utilize quantum error correcting code [68, 69]. The other promising and efficient method of preventing decoherence is the so-called bang-bang control by shining repetitive intense laser pulses on the target quantum system [70].

Although the methods mentioned earlier are proposed to be applied to simple two-level quantum systems (qubits), most quantum systems are composed of many eigenstates (qudits), e.g., molecular internal degrees of freedom. Therefore, the analytical approaches of the error correcting code and the bang-bang control cannot easily be extended to qudits such as molecular modes. If this is the case, one has to resort to other methods for the purpose of decoherence suppression of realistic quantum systems. One of the advantageous methods will be to OCT and apply it to concrete calculations of realistic multilevel quantum systems in order to control the dissipative quantum dynamics most efficiently.

In fact, OCT for dissipative quantum dynamics has attracted much attention in recent years. This is because it is possible to construct laser pulses that can manipulate quantum dynamics efficiently in the presence of the surrounding environment and because it is difficult to predict by intuition what kind of laser pulses are the most appropriate for achieving the target dissipative quantum dynamics. OCT for the dissipative quantum dynamics has been developed and improved by many researchers. For example, the OCT for dissipative quantum systems was constructed in a fully systematic and rigorous fashion by Cao and coworkers for the first time [71]. However, their theory can only be applied to the weak response regime. Almost at the same time, the OCT in the strong response regime was developed in terms of the Liouville-space density matrix [72]. Ohtsuki and coworkers developed a monotonically convergent algorithm for dissipative quantum systems [73] and applied their theory to the control of wave packet dynamics under the influence of dissipation [74]. Recently, there have appeared several numerical applications of OCT in realistic dissipative media for a variety of purposes. For example, simulations of molecular quantum computers using the vibrational modes of molecules including dissipation have been performed by Ndong and coworkers [27]. Seideman and coworkers have applied dissipative OCT to manipulate rotational wave packet dynamics in a dissipative environment [75, 76]. From the experimental viewpoint, dissipative OCT was used for the quantum control of I_2 in the gas phase and in condensed phase solid Kr matrix [77].

Also for the quantum control in the dissipative environment, only FIFP-OCTs have been developed. Dissipative quantum dynamics can be regarded as one of the most time-sensitive processes. The reason is that the decoherence rate Γ governs the decoherence degree versus time. Therefore, FRFP-OCT also has a significant importance for dynamical control of dissipative quantum dynamics. If this is the case for the quantum system under investigation, the equation of motion should be replaced by, e.g., the Liouville–von Neumann equation in the framework of the density matrix representation. Consequently, one of the main purposes here is to generalize FRFP-OCT suitable only for pure states to *mixed state* FRFP-OCT following the general Master equation in both Markov approximation and without any approximations.

4.1 FRFP-OCT in Pure State [64]

We assume that the quantum system of our interest is separated from the surrounding environment so that our system can adequately be described by the Schrödinger equation. The objective functional of our problem to be maximized is just given by

$$J = \left| \langle \Psi_i(T) | \Phi_f \rangle \right|^2, \tag{31}$$

where $|\Psi_i(t)\rangle$ is time-dependent wavefunction at time t and $|\Psi_i(T)\rangle$ is the time-dependent wavefunction at the target final time $t = T$. On the other hand, $|\Phi_f\rangle$ is the final target wavefunction at time $t = T$. Our purpose is to maximize the objective function, J, at some time T. Note that we *do not fix T* while J should be maximized. This kind of problem has not yet been investigated in control problems in quantum mechanics so far. It should be noticed that the objective functional given by Eq. (31) is different from that of the optimal control theory investigated so far. In the conventional FIFP-OCT, the objective functional is usually given by

$$J = \left|\langle \Psi_i(T)|\Phi_f\rangle\right|^2 - \alpha \int_0^T E(t)^2 dt, \tag{32}$$

where $E(t)$ is the external laser fields and α is usually called penalty factor that is added to minimize the strength of the external laser fields. Defining the objective functional as Eq. (32) and adding the constraints that the system obeys, Rabitz and coworkers proposed, e.g., monotonically convergent OCT [52].

Let us now derive the quantum mechanical FRFP-OCT that is necessary, e.g., for entanglement generation as mentioned earlier. First, we introduce *real* time t and *fictitious*-time τ, which are related by the following equality:

$$t = T(\tau)\tau, \tag{33}$$

where τ is a dimensionless parameter that ranges from zero to unity. In addition, we have included the implicit dependence of T on dimensionless parameter τ in Eq. (33). The time-dependent equation for $|\Psi_i(t)\rangle$ is given by the conventional *real-time* Schrödinger equation:

$$i\hbar \frac{\partial |\Psi_i(t)\rangle}{\partial t} = \left\{\hat{H} - \vec{\mu} \cdot \vec{E}(t)\right\}|\Psi_i(t)\rangle, \tag{34}$$

where $\hat{H}$ is the 0th-order Hamiltonian and $-\vec{\mu} \cdot \vec{E}(t)$ is the laser–molecule interaction. Using the relationship of Eq. (33) for Eq. (34), we obtain

$$i\hbar \frac{\partial |\Psi_i(\tau)\rangle}{\partial \tau} = \left\{\hat{H} - \vec{\mu} \cdot \vec{E}(\tau)\right\}|\Psi_i(\tau)\rangle T(\tau). \tag{35}$$

We call Eq. (35) as *fictitious-time* Schrödinger equation.

Usually, the objective functional to be maximized or minimized is constrained by some of the factors, e.g., the equation of dynamics that the problem in mind follows. In this case, we can add such constraints into Eq. (31) using Lagrange multipliers and we obtain the new objective functional,

$$\hat{J} = \left|\langle \Psi_i(\tau=1)|\Phi_f\rangle\right|^2 - 2\mathrm{Re}\left[\int_0^1 \langle \Psi_f(\tau)|\left\{\frac{i}{\hbar}(\hat{H} - \vec{\mu}\cdot\vec{E}(\tau)) + \frac{\partial}{T(\tau)\partial\tau}\right\}|\Psi_i(\tau)\rangle T(\tau)d\tau\right]$$
$$- \int_0^1 \nu_T(\tau)\frac{\partial T(\tau)}{\partial\tau}d\tau. \tag{36}$$

Then, we introduce the variational principle for Eq. (36). In order for $\hat{J}$ to be maximized, we can deduce the following equations:

$$i\hbar\frac{\partial|\Psi_i(\tau)\rangle}{\partial\tau} = \{\hat{H} - \vec{\mu}\cdot\vec{E}(\tau)\}|\Psi_i(\tau)\rangle T(\tau) \quad \text{subject to the initial condition } |\Psi_i(\tau=0)\rangle$$

$$= |\Phi_i\rangle,$$

$$(37)$$

where $|\Phi_i\rangle$ is the initial given state.

$$i\hbar\frac{\partial|\Psi_f(\tau)\rangle}{\partial\tau} = \{\hat{H} - \vec{\mu}\cdot\vec{E}(\tau)\}|\Psi_f(\tau)\rangle T(\tau) \quad \text{subject to the initial condition } |\Psi_f(\tau=1)\rangle = |\Phi_f\rangle,$$

$$(38)$$

$$\frac{\partial v_T(\tau)}{\partial\tau} = -\frac{2}{\hbar}\text{Im}\{\langle\Psi_f(\tau)|[\hat{H} - \vec{\mu}\cdot\vec{E}(\tau)]|\Psi_i(\tau)\rangle\} \quad \text{subject to the initial condition}$$

$$v_T(\tau=1) = 2\text{Re}\left\{\langle\Psi_i(\tau=1)|\Phi_f\rangle\left\langle\Phi_f\left|\frac{\partial\Psi_i(\tau=1)}{T(\tau=1)\partial\tau}\right.\right\rangle\right\}, \quad (39)$$

When Eqs. (37)–(39) are satisfied, we have

$$\delta\hat{J} = \int_0^1 d\tau g(\tau)\delta E(\tau) + v_T(\tau=0)\delta T(\tau=0), \quad (40)$$

where we have defined

$$g(\tau) = -\frac{2}{\hbar}\text{Im}\{\langle\Psi_f(\tau)|\mu|\Psi_i(\tau)\rangle\}T(\tau). \quad (41)$$

If the correction of the laser amplitude $E(\tau)$ is represented as $\delta E(\tau)$, we define

$$\delta E(\tau) = \alpha g(\tau). \quad (42)$$

On the other hand, if we defined the correction of $T(\tau)$ as $\delta T(\tau)$, we choose

$$\delta T(\tau) = \beta v_T(\tau=0). \quad (43)$$

When Eqs. (42) and (43) are inserted into Eq. (40), we find

$$\delta\hat{J} = \int_0^1 d\tau\alpha g(\tau)^2 + \beta v_T(\tau=0)^2. \quad (44)$$

If both α and β are positive, it is expected that the objective reaches maximum monotonically as is clearly understood from Eq. (44). On the other hand, if both α and β are negative, it is expected that the objective reaches minimum monotonically.

Based on the earlier equations, we have constructed the following FRFP-OCT in pure state following the Schrödinger equation. In what follows, the superscript (j) is used to denote the quantities for the jth iteration.

1. One chooses initial guess external fields $E^{(0)}(\tau)$ and nominal $T^{(0)}$ that is the final time of quantum dynamics. Here and in the following, the superscript (j) is used to denote the quantity of the jth iteration. In addition, the trial positive parameters α and β are given because our purpose is to maximize Eq. (31).

2. The Schrödinger equation (Eq. (37)) is propagated forwardly in time from $\tau = 0$ to $\tau = 1$ and the obtained wavefunction $|\Psi_i^{(j)}(\tau)\rangle$ is stored. At the same time, the objective functional $J^{(j)} = \left| \left\langle \Psi_i^{(j)}(T) | \Phi_f \right\rangle \right|^2$ is calculated.

3. Equations (38) and (39) are propagated backwardly in time from $\tau = 1$ to $\tau = 0$ and the wavefunction $|\Psi_f^{(j)}(\tau)\rangle$ is stored. In addition, $\nu_T(\tau = 0)$ is calculated.

4. Using Eqs. (42) and (43), the laser amplitude $E^{(j)}(\tau)$ and $T^{(j)}$ are updated as follows,

$$E^{(j+1)}(\tau) = E^{(j)}(\tau) + \alpha g(\tau), \tag{45}$$

and

$$T^{(j+1)} = T^{(j)} + \beta \nu_T(\tau = 0). \tag{46}$$

5. One sets the convergence criterion η and if the following criterion

$$\left| J^{(j+1)} - J^{(j)} \right| \leq \eta \tag{47}$$

is met, the calculation is terminated.

6. If the convergence is not sufficient, one updates $E^{(j)}(\tau)$ and $T^{(j)}$ to $E^{(j+1)}(\tau)$ and $T^{(j+1)}$, and loops back to the step (2).

To show how our theory works concretely, we have applied the above algorithm to tailoring optimal laser pulses that can create the maximally entangled Bell states. One of the calculation examples is shown in Fig. 11.

In Fig. 11, we show the numerical results for the optimization of the quantum transfer $|0, 0\rangle \rightarrow (|0, 0\rangle + |1, 1\rangle)/\sqrt{2}$ with the nominal $T^{(0)} = 300$ ps. From panel (a), we can see that the rate of the monotonic convergence of the transition probability is better for FRFP-OCT than that for FIFP-OCT. In addition, the finally obtained transition probability is better for FRFP-OCT. On the other hand, from panel (b), it is seen that the temporal duration of the laser pulse becomes longer with the optimization iteration. This reflects the fact that the longer temporal duration of the laser pulse is more favorable than the shorter one because the nominal $T^{(0)}$ was too short to reach a high transition probability. It is clear from panels (d) and (f), the maximally entangled Bell state cannot be created by both FRFP-OCT and FIFP-

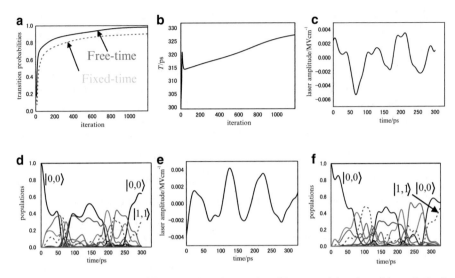

Fig. 11 (**a**) Transition probability versus iteration number, (**b**) temporal duration of the optimized laser pulse versus iteration number, (**c**) optimized laser pulse with α and β being equal to 2×10^{-16} a.u. and 0.0 a.u., respectively, (**d**) population transfer for panel (**c**), (**e**) optimized laser pulse with α and β being equal to 2×10^{-16} a.u. and 2×10^{11} a.u., respectively, and (**f**) population transfer for panel (**e**). The nominal $T^{(0)}$ was set to be 300 ps. The intermolecular distance R is equal to 5.0 nm. In this figure, the target transition $|0, 0\rangle \rightarrow (|0, 0\rangle + |1, 1\rangle)/\sqrt{2}$ was optimized

OCT. This is because the tailored laser pulses have a short temporal duration so that it is difficult to reach the maximally entangled state as mentioned earlier. However, it is clearly seen that FRFP-OCT has attained much higher transition probability than FIFP-OCT has (see panel (f)). The optimal time duration of the laser pulse obtained by FRFP-OCT was 327.95 ps. It is expected that the behaviors shown in these figures are also universal to controls of other physical and chemical phenomena.

From the above numerical results, we can conclude that our FRFP-OCT is much more efficient than the conventional FIFP-OCT because the temporal duration of the laser pulse can also be optimized accurately, which makes OCT more flexible.

4.2 FRFP-OCT in Dissipative Media [65]

Next, we are interested in the situation where the quantum system of interest is affected by the surrounding environment so that it is necessary to describe the quantum system in the density-matrix representation. In such a case, we start from the assumption that the objective functional to be maximized is simply given by

$$J = \langle\langle \hat{W} | \hat{\rho}(T) \rangle\rangle, \tag{48}$$

where $\hat{\rho}(t)$ represents the time-dependent reduced density matrix at time t, $\hat{\rho}(T)$ is the time-dependent reduced density matrix at the target final time $t = T$, and $\hat{W}$ is the objective reduced density matrix. The notation in Eq. (48), $\langle\langle \hat{B}\hat{C} \rangle\rangle$ for arbitrary matrices $\hat{B}$ and $\hat{C}$, is defined by

$$\langle\langle \hat{B}\hat{C} \rangle\rangle = \mathrm{Tr}\left(\hat{B}^{\dagger}\hat{C} \right). \tag{49}$$

Equation (49) measures the degree of closeness between the matrices $\hat{B}$ and $\hat{C}$. Then, our purpose is to maximize the objective function, J, at some time T. Note that we *do not fix* T while J should be maximized. It should be noticed that the objective functional given by Eq. (48) is different from that of the conventional FIFP-OCT. In the theory, the objective functional is usually given by [73]

$$J = \langle\langle \hat{W} | \hat{\rho}(T) \rangle\rangle - \frac{1}{\hbar A} \int_0^T E(t)^2 dt, \tag{50}$$

where $E(t)$ is the external laser field and the positive constant A is the penalty factor to weigh the significance of the pulse fluence. Because of this difference, our derivation of the OCT in dissipative media is also quite different from theirs.

For the FRFP-OCT, we have also introduced the fictitious time defined by Eq. (33). In real time, the time-dependent equation for the reduced density matrix, $\hat{\rho}(t)$, is expressed as:

$$i\hbar \frac{\partial \hat{\rho}(t)}{\partial t} = \left(\hat{L}_0 + \hat{L}_{el}(t) - i\hbar\hat{\Gamma} \right)\hat{\rho}(t), \tag{51}$$

where

$$\hat{L}_0\hat{\rho}(t) = [\hat{H}_0, \hat{\rho}(t)], \quad \hat{L}_{el}(t)\hat{\rho}(t) = [\hat{H}_{el}(t), \hat{\rho}(t)], \tag{52}$$

and $\hat{\Gamma}$ is the damping operator due to the interaction between the system of interest and the surrounding environment. $\hat{H}_0$ is the 0th-order Hamiltonian and $\hat{H}_{el}(t) = -\vec{\mu} \cdot \vec{E}(t)$ is the laser–molecule interaction with $\vec{\mu}$ being the transition dipole moment. Using the relationship of Eq. (33) for Eq. (51), we obtain the *fictitious time* Master equation,

$$i\hbar \frac{\partial \hat{\rho}(\tau)}{\partial \tau} = \left(\hat{L}_0 + \hat{L}_{el}(\tau) - i\hbar\hat{\Gamma} \right)\hat{\rho}(\tau)T(\tau). \tag{53}$$

When the objective functional to be optimized is constrained by some equations, we should sum up such constraints into Eq. (48) using Lagrange multipliers. Then, we obtain the following new objective function,

$$\bar{J} = \langle\langle \hat{W} | \hat{\rho}(\tau = 1)\rangle\rangle - \int_0^1 \langle\langle \hat{\sigma}(\tau) | \left\{ \frac{i}{\hbar}\left(\hat{L}_0 + \hat{L}_{el}(\tau) - i\hbar\hat{\Gamma}\right) + \frac{\partial}{T(\tau)\partial\tau} \right\} T(\tau) | \hat{\rho}(\tau)\rangle\rangle d\tau$$
$$- \int_0^1 \nu_T(\tau) \frac{\partial T(\tau)}{\partial\tau} d\tau.$$

(54)

For $\bar{J}$ to be maximized, it is possible to deduce the following equations by applying variational principle to Eq. (54):

$i\hbar\frac{\partial\hat{\rho}(\tau)}{\partial\tau} = \left(\hat{L}_0 + \hat{L}_{el}(\tau) - i\hbar\hat{\Gamma}\right)\hat{\rho}(\tau)T(\tau)$ subject to the initial condition

$\hat{\rho}(\tau = 0) = \hat{W}_0$, where $\hat{W}_0$ is the initial fixed reduced density matrix, (55)

$i\hbar\frac{\partial\hat{\sigma}(\tau)}{\partial\tau} = \left(\hat{L}_0 + \hat{L}_{el}(\tau) - i\hbar\hat{\Gamma}\right)^\dagger\hat{\sigma}(\tau)T(\tau)$ subject to the initial condition

$$\hat{\sigma}(\tau = 1) = \hat{W},$$

(56)

where the superscript, †, denotes Hermitian conjugation,

$\frac{\partial\nu_T(\tau)}{\partial\tau} = \langle\langle\hat{\sigma}(\tau)|\frac{i}{\hbar}\left(\hat{L}_0 + \hat{L}_{el}(\tau) - i\hbar\hat{\Gamma}\right)|\hat{\rho}(\tau)\rangle\rangle$ subject to the initial condition

$$\nu_T(\tau = 1) = \frac{1}{T(\tau = 1)}\langle\langle\hat{W}|\partial\hat{\rho}(\tau = 1)/\partial\tau\rangle\rangle.$$

(57)

When Eqs. (55)–(57) are satisfied, we have

$$\delta\bar{J} = \int_0^1 d\tau g(\tau)\delta E(\tau) + \nu_T(\tau = 0)\delta T(\tau = 0),$$

(58)

where we have defined

$$g(\tau) = \frac{\frac{i}{\hbar}\langle\langle\hat{\sigma}(\tau)|\partial\hat{L}_{el}(\tau)}{\partial E(\tau)}|\hat{\rho}(\tau)\rangle\rangle T(\tau).$$

(59)

Note that $g(\tau)$ is real. If the correction to the laser amplitude $E(\tau)$ is expressed as $\delta E(\tau)$, we define

$$\delta E(\tau) = \alpha g(\tau). \tag{60}$$

On the other hand, if we define the correction to $T(\tau)$ as $\delta T(\tau)$, we put

$$\delta T(\tau = 0) = \beta v_T(\tau = 0). \tag{61}$$

By inserting Eqs. (60) and (61) into Eq. (58), we obtain

$$\delta \bar{J} = -\int_0^1 d\tau \alpha g(\tau)^2 + \beta v_T(\tau = 0)^2. \tag{62}$$

From this equation, it is clear that if α is negative and β is positive, the objective function reaches a maximum monotonically. On the other hand, if α is positive and β is negative, the objective functional reaches minimum monotonically. Here, it should be noted that the units of α and β are Wcm^{-2} and fs^2, respectively.

From the earlier derivation, we have constructed the following FRFP-OCT in dissipative media following the Master equation. In what follows, the superscript (j) is used to denote the quantity for the jth iteration.

1. An initial guess is selected for the external field $E^{(0)}(\tau)$ and initial $T^{(0)}$ that is the final time of the quantum dynamics. In addition, the trial negative and positive parameters, α and β, are given because our purpose is to maximize Eq. (48).
2. The Liouville–von Neumann equation of Eq. (55) is propagated forward in time from $\tau = 0$ to $\tau = 1$ and the obtained density matrix $\hat{\rho}^{(j)}(\tau)$ is stored. At the same time, the objective function $J^{(j)} = \langle\langle \hat{W} | \hat{\rho}^{(j)}(\tau = 1) \rangle\rangle$ is calculated.
3. Equations (56) and (57) are propagated backward in time from $\tau = 1$ to $\tau = 0$ and the density matrix $\hat{\sigma}^{(j)}(\tau)$ is stored. At the same time, $v_T(\tau = 0)$ is calculated.
4. The laser amplitude $E^{(j)}(\tau)$ and the temporal duration of the external field $T^{(j)}$ are updated as follows,

$$E^{(j+1)}(\tau) = E^{(j)}(\tau) + \alpha g(\tau), \tag{63}$$

and

$$T^{(j+1)} = T^{(j)} + \beta v_T(\tau = 0). \tag{64}$$

5. One sets the convergence criterion η and when the following criterion

$$\left| J^{(j+1)} - J^{(j)} \right| \le \eta \tag{65}$$

is met, the calculation is terminated.
6. If the convergence criterion of Eq. (65) is not satisfied, $E^{(j)}(\tau)$ and $T^{(j)}$ are updated to $E^{(j+1)}(\tau)$ and $T^{(j+1)}$, respectively, and loop back to step (2).

To apply the theory and the algorithm developed earlier and demonstrate numerical tests, we shall employ the vibrational degrees of freedom of carbon monoxide adsorbed on the copper (100) surface, CO/Cu(100). In this case, the total Hamiltonian $\hat{H}$ in the absence of the laser fields is expressed as

$$\hat{H} = \hat{H}_0 + \hat{V}, \tag{66}$$

where $\hat{H}_0$ is the kinetic energy operator and $\hat{V}$ is the potential energy operator defined in the next section. When we introduce three coordinates r, Z, and X for CO stretch, CO-surface stretch, and frustrated translation modes, respectively, $\hat{H}_0$ is given by

$$\hat{H}_0 = -\frac{\hbar^2}{2\mu_{CO}}\frac{\partial^2}{\partial r^2} - \frac{\hbar^2}{2m_{CO}}\frac{\partial^2}{\partial Z^2} - \frac{\hbar^2}{2m_{CO}}\frac{\partial^2}{\partial X^2} \tag{67}$$

where the masses are

$$\mu_{CO} = \frac{m_C m_O}{m_C + m_O} = 6.856 \text{ amu}, \quad m_{CO} = m_C + m_O = 27.995 \text{ amu}. \tag{68}$$

The eigenstates and eigenenergies of the Hamiltonian, $\hat{H}$, are calculated from

$$\hat{H}|n_r, n_Z, n_X\rangle = E_n|n_r, n_Z, n_X\rangle, \tag{69}$$

where we have used the abbreviation $|n\rangle \equiv |n_r, n_Z, n_X\rangle$ and E_n is the eigenenergy of the state $|n\rangle$. Here, n_r, n_Z, and n_X denote the quanta of vibrational modes, CO stretch, CO-surface stretch, and frustrated translation, respectively.

The Liouville–von Neumann equation in the Markov approximation in the energy representation is explicitly expressed as

$$\frac{d\rho_{nn}(t)}{dt} = -\frac{i}{\hbar}E_z(t)\sum_{i=1}^{N}\{\mu_{ni}\rho_{in}(t) - \rho_{ni}(t)\mu_{in}\} + \sum_{i=1}^{N}\{\Gamma_{i\to n}\rho_{ii}(t) - \Gamma_{n\to i}\rho_{nn}(t)\} \tag{70}$$

for the diagonal elements (populations) of the reduced density matrix and

$$\frac{d\rho_{mn}(t)}{dt} = -i\omega_{mn}\rho_{mn}(t) - \frac{i}{\hbar}E_z(t)\sum_{i=1}^{N}\{\mu_{mi}\rho_{in}(t) - \rho_{mi}(t)\mu_{in}\} - \gamma_{m\to n}\rho_{mn}(t) \tag{71}$$

for the off-diagonal elements (coherences). Here, we have defined the energy gap,

$$\omega_{nm} = (E_n - E_m)/\hbar. \tag{72}$$

The total dephasing rate is given by

$$\gamma_{mn} = \sum_{i=1}^{N} (\Gamma_{m \to i} + \Gamma_{n \to i})/2 + \gamma^*_{m \to n}, \tag{73}$$

where $\gamma^*_{m \to n}$ is the pure dephasing rate and $\Gamma_{m \to n}$ is the population transfer rate from the state m to the state n. In the next section, the values of these parameters were taken from [78]. For the pure dephasing rate, we have taken into account $\gamma^*_{(0,0,0) \to (1,0,0)} \approx \gamma^*_{(1,0,0) \to (2,0,0)} \approx \gamma^*_{(0,0,0) \to (2,0,0)}/4$ with values taken from Table IV of [78]. For the same reason as mentioned in [78], the precise values of the pure dephasing rates are of no concern in the present calculations.

To check the mixedness of the reduced density matrix in the Hilbert space of our interest (CO stretch and CO-surface stretch modes), we explicitly define it by

$$\text{mixedness} = 1 - \text{Tr}_{\text{frust}}\left\{\rho(t)^2\right\}, \tag{74}$$

where Tr_{frust} denotes the trace over the frustrated translation mode that is of no concern.

Note that we can apply our algorithm to other types of Master equations in addition to the Liouville–von Neumann equation.

We have investigated the configuration of the CO/Cu(100) system shown in Fig. 12. We have taken into account two layers of copper atoms and in each layer the nearest nine Cu atoms in the same manner as in [79].

The purpose here is twofold. First, we shall tailor the optimal laser pulses that create maximally entangled Bell state $(|0,0,0\rangle + |1,1,0\rangle)/\sqrt{2}$ from the separable

Fig. 12 Schematic of the dissipative CO/Cu(100) system used to apply FRFP-OCT in dissipative media. The solid circles represent Cu atoms

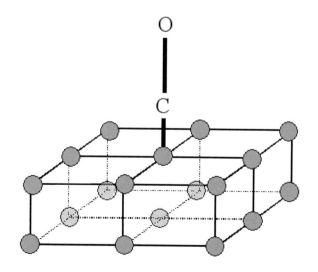

state $|0, 0, 0\rangle$. Of course, this is of fundamental importance for quantum computing and quantum information science. Second, we assume that the maximally entangled state, $(|0, 0, 0\rangle + |1, 1, 0\rangle)/\sqrt{2}$, is prepared at $t = 0$ fs. We shall examine by what kinds of laser pulses this state is maintained in the presence of dissipation. That is, our target transition is $(|0, 0, 0\rangle + |1, 1, 0\rangle)/\sqrt{2} \rightarrow (|0, 0, 0\rangle + |1, 1, 0\rangle)/\sqrt{2}$. This problem seems to be important to study in detail because it may be necessary to maintain some specific entangled sates during other processes in large-scale quantum computers composed of many qubits. Because the effect of decoherence generally seems to be negligible in low temperatures, it may be difficult to show the influence of dissipation on the optimal control. Therefore, we shall mainly present numerical results at high temperatures in the following.

In Fig. 13, we show the case where the initial temporal duration of the laser pulse, $T^{(0)}$, is 1000 fs. The maximum transition probability is attained at $T = 996.219$ fs, as shown in panel (c). In this case, the incident laser pulse has a shape quite different from that of the other cases. As is clear from panel (a), the laser amplitude from the initial time $t = 0$ fs to around the time $t = 800$ fs is quite small (~4 MVcm^{-1}). Therefore, we can hardly observe the population transfer due

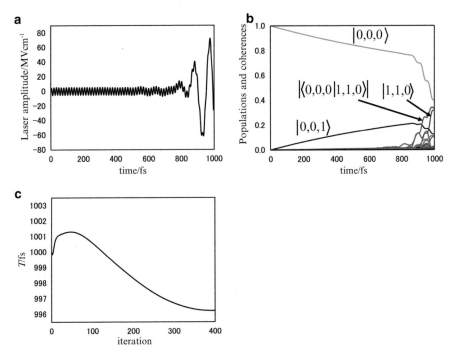

Fig. 13 (a) Optimized laser pulse with α and β being equal to -1.755×10^9 W cm^{-2} and 5.851×10^2 fs^2, respectively, (b) population transfer induced by the optimized laser pulse of panel (a), (c) temporal duration of the optimized laser pulse versus iteration number. The initial $T^{(0)}$ was set to be 1000 fs. The temperature was 300 K. The target transition $|0, 0, 0\rangle \rightarrow (|0, 0, 0\rangle + |1, 1, 0\rangle)/\sqrt{2}$ was optimized

to the laser pulse. Instead, we can see a significant population transfer from the state $|0,0,0\rangle$ to the state $|0,0,1\rangle$ because of the large population transfer rate, $1/\Gamma_{(0,0,0)\rightarrow(0,0,1)} = 3.3$ ps. This transition represents the absorption of the single reservoir quantum by the frustrated translation mode. From the time $t = 800$ fs to the optimal final time $T = 996.219$ fs, the amplitude of the optimized laser pulse is quite large (~ 60 MVcm^{-1}) so that a significant population transfer from the state $|0,0,0\rangle$ to the target state $|1,1,0\rangle$ takes place and coherence between the states, $|0,0,0\rangle$ and $|1,1,0\rangle$, builds up during this period. These trends are reasonable because if the transition to the target state $|1,1,0\rangle$ occurred much earlier as the result of intense laser pulses, the damping of the population of the state $|1,1,0\rangle$ to other states and the decoherence could be quite significant, which would lead to much larger mixedness and a lower transition probability.

When the initial temporal duration, $T^{(0)}$, is 1000 fs and the temperature is 300 K, we observe that the temporal duration becomes a little bit longer, $T = 1040.56$ fs, as can be seen in Fig. 14. The transition probability and the mixedness at the final time are 66.3430 % and 0.50711 for the free-time case and are 65.8890 % and 0.50515

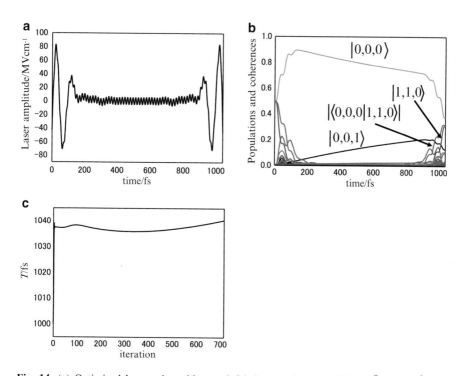

Fig. 14 (a) Optimized laser pulse with α and β being equal to -1.755×10^9 W cm^{-2} and 5.851×10^2 fs^2, respectively, (b) population transfer induced by the optimized laser pulse of panel (a), and temporal duration of the optimized laser pulse versus iteration number. The initial $T^{(0)}$ was set to be 1000 fs. The temperature was 300 K. The target transition $(|0,0,0\rangle + |1,1,0\rangle)/\sqrt{2} \rightarrow (|0,0,0\rangle + |1,1,0\rangle)/\sqrt{2}$ was optimized

for the fixed-time case, respectively. In both the free-time and fixed-time cases, the shape of the optimized laser pulses is interesting (here, we do not show the results for the fixed-time case). For the initial half time of total duration, the amplitude of the laser pulse is strong. In the middle of the temporal duration, it becomes weak. After that, the amplitude of the laser pulse becomes stronger with time. This tendency can be explained as follows. Because it is known that the population of the state $|0,0,0\rangle$ can be excited to the state $|0,0,1\rangle$ during the time evolution because of the dissipative effect as mentioned earlier, the population of the state $|0,0,0\rangle$ has to increase for the initial half time of total duration using the large intensity of the laser pulse. During this period, almost all the population of the state $|1,1,0\rangle$ contributes to the population increase of the state $|0,0,0\rangle$. For the last half period of the total duration, because of the large intensity of the laser pulse, almost all the population of the state $|0,0,0\rangle$ is excited to the state $|1,1,0\rangle$, as in the cases shown earlier, and the optimized laser pulse tries to recover the initial maximally entangled state, $(|0,0,0\rangle + |1,1,0\rangle)/\sqrt{2}$, as much as possible. The reason for the lengthening of the temporal duration compared with the initial guess is that the additional time duration required by the initial recovery of the state $|0,0,0\rangle$ was absent for the target transition $|0,0,0\rangle \rightarrow (|0,0,0\rangle + |1,1,0\rangle)/\sqrt{2}$ shown in Fig. 13.

Figure 15 shows the case where $T^{(0)}$ is 1000 fs and the temperature is 10 K. Comparing panel (a) with panel (a) of Fig. 14, the pulse shapes are rather similar although the temperatures are quite different. However, because of their small difference, the optimized laser pulse in Fig. 15 creates the population of the state $|0,0,0\rangle$ as much as possible until around $t = 200$ fs. Unlike panel (b) of Fig. 14, that of Fig. 15 does not show any significant change of population of the state $|0,0,0\rangle$ during the period when the laser pulse is almost off (from around $t = 200$ fs to around $t = 900$ fs). This is also due to the small population transfer rate, $1/\Gamma_{(0,0,0)\rightarrow(0,0,1)} = 85300.0$ ps. Therefore, the transition probability is much larger

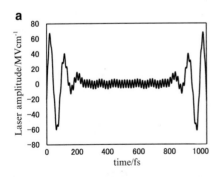
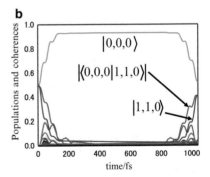

Fig. 15 (a) Optimized laser pulse with α and β being equal to -1.755×10^9 W cm^{-2} and 2.340×10^1 fs^2, respectively, (b) population transfer induced by the optimized laser pulse of panel (a). The initial $T^{(0)}$ was set to be 1000 fs. The temperature was 10 K. The target transition $(|0,0,0\rangle + |1,1,0\rangle)/\sqrt{2} \rightarrow (|0,0,0\rangle + |1,1,0\rangle)/\sqrt{2}$ was optimized

and the mixedness is much smaller than in the case of Fig. 14. That is, the transition probability and the mixedness at the final time are 86.9429 % and 0.22626 for the free-time case and are 86.7598 % and 0.23058 for the fixed-time case, respectively. In addition, the optimal temporal duration is also longer than the initial guess: $T = 1041.12$ fs. The reason is the same as that for Fig. 14.

5 Concluding Remarks

In the present article, we have reviewed our recent main theoretical and numerical contributions to the development of molecular quantum computing and quantum information science. In particular, we have paved a new way for applying molecular internal degrees of freedom (electronic, vibrational, and rotational states) to quantum computing and quantum information science by theoretical and numerical methods.

Now, quantum computing and quantum information science have become an unshakeable important research topics, ranging among a variety of disciplines. However, some basics of the theoretical aspects have not yet been solved and are still debatable. For instance, the definition of multipartite entanglement degree in pure and mixed states is still discussed in the recently published papers. In addition, scalability and decoherence of quantum states in quantum computers have gradually become obvious to be extremely challenging with the rapid development of experiments and theories. At the same time, the experimental realization of quantum computers based on the theories is also very important in order to extremely outperform the present-day classical computers. Although there are a number of experimental data for physical systems, at present there are few experimental evidences for molecules which chemists are interested in. Therefore, we suspect that there may be a number of rooms for improvement in molecular quantum computers. We chemists hope that molecular quantum computing will be investigated in more detail from the chemical viewpoint in future. In particular, we expect that our and other's theoretical and numerical results will provide important guides to experimental realization of quantum computers and quantum information processing.

Although we have applied our FRFP-OCT to two specific control problems as shown in Sect. 4, the theory is so general that it may be possible to apply it to a variety of quantum dynamics with and without dissipation in future. An experimental application of FRFP-OCTs developed by us for the first time could be expected in the same manner as closed-loop quantum learning control experiments [80–83].

Finally, although we have not covered such topics in the present review article, we would like to recommend the readers to refer to our recent studies on entanglement of angular momenta of atoms and molecules [84], decoherence of vibrational entanglement by intramolecular vibrational relaxation (IVR) in polyatomic molecules [85], and quantum computing using molecular vibrational and rotational modes of open-shell $^{14}N^{16}O$ molecule [60]. In addition, it will be useful to refer to our previous researches on the simulation of two-qubit operations in semiconductor quantum dots using the *spatial phase* of the incident laser pulse [86], entanglement generation in the scattering processes [87], and time-resolved entanglement of bound and dissociative atoms and molecules [88].

References

1. M.A. Nielsen, I. Chuang, *Quantum Computation and Quantum Information* (Cambridge University Press, Cambridge, 2000)
2. C.H. Bennett, G. Brassard, C. Crepeau, R. Jozsa, A. Peres, W.K. Wootters, Phys. Rev. Lett. **70**, 1895 (1993)
3. C. Bennett, S.J. Wiesner, Phys. Rev. Lett. **69**, 2881 (1992)
4. M. Brune, F. Schnidt-Kaler, A. Maali, J. Dreyer, E. Hagley, J. Raimond, S. Haroche, Phys. Rev. Lett. **76**, 1800 (1996)
5. D.L. Moehring, P. Maunz, S. Olmschenk, K.C. Younge, D.N. Matsukevich, L.-M. Duan, C. Monroe, Nature **449**, 68 (2007)
6. J. Benhelm, G. Kirchmair, C.F. Roos, R. Blatt, Nat. Phys. **4**, 463 (2008)
7. A. Friedenauer, H. Schmitz, J.T. Glueckert, D. Porras, T. Schaetz, Nat. Phys. **4**, 757 (2008)
8. G.K. Brennen, C.M. Caves, P.S. Jessen, I.H. Deutsch, Phys. Rev. Lett. **82**, 1060 (1999)
9. I.L. Chuang, L.M.K. Vandersypen, X. Zhou, D.W. Leung, S. Lloyd, Nature **393**, 143 (1998)
10. J.A. Jones, M. Mosca, J. Chem. Phys. **109**, 1648 (1998)
11. J. Clarke, F.K. Wilhelm, Nature **453**, 1031 (2008)
12. B.E. Kane, Nature **393**, 133 (1998)
13. A.P. Nizovtsev, S.Y. Killin, F. Jelezko, T. Gaebal, I. Popa, A. Gruber, J. Wrachtrup, Opt. Spectrosc. **99**, 248 (2004)
14. P. Neumann, N. Mizouchi, F. Rempp, P. Hemmer, H. Watanabe, S. Yamasaki, V. Jacques, T. Gaebel, Science **320**, 1326 (2008)
15. C.M. Tesch, L. Kurtz, R. de Vivie-Riedle, Chem. Phys. Lett. **343**, 633 (2001)
16. C.M. Tesch, R. de Vivie-Riedle, Phys. Rev. Lett. **89**, 157901 (2002)
17. C.M. Tesch, R. de Vivie-Riedle, J. Chem. Phys. **121**, 12158 (2004)
18. U. Troppmann, C.M. Tesch, R. de Vivie-Riedle, Chem. Phys. Lett. **378**, 273 (2003)
19. B.M.R. Korff, U. Troppmann, K.L. Kompa, R. de Vivie-Riedle, J. Chem. Phys. **123**, 244509 (2005)
20. U. Troppmann, C. Gollub, R. de Vivie-Riedle, New J. Phys. **8**, 100 (2006)
21. C. Gollub, R. de Vivie-Riedle, J. Chem. Phys. **128**, 167101 (2008)
22. D. Babikov, J. Chem. Phys. **121**, 7577 (2004)
23. M. Zhao, D. Babikov, J. Chem. Phys. **125**, 024105 (2006)
24. M. Zhao, D. Babikov, J. Chem. Phys. **126**, 204102 (2007)
25. D. Babikov, M. Zhao, J. Chem. Phys. **128**, 167102 (2008)
26. T. Cheng, A. Brown, J. Chem. Phys. **124**, 034111 (2006)
27. M. Ndong, D. Lauvergnat, X. Chapuisat, M. Desouter-Lecomte, J. Chem. Phys. **126**, 244505 (2007)
28. L. Bomble, D. Lauvergnat, F. Remacle, M. Desouter-Lecomte, J. Chem. Phys. **128**, 064110 (2008)
29. S. Suzuki, K. Mishima, K. Yamashita, Chem. Phys. Lett. **410**, 358 (2005)
30. M. Schröder, A. Brown, J. Chem. Phys. **131**, 034101 (2009)
31. S.A. Rice, M. Zhao, *Optical Control of Molecular Dynamics* (Wiley-Interscience, New York, 2000)

32. Y. Teranishi, Y. Ohtsuki, K. Hosaka, H. Chiba, H. Katsuki, K. Ohmori, J. Chem. Phys. **124**, 114110 (2006)
33. E.A. Shapiro, I. Khavkine, M. Spanner, M.Y. Ivanov, Phys. Rev. A **67**, 013406 (2003)
34. M. Tsubouchi, T. Momose, Phys. Rev. A **77**, 052326 (2008)
35. E. Charron, P. Milman, A. Keller, O. Atabek, Phys. Rev. A **75**, 033414 (2007)
36. K. Mishima, K. Yamashita, Chem. Phys. **361**, 106 (2009)
37. J. Vala, Z. Amitay, B. Zhang, S.R. Leone, R. Kosloff, Phys. Rev. A **66**, 062316 (2002)
38. M. Tsubouchi, T. Momose, J. Opt. Soc. Am. B **24**, 1886 (2007)
39. H. Katsuki, H. Chiba, B. Girard, C. Meier, K. Ohmori, Science **311**, 1589 (2006)
40. K. Ohmori, H. Katsuki, H. Chiba, M. Honda, Y. Hagihara, K. Fujiwara, Y. Sato, K. Ueda, Phys. Rev. Lett. **96**, 093002 (2006)
41. H. Katuski, K. Hosaka, H. Chiba, K. Ohmori, Phys. Rev. A **76**, 013403 (2007)
42. H. Katsuki, H. Chiba, C. Meier, B. Girard, K. Ohmori, Phys. Rev. Lett. **102**, 103602 (2009)
43. K. Ohmori, Annu. Rev. Phys. Chem. **60**, 487 (2009)
44. K. Mishima, K. Shioya, K. Yamashita, Chem. Phys. Lett. **442**, 58 (2007)
45. L.D. Landau, Phys. Z. Sowj. **2**, 46 (1932)
46. C. Zener, Proc. R. Soc. Lond. A **137**, 696 (1932)
47. V.S. Malinovsky, J.L. Krause, Eur. Phys. J. D **14**, 147 (2001)
48. D.P. DiVincenzo, Phys. Rev. A **51**, 1015 (1995)
49. D. Deutsch, Proc. R. Soc. Lond. A **400**, 97 (1985)
50. D. Deutsch, R. Jozsa, Proc. R. Soc. Lond. A **439**, 553 (1992)
51. P. Shor, *Proceedings 35th Annual Symposium on Foundations of Computer Science*, 124. (1994)
52. W. Zhu, J. Botina, H. Rabitz, J. Chem. Phys. **108**, 1953 (1998)
53. K. Sundermann, R. de Vivie-Riedle, J. Chem. Phys. **110**, 1896 (1999)
54. Y. Ohtsuki, K. Nakagami, Y. Fujimura, W. Zhu, H. Rabitz, J. Chem. Phys. **114**, 8867 (2001)
55. K. Mishima, K. Tokumo, K. Yamashita, Chem. Phys. **343**, 61 (2008)
56. K. Shioya, K. Mishima, K. Yamashita, Mol. Phys. **105**, 1283 (2007)
57. J.I. Cirac, P. Zoller, Phys. Rev. Lett. **74**, 4091 (1995)
58. S.F. Yelin, K. Kirby, R. Cote, Phys. Rev. A **74**, 050301(R) (2006)
59. G.V. Varada, G.S. Agarwal, Phys. Rev. A **45**, 6721 (1992)
60. K. Mishima, K. Yamashita, Chem. Phys. **379**, 13 (2011)
61. K. Mishima, K. Yamashita, Chem. Phys. **342**, 141 (2007)
62. K. Mishima, K. Yamashita, Chem. Phys. **352**, 281 (2008)
63. M. Shapiro, P. Brumer, *Principles of the Quantum Control of Molecular Processes* (Wiley-Interscience, Hoboken, NJ, 2003)
64. K. Mishima, K. Yamashita, J. Chem. Phys. **130**, 034108 (2009)
65. K. Mishima, K. Yamashita, J. Chem. Phys. **131**, 014109 (2009)
66. W.G. Unruh, Phys. Rev. A **51**, 992 (1995)
67. G.M. Palma, K.-A. Suominen, A.K. Ekert, Proc. R. Soc. London, Ser. A **452**, 567 (1996)
68. P.W. Shor, Phys. Rev. A **52**, R2493 (1995)
69. A.R. Calderbank, P.W. Shor, Phys. Rev. A **54**, 1098 (1996)
70. L. Viola, S. Lloyd, Phys. Rev. A **58**, 2733 (1998)
71. J. Cao, M. Messina, K.R. Wilson, J. Chem. Phys. **106**, 5239 (1997)
72. J. Cheng, Z. Shen, Y. Yan, J. Chem. Phys. **109**, 1654 (1998)
73. Y. Ohtsuki, W. Zhu, H. Rabitz, J. Chem. Phys. **110**, 9825 (1999)
74. Y. Ohtsuki, K. Nakagami, W. Zhu, H. Rabitz, Chem. Phys. **287**, 197 (2003)
75. S. Ramakrishna, T. Seideman, J. Chem. Phys. **124**, 034101 (2006)
76. A. Pelzer, S. Ramakrishna, T. Seideman, J. Chem. Phys. **129**, 134301 (2008)
77. C.J. Bardeen, J. Che, K.R. Wilson, V.V. Yakovlev, V.A. Apkarian, C.C. Martens, R. Zadoyan, B. Kohler, M. Messina, J. Chem. Phys. **106**, 8486 (1997)
78. S. Beyvers, Y. Ohtsuki, P. Saalfrank, J. Chem. Phys. **124**, 234706 (2006)
79. C. Cattarius, H.-D. Meyer, J. Chem. Phys. **121**, 9283 (2004)

80. D. Cardoza, C. Trallero-Herrero, F. Langhojer, H. Rabitz, T. Weinacht, J. Chem. Phys. **122**, 124306 (2005)
81. P. Gross, D. Neuhauser, H. Rabitz, J. Chem. Phys. **98**, 4557 (1993)
82. R.S. Judson, H. Rabitz, Phys. Rev. Lett. **68**, 1500 (1992)
83. R.J. Levis, H.A. Rabitz, J. Phys. Chem. A **106**, 6427 (2002)
84. K. Mishima, K. Yamashita, Int. J. Quant. Chem. **108**, 1352 (2008)
85. K. Mishima, K. Yamashita, Int. J. Quant. Chem. [Hirao Special Issue] **109**, 1827 (2009)
86. K. Mishima, M. Hayashi, S.H. Lin, Phys. Lett. **315**, 16 (2003)
87. K. Mishima, M. Hayashi, S.H. Lin, Phys. Lett. **333**, 371 (2004)
88. K. Mishima, M. Hayashi, S.H. Lin, Chem. Phys. **306**, 219 (2004)

Preface

This review article consists of three major parts: generation of entanglement and arbitrary superposition states using vibrational and rotational modes of molecules (Sect. 2), introduction of fundamental theory of quantum algorithms and numerical demonstrations of their efficiencies using molecular internal degrees of freedom (Sect. 3), and construction of numerical algorithms of free-time and fixed end-point optimal control theory (FRFP-OCT) with and without dissipation and its application to entanglement generation and maintenance (Sect. 4). The current status of quantum computing and quantum information science is outlined in "Introduction." The sections in this article are based on the following published and/or submitted materials: K. Mishima, K. Shioya, and K. Yamashita, Chem. Phys. Lett. **442**, 58 (2007), K. Mishima, K. Tokumo, and K. Yamashita. Chem. Phys. **343**, 61 (2008), K. Shioya, K. Mishima, and K. Yamashita, Mol. Phys. **105**, 1283 (2007), K. Mishima and K. Yamashita, Chem. Phys. **379**, 13 (2011), K. Mishima and K. Yamashita, Chem. Phys. **361**, 106 (2009), K. Mishima and K. Yamashita, J. Chem. Phys. **130**, 034108 (2009), and K. Mishima and K. Yamashita, J. Chem. Phys. **131**, 014109 (2009).

Finally, we would like to thank CREST, JST for funding. We would also like to express gratitude to Professors T. Momose (The University of British Columbia), H. Kanamori (Tokyo Institute of Technology), K. Ohmori (Institute for Molecular Science), and Y. Ohtsuki (Tohoku University) for stimulating and useful discussions.

Introduction

Quantum computing and quantum information science are expected to be one of the newest technologies in the next generation. In this article, we focus on theoretical and numerical studies on quantum computing and entanglement generation using molecular internal degrees of freedom (electronic, vibrational, and rotational). We have proposed one method of creating the Bell states and arbitrary linear superposition states in molecular vibrational–rotational modes by using sequential chirped laser pulses. In addition, the numerical simulations of Deutsch–Jozsa algorithm using several combinations of the molecular internal states are reported and compared them from the viewpoint of fidelity of the measurement results of the sender. It turned out that rotational modes of polar molecules coupled by dipole–dipole interaction are the most promising candidates for molecular quantum computing. In connection with quantum computing and entanglement manipulation by external laser fields, we have constructed free-time and fixed end-point optimal control theories (FRFP-OCTs) for the quantum systems with and without dissipation. Using the theories, we have performed simulations of entanglement generation and maintenance. From the numerical results, we have found that FRFP-OCT is more efficient than the conventional fixed-time and fixed end-point optimal control theory (FIFP-OCT) because the optimal time duration of the external laser fields can also be determined exactly using FRFP-OCT.

Gateway Schemes of Quantum Control for Spin Networks

Koji Maruyama and Daniel Burgarth

Abstract Towards the full-fledged quantum computing, what do we need? Obviously, the first thing we need is a (many-body) quantum system, which is reasonably isolated from its environment in order to reduce the unwanted effect of noise, and the second might be a good technique to fully control it. Although we would also need a well-designed quantum code for information processing for fault-tolerant computation, from a physical point of view, the primary requisites are a system and a full control for it. Designing and fabricating a controllable quantum system is a hard work in the first place, however, we shall focus on the subsequent steps that cannot be skipped and are highly nontrivial.

Keywords Quantum control • Spin networks • Quantum computing • Lie algebra

1 Motivation and Overview

Towards the full-fledged quantum computing, what do we need? Obviously, the first thing we need is a (many-body) quantum system, which is reasonably isolated from its environment in order to reduce the unwanted effect of noise, and the second might be a good technique to fully control it. Although we would also need a well-designed quantum code for information processing for fault-tolerant computation, from a physical point of view, the primary requisites are a system and a full control for it. Designing and fabricating a controllable quantum system is a hard work in the first place, however, we shall focus on the subsequent steps that cannot be skipped and are highly nontrivial.

Typically, when attempting to control a many-body quantum system, every subsystem of it has to be a subject of accurate and individual access to apply operations and to perform measurements. Such a (near-) full accessibility leads to

K. Maruyama (✉)
Department of Chemistry and Materials Science, Osaka City University,
Osaka 558-8585, Japan
e-mail: maruyama@sci.osaka-cu.ac.jp; kochan.maruchan@gmail.com

D. Burgarth
Institute of Mathematics and Physics, Aberystwyth University, Aberystwyth SY23 3BZ, UK

© Springer New York 2016
T. Takui et al. (eds.), *Electron Spin Resonance (ESR) Based Quantum Computing*,
Biological Magnetic Resonance 31, DOI 10.1007/978-1-4939-3658-8_6

a problem of not only technical difficulties, but also noise (decoherence), as the system can readily interact with its surrounding environment. In a sense, we are wishing for two inconsistent demands, namely being able to manipulate a quantum system fully by controlling the field parameters while suppressing its interaction with the field.

A good news is that the technological progress over the last decades has been so great that we are now able to access and control quantum systems quite well, provided they are not too large. The coherent manipulations of small quantum systems, in addition to the observations of quantum behaviours, have been reported for various systems, e.g., NMR/ESR [1–4], semiconductor quantum dots [5–7], superconducting quantum bits (*qubits*) [8–10], and NV-centres in diamonds [11, 12].

Here, we discuss a possible scheme to bridge the gap between what we wish to achieve and what we can realise today. Namely, we aim at controlling a given many-body quantum system and identifying it by accessing only a small subsystem, i.e., *gateway*. Restricting the size of accessible gateway and minimising the number of control parameters should be of help in suppressing the effects of noise.

This chapter consists of two parts, each of which is devoted to these two topics, full quantum control through a gateway and Hamiltonian identification, respectively. Such situations, in which only a subsystem is accessible, arise, for example, in networks of "dark spins" in diamond and solid state quantum devices[12–14] as well as spin networks in NMR and ESR setups [1, 4, 15].

In the first part, we present how a system can be controlled through access to a small gateway. Starting with a general argument on the controllability of a quantum system, we show a possible scheme to control spin networks under limited access. The two major issues of our interest in terms of the controllability concern the algebraic criterion for the form of Hamiltonians and the topological (or graph theoretical) condition for the choice of gateway. While the consideration about these aspects will lead to clear insights into the control of spin-1/2 systems, the theory is general enough to be applied to other systems we encounter in the lab. We shall also discuss a few issues related to efficiency, such as, can we compute a pulse sequence for a certain unitary on the chain by a classical computer within polynomial time? Or how much time would a unitary require to be performed?

All these discussions on the controllability assume the complete knowledge of the system Hamiltonian. The second part of this chapter is devoted to the discussions on how the Hamiltonian can be identified despite the limited access. Without the knowledge of Hamiltonian, we can never control a quantum system at will: it will be like going for treasure hunting without a map and a compass. Having learned the details of the system Hamiltonian, we then attempt to fully control it, enjoying the quantumness of the dynamics. Nonetheless, both the full information acquisition and the full control are still very hard. In addition, the operational complexity of information acquisition (state and process tomographies) grows rapidly (exponentially) with respect to the system size.

Presumably the most straightforward way to estimate the quantum dynamics is to apply quantum process tomography (QPT), which is a method to determine a completely positive map $\mathcal{E}$ on quantum states. The map $\mathcal{E}$ on a state ρ can be written as $\mathcal{E}(\rho) = \sum_i E_i \rho E_i^\dagger$, where the operators E_i satisfy $\sum_i E_i^\dagger E_i = I$ (if $\mathcal{E}$ occurs with unit probability) [16]. The complexity of QPT grows exponentially with respect to the system size; for an N qubit system, we need to specify 2^{4N} parameters for $\mathcal{E}$ and it is an overwhelming task even for small qubit systems [17–19]. Moreover, QPT necessitates estimating all the matrix elements of ρ, the state of the whole system, which is impossible under a restricted access with zero or little knowledge on the Hamiltonian.

The hardness of the task stems from our complete ignorance about the nature of the dynamics. However, here we will consider the cases in which some a priori knowledge or good plausible assumptions are available to us. In reality, it is natural to have substantial knowledge on a fabricated physical system, which is the subject of our control, due to the underlying physics we intend to exploit. Thus, here we will see how such a priori information on the system can help reduce the complexity of Hamiltonian identification. We will primarily focus on the systems consisting of spin-1/2 particles. This is largely because they have been attracting much attention recently as a promising candidate for the implementation of quantum computers.

Yet, it would not make much sense if the size of the gateway is comparable to that of the entire system. From the viewpoint of noise suppression, the smaller the gateway size, the better. Then how can we find a minimal gateway that suffices to obtain full knowledge on the system? As we will see below, the same graph property we introduce in the first part, i.e., the study of spin network control, comes in to the discussion as a criterion for estimability of the spin network Hamiltonian.

This chapter is based on the results from [20–24] as well as some new results.

2   Indirect Control of Spin Networks

2.1   Reachability in Quantum Control

A central question in control theory is provided a system, typically described by states, interactions, and our influence on them, to characterise the operations that can be achieved by suitable controls. In (unitary) quantum dynamics, the usual setup is a time dependent Hamiltonian of the form

$$H(t) = H_0 + \sum_k f_k(t) H_k, \tag{1}$$

where the time dependence $f_k(t)$ can be chosen by the experimentator. While in usual quantum mechanics we solve the Schrödinger equation for a given $f_k(t)$ to obtain a time evolution unitary U, the question of control is exactly the inverse: provided a unitary U, is there a control $f_k(t)$ which achieves it? The unitaries for which this is true are called *reachable*.

Given a system (1), how do we characterise the reachable unitaries? It turns out that it is easier to include those unitaries which are reachable *arbitrarily well* into our consideration, and to describe things in terms of *simulable Hamiltonians:* we call a Hamiltonian iH simulable if $\exp(-iHt)$ is reachable arbitrarily well for any $t \geq 0$. Clearly, iH_0 is effectively reachable by setting $f_k \equiv 0$ and letting the system evolve for a suitable time t. We could also set $f_1 \equiv 1$ and all others zero, and simulate $iH_0 + iH_1$, and so on. Let us call the simulable set $\mathcal{L}$ and see which rules it obeys:

1. $A, B \in \mathcal{L} \Rightarrow A + B \in \mathcal{L}$: this is a simple consequence of Trotter's formula, which says that by switching quickly between A and B the system evolves under the average of A and B.
2. $A \in \mathcal{L}, \alpha > 0 \Rightarrow \alpha A \in \mathcal{L}$: this follows simply from letting a weaker interaction evolve longer to simulate a stronger one, and vice versa.
3. $A, -A, B, -B \in L \Rightarrow [A, B] \in \mathcal{L}$: this follows from a not so well-known variant of Trotter's formula given by

$$\lim_{n \to \infty} \left(e^{Bt/n} e^{At/n} e^{-Bt/n} e^{-At/n} \right)^{n^2} = e^{-[A,B]t^2} \tag{2}$$

4. $A \in \mathcal{L} \Rightarrow -A \in \mathcal{L}$: This is a property which heavily relies on finite dimensions, where the quantum recurrence theorem holds,

$$\forall \epsilon, t > 0 \exists T > t : \quad ||e^{-AT} - 1|| \leq \epsilon \tag{3}$$

which implies $e^{-A(T-t)} \approx e^{+At}$.

If we combine all the above properties, we find that the simulable set obeys exactly the properties of a Lie algebra over the reals. This is very useful; in particular, if through rules 1–4 *arbitrary* Hamiltonians can be simulated, then likewise arbitrary unitaries are reachable: the system is *fully controllable* [25–27] (in fact, this condition is necessary and sufficient). It was shown by Lloyd that it is a generic property: in fact two randomly chosen Hamiltonians are universal for quantum computing almost surely. We will not prove this here as we are going to show something stronger: a randomly chosen pair of two-body qubit Hamiltonians is universal for quantum computing almost surely. That is, Lloyd's result holds even when restricting ourselves to *physical* Hamiltonians.

2.2 Indirect Control

The above equations do not yet take into account the structure of the controls. As discussed in the introduction, it is interesting to consider the case of composite system $V = C \bigcup \overline{C}$ where only a part C of the system is controlled, while the remainder $\overline{C}$ is completely untouched. In the light of Eq. (1) this means that $H_k = h_C^{(k)} \otimes 1_{\overline{C}}$. Control is mediated to $\overline{C}$ only through the *drift* $H_0 = H_V$, which acts on C and $\overline{C}$. If through H_V the whole system is controllable, it means that we have a case of *weak* controllability: the controls H_k do not themselves generate all Hamiltonians, the drift evolution is necessary. This implies that H_V sets a time limit for how quickly the system can be controlled. It also reveals many-body properties of H_V and is therefore interesting from a fundamental perspective.

The question is, given H_V and a split of the system into $C\overline{C}$, how can we decide if the system is controllable? Is the general result by Lloyd still correct when restricting ourselves to such a split, and to a physically realistic H_V? In the following, we will aim to answer both questions.

Using the results from the last section, V is controllable if and only if

$$\langle iH_V, \mathcal{L}(C)\rangle = \mathcal{L}(V), \tag{4}$$

where, for the sake of simplicity, we have assumed the $ih_C^{(k)}$'s to be generators of the local Lie algebra $\mathcal{L}(C)$ of C and where we use the symbol $\langle \mathcal{A}, \mathcal{B}\rangle$ to represent the algebraic closure of the operator sets $\mathcal{A}$ and $\mathcal{B}$. $\mathcal{L}(V)$ denotes the full Lie algebra of the composite system V. The condition (4) can be tested numerically only for relatively small systems. It becomes impractical instead when applied to large many-body systems where V is a collection of quantum sites (e.g. spins) whose Hamiltonian is described as a summation of two-sites terms. For such configurations, a graph theoretical approach is more fruitful.

2.3 Graph Infection

The proposed method exploits the topological properties of the graph defined by the coupling terms entering the many-body Hamiltonian H_V. This allows us to translate the controllability problem into a simple graph property, *infection* [28–30]. In many-body quantum mechanics this property has many interesting consequences on the controllability and on relaxation properties of the system [20, 28]. Also, the same property, also called *zero-forcing*, has been studied in fields of mathematics, e.g., graph theory, in a different context [31]. Let us start reviewing this infection property for the most general setup, which will show more clearly where the topological properties come from.

The infection process can be described as follows. Suppose that a subset C of nodes of the graph is "infected" with some property. This property then spreads, infecting other nodes, by the following rule: an infected node infects a "healthy" (uninfected) neighbour if and only if it is its *unique* healthy neighbour. If eventually all nodes are infected, the initial set C is called *infecting*. Figure 1 would be helpful to grasp the picture.

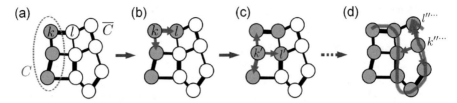

Fig. 1 An example of graph infection. (**a**) Initially, three coloured nodes in the region C are "infected". As the node l is the only one uninfected node among the neighbours of k, it becomes infected as in (**b**). (**c**) Similarly, l' becomes infected by k'. (**d**) Eventually all nodes will be infected one by one

Note that the choice of C that infects V is not unique. Though we are interested in small C, finding the smallest one is a nontrivial, and indeed hard, problem. Nevertheless, from a pragmatic point of view, the number of nodes we consider for the purpose of quantum computing would not be too large to deal with as a graph problem.

2.4 Controllability of Spin Networks

The link to quantum mechanics is that each node n of the graph has a quantum degree of freedom associated with the Hilbert space $\mathcal{H}_n$, which describes the nth site of the many-body system V we wish to control. The coupling Hamiltonian determines the edges through

$$H_V = \sum_{(n,m) \in E} H_{nm} \,, \tag{5}$$

where $H_{nm} = H_{mn}$ are some arbitrary Hermitian operators acting on $\mathcal{H}_n \otimes \mathcal{H}_m$. Within this context we call the Hamiltonian (5) *algebraically propagating* iff for all $n \in V$ and $(n,m) \in E$ one has

$$\langle [iH_{nm}, \mathcal{L}(n)], \mathcal{L}(n) \rangle = \mathcal{L}(n,m), \tag{6}$$

where for a generic set of nodes $P \subseteq V$, $\mathcal{L}(P)$ is the Lie algebra associated with the Hilbert space $\otimes_{n \in P} \mathcal{H}_n$[1]. The graph criterion can then be expressed as follows:

Theorem *Assume that the Hamiltonian* (5) *of the composed system V is algebraically propagating and that $C \subseteq V$ infects V. Then V is controllable acting on its subset C.*

---

[1] Note that the condition (6) is a stronger property than the condition of controlling n, m by acting on n. According to Eq. (4) the latter in fact reads $\langle iH_{nm}, \mathcal{L}(n) \rangle = \mathcal{L}(n,m)$, which is implied by Eq. (6).

Proof. To prove the theorem we have to show that Eq. (4) holds, or equivalently that $\mathcal{L}(V) \subseteq \langle iH_V, \mathcal{L}(C) \rangle$ (the opposite inclusion being always verified). By infection there exists an ordered sequence $\{P_k; k = 1, 2, \ldots, K\}$ of K subsets of V

$$C = P_1 \subseteq P_2 \subseteq \cdots \subseteq P_k \subseteq \cdots \subseteq P_K = V , \tag{7}$$

such that each set is exactly one node larger than the previous one,

$$P_{k+1} \backslash P_k = \{m_k\}, \tag{8}$$

and there exists an $n_k \in P_k$ such that m_k is its unique neighbour *outside* P_k:

$$N_G(n_k) \cap V \backslash P_k = \{m_k\}, \tag{9}$$

with $N_G(n_k) \equiv \{n \in V | (n, n_k) \in E\}$ being the set of nodes of V which are connected to n_k through an element of E. The sequence P_k provides a natural structure on the graph which allows us to treat it almost as a chain. In particular, it gives us an index k over which we will be able to perform inductive proofs showing that $\mathcal{L}(P_k) \subseteq \langle iH_V, \mathcal{L}(C) \rangle$.

Basis. By Eq. (7) we have $\mathcal{L}(P_1) = \mathcal{L}(C) \subseteq \langle iH_V, \mathcal{L}(C) \rangle$. Inductive step: assume that for some $k < K$

$$\mathcal{L}(P_k) \subseteq \langle iH_V, \mathcal{L}(C) \rangle. \tag{10}$$

We now consider n_k from Eq. (9). We have $\mathcal{L}(n_k) \subset \mathcal{L}(P_k) \subseteq \langle iH_V, \mathcal{L}(C) \rangle$ and

$$[iH_{n_k,m_k}, \mathcal{L}(n_k)] = [iH_V, \mathcal{L}(n_k)] - \sum_m [iH_{n_k,m}, \mathcal{L}(n_k)],$$

where the sum on the right-hand side contains only nodes from P_k by Eq. (9). It is therefore an element of $\mathcal{L}(P_k)$. The first term on the right-hand side is a commutator of an element of $\mathcal{L}(P_k)$ and iH_V and thus an element of $\langle iH_V, \mathcal{L}(C) \rangle$ by Eq. (10). Therefore $[iH_{n_k,m_k}, \mathcal{L}(n_k)] \subseteq \langle iH_V, \mathcal{L}(C) \rangle$ and by algebraic propagation Eq. (6) we have

$$\langle [iH_{n_k,m_k}, \mathcal{L}(n_k)], \mathcal{L}(n_k) \rangle = \mathcal{L}(n_k, m_k) \subseteq \langle iH_V, \mathcal{L}(C) \rangle.$$

But $\langle \mathcal{L}(P_k), \mathcal{L}(n_k, m_k) \rangle = \mathcal{L}(P_{k+1})$ by Eq. (8) so $\mathcal{L}(P_{k+1}) \subseteq \langle iH_V, \mathcal{L}(C) \rangle$. Thus by induction

$$\mathcal{L}(P_K) = \mathcal{L}(V) \subseteq \langle iH_V, \mathcal{L}(C) \rangle \subseteq \mathcal{L}(V). \quad \blacksquare \tag{11}$$

The above theorem has split the question of algebraic control into two separate aspects. The first part, the algebraic propagation Eq. (6) is a property of the coupling that lives on a small Hilbert space $\mathcal{H}_n \otimes \mathcal{H}_m$ and can therefore be checked easily numerically. The second part is a topological property of the (classical) graph. An important question arises here if this may be not only a sufficient but also necessary criterion. As we will see below, there are systems where C does not infect V but the system is controllable *for specific coupling strengths*. However the topological stability with respect to the choice of coupling strengths is no longer given.

An important example of the above theorem are systems of coupled spin-1/2 systems (qubits). We consider the two-body Hamiltonian given by the following Heisenberg-like coupling,

$$H_{nm} = c_{nm}(X_n X_m + Y_n Y_m + \Delta Z_n Z_m), \tag{12}$$

where the c_{nm} are arbitrary coupling constants, Δ is an anisotropy parameter, and X, Y, Z are the standard Pauli matrices. The edges of the graph are those (n, m) for which $c_{nm} \neq 0$.

To apply our method we have first shown that the Heisenberg interaction is algebraically propagating. In this case the Lie algebra $\mathcal{L}(n)$ is associated with the group su(2) and it is generated by the operators $\{iX_n, iY_n, iZ_n\}$. Similarly the algebra $\mathcal{L}(n, m)$ is associated with su(4) and it is generated by the operators $\{iX_n I_m, iX_n X_m, iX_n Y_m, \ldots, iZ_n Z_m\}$. The identity (6) can thus be verified by observing that

$$
\begin{aligned}
[X_n, H_{nm}] &= Z_n Y_m - Y_n Z_m \\
[Z_n, Z_n Y_m - Y_n Z_m] &= X_n Z_m \\
[Y_n, X_n Z_m] &= Z_n Z_m \\
[X_n, Z_n Z_m] &= Y_n Z_m,
\end{aligned}
$$

where for the sake of simplicity irrelevant constants have been removed. Similarly using the cyclicity $X \to Y \to Z \to X$ of the Pauli matrices we get

$$
\begin{aligned}
X_n Z_m &\to Y_n X_m \to Z_n Y_m \\
Z_n Z_m &\to X_n X_m \to Y_n Y_m \\
Y_n Z_m &\to Z_n X_m \to X_n Y_m.
\end{aligned}
$$

Finally, using

$$[Z_n Z_m, Z_n Y_m] = X_m,$$

and cyclicity, we obtain all 15 basis elements of $\mathcal{L}(n, m)$ concluding the proof. According to our Theorem we can thus conclude that *any* network of spins coupled through Heisenberg-like interaction is controllable when operating on the subset C if the associated graph can be infected. In particular, this shows that Heisenberg-like chains with arbitrary coupling strengths admit controllability when operated at one end (or, borrowing from [25], that the end of such a chain is a universal quantum interface for the whole system).

2.5   General Two-Body Qubit Hamiltonians

Using the graph criterion we found that the dynamical Lie algebra for a Heisenberg spin chain with full local control on the first site

$$H_{Hsbg} + g(t)Y_1 + f(t)Z_1 \tag{13}$$

is su(2^N), where H_{Hsbg} is the Hamiltonian describing the Heisenberg-type interaction, $H_{Hsbg} = \sum_{(n,m)\in E} H_{nm}$ with H_{nm} in Eq. (12). We can also see that the algebra generated by

$$H_{Hsbg} + Y_1 + f(t)Z_1 \tag{14}$$

is su(2^N).

Extending further, we can consider the Lie algebra generated by $A = H_{Hsbg} + Y_1$ and $B = Z_1 + 1$. Because $X_1 = p(A, Z_1)$, where p is a (Lie) polynomial in A and Z_1, replacing Z_1 with $Z_1 + 1$ we obtain $p(A, Z_1 + 1) = X_1 + c1$. Commuting with B we find that Y_1 and therefore also Z_1 and 1 separately are in the algebra generated by A and B. This has an interesting implication—namely, that the two Hamiltonians $A = H_{Hsbg} + Y_1$ and $B = Z_1 + 1$ generate $u(2^N)$. These are *physical* Hamiltonians, because they consist of two-body interactions only. The fact that such pair exists can be used to prove that *almost all pairs of two-body qubit Hamiltonians* are universal: to do so, we first observe that we can construct a basis of $u(2^N)$ through repeated commutators and linear combinations of A and B:

$$u(2^N) = \text{span}\{p_1(A, B), \ldots, p_{2^{2N}}(A, B)\}$$

where the p_k are (Lie) polynomials in A and B. The fact that this is a basis can be expressed equivalently through

$$D \equiv \det\{|p_1\rangle, \ldots, |p_{2^{2N}}\rangle\} \neq 0, \tag{15}$$

where $|p_k\rangle$ is the vector corresponding to the matrix $p_k(A, B)$. Now, parametrising A and B through

$$A = \sum_{n, m, \alpha, \beta} a_{\alpha\beta nm} \sigma_n^\alpha \sigma_m^\beta \tag{16}$$

$$B = \sum_{n, m, \alpha, \beta} b_{\alpha\beta nm} \sigma_n^\alpha \sigma_m^\beta \tag{17}$$

with $\sigma_n^{(0,1,2,3)} \equiv (1_n, X_n, Y_n, Z_n)$ we can expand D in Eq. (15) as a multinomial in $a_{\alpha\beta nm}$ and $b_{\alpha\beta nm}$. Our result implies that this multinomial is not identical to zero, and therefore its roots have measure zero. Therefore the set of parameters $(a_{\alpha\beta nm}, b_{\alpha\beta nm})$

for which the system is not controllable is of measure zero. But the parametrisation (16) holds for arbitrary two-body qubit Hamiltonians, which concludes the argument. We note that this argument is easily extended to general many-body Hamiltonians.

2.6 Efficiency Considerations

The above results are interesting from the theoretical point of view; however, can they be practically useful from the quantum computing perspective? The two main problems we need to contemplate before attempting to build a large quantum computer using quantum control are as follows. First, the precise sequence of actual controls (or "control pulses") is generally not computable without already simulating the whole dynamics. We need to find an *efficient* mapping from the quantum algorithm (usually presented in the gate model) to the control pulse. Second, even if such a mapping can be found, the theory of control tells us nothing about the overall *duration* of the control pulses to achieve a given task, and it might take far too long to be practically relevant.

One approach to circumvent these scaling problems focuses on systems that are sufficiently small, so that we do not already require a quantum computer to check their controllability and to design control pulses. In such a case, the theory of time optimal control [32] can be used to achieve impressive improvements in terms of total time or type of pulses required in comparison with the standard gate model. More complicated desired operations on larger systems are then decomposed ("compiled") into sequences of smaller ones. Yet, the feasibility of this approach is ultimately limited by the power of our classical computers, therefore constrained to low-dimensional many-body systems only.

The goal of this section is to provide an example where one can efficiently compute control pulses for a large system, using the full Hilbert space, and to show that the duration of the pulses scales efficiently (i.e., polynomially) with the system size. We will use a Hamiltonian that can be efficiently diagonalised for large systems through the Jordan–Wigner transformation. A similar scheme was developed independently in [33]. The control pulses are applied only to the *first two* spins of a chain (see Fig. 2). The control consists of two parts: one where we will use the Jordan–Wigner transformation to efficiently compute and control the information transfer through the chain (thus using it as a quantum data bus), and a second part where we will use some local gates acting on the chain end to implement two-qubit operations. To be efficiently computable, these local gates need to be fast with respect to the natural dynamics of the chain. Combining the two actions allows us to implement any unitary operation described in the gate model.

More specifically, we consider a chain of N spin-$1/2$ particles coupled by the Hamiltonian

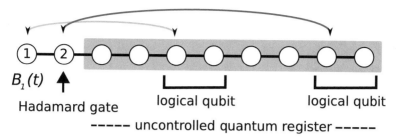

Fig. 2 Our approach for universal quantum computation works on a chain of N spins. By modulating the magnetic field $B_1(t)$ on qubit 1, we induce information transfer and swap gates on the chain (*red* and *green lines*). The states of the qubits from the uncontrolled register can be brought to the controlled part. There, the gates from a quantum algorithm are performed by local operations. Afterward, the (modified) states are swapped back into their original position

$$H = \frac{1}{2}\sum_{n=1}^{N-1} c_n[(1+\gamma)XX + (1-\gamma)YY]_{n,n+1} + \sum_{n=1}^{N} B_n Z_n,$$

where X, Y, Z are the Pauli matrices, the c_n are generic coupling constants, and the B_n represent a magnetic field. Variation of the parameter γ encompasses a wide range of Hamiltonians, including the transverse Ising model ($\gamma = 1$; for this case, we require the fields $B_n \neq 0$) and the XX model ($\gamma = 0$). We assume that the value of B_1 can be controlled externally. This control will be used to induce information transfer on the chain and realise swap gates between arbitrary spins and the two "control" spins $1, 2$ at one chain end. Hence such swap gates are steered *indirectly* by only acting on the first qubit.

In order to focus on the main idea we now present our method for $\gamma = 0$ and $B_n = 0$ for $n > 1$. The general case follows along the same lines, though more technically involved. Our first task is to show that by only tuning $B_1(t)$, we can perform swap gates between arbitrary pairs of qubits. First we rewrite the Hamiltonian using the Jordan–Wigner transformation $a_n = \sigma_n^+ \prod_{m<n} Z_m$, into $H = \sum_{n=1}^{N-1} c_n\{a_n^\dagger a_{n+1} + a_{n+1}^\dagger a_n\}$. The operators a_n obey the canonical anticommutation relations $\{a_n, a_m^\dagger\} = \delta_{nm}$ and $\{a_n, a_m\} = 0$. The term we control by modulating $B_1(t)$ is $h_1 = Z_1 = 1 - 2a_1^\dagger a_1$. From Sect. 2.1, we know that the reachable set of unitary time-evolution operators on the chain can be obtained from computing the *dynamical Lie algebra* generated by ih_1 and iH. It contains all possible commutators of these operators, of any order, and their real linear combinations. For example, it contains the anti-Hermitian operators $ih_{12} \equiv [ih_1, [ih_1, iH]]/(4c_1) = i(a_1^\dagger a_2 + a_2^\dagger a_1)$, $ih_{13} \equiv [iH, ih_{12}]/c_2 = a_1^\dagger a_3 - a_3^\dagger a_1$ and $ih_{23} \equiv [ih_{12}, ih_{13}] = i(a_2^\dagger a_3 + a_3^\dagger a_2)$. We observe that taking the commutator with h_{12} exchanges the index 1 of h_{13} with 2. Taking the commutator with iH we find that $ih_{14} \equiv [ih_{13}, iH] + ic_1 h_{23} - ic_2 h_{12} = i(a_1^\dagger a_4 + a_4^\dagger a_1)$ and $ih_{24} \equiv a_2^\dagger a_4 - a_4^\dagger a_2$ are

also elements of the dynamical Lie algebra. Hence the effect of taking the commutator with H is raising the index of the h_{kl}. Generalising this, we find that the algebra contains the elements ih_{kl}, with $k < l$, $ih_{kl} \equiv a_k^\dagger a_l - a_l^\dagger a_k$ for $(k - l)$ even, $ih_{kl} \equiv i(a_k^\dagger a_l + a_l^\dagger a_k)$ for $(k - l)$ odd, and $h_k = Z_k = 1 - 2a_k^\dagger a_k$. We thus know that the time evolution operators $\exp(-\pi ih_{kl}/2)$ (which will turn out to be very similar to swap gates) can be achieved through tuning $B_1(t)$. The main point is that because both h_1 and H are free-Fermion Hamiltonians, the corresponding control functions can be computed *efficiently* in a $2N$-dimensional space (we will do so explicitly later). Ultimately, we need to transform the operators back to the canonical spin representation. Using $a_k^\dagger a_l = \sigma_k^- \sigma_l^+ \prod_{k<j<l} Z_j$, we find $\exp(-\pi ih_{kl}/2) = (|00\rangle_{kl}\langle 00| + |11\rangle_{kl}\langle 11$

$|) \otimes 1 + (|01\rangle_{kl}\langle 10| - |10\rangle_{kl}\langle 01|) \otimes L_{kl}$ for $(k - l)$ even. The operator $L_{kl} = \prod_{k<j<l} Z_j$

arises from the non-local tail of the Jordan–Wigner transformation and acts only on the state of the spins *between* k and l, *controlled* by the state of the qubits k, j in the odd parity sector.

In order to use the chain as a quantum data bus, our goal is to implement *swap gates* $S_{kl} = |00\rangle_{kl}\langle 00| + |11\rangle_{kl}\langle 11| + |10\rangle_{kl}\langle 01| + |01\rangle_{kl}\langle 10|$, so the fact that we have achieved some modified operators with different phases on k, l instead, and also the controlled non-local phases L_{kl}, could potentially be worrisome. We will use a method suggested in [33] that allows us to tackle these complications. That is, rather than using the physical qubits, we encode in *logical* qubits, consisting of two neighbouring physical qubits each. They are encoded in the odd parity subspace $|01\rangle, |10\rangle$. Although this encoding sacrifices half of the qubits, the Hilbert space remains large enough for quantum computation, and the encoding has the further advantage of avoiding macroscopic superpositions of magnetisation, which would be very unstable. Swapping a logical qubit n to the control end of the chain then consists of two physical swaps $\exp(-\pi ih_{1\ 2n-1}/2)$ and $\exp(-\pi ih_{2\ 2n}/2)$. Since both physical swaps give the same phases, the resulting operation is indeed a full logical swap. Any single-qubit operation on the logical qubits can be implemented by bringing the target qubit to the control end, performing the gate there, and bringing it back again. We could equally decide to perform single logical qubit gates directly, without bringing them to the control end. This is possible because $\exp(-ih_{2n-1\ 2n}t)$ in the physical picture translates to $\exp(-iX_{L,n}t)$ in the logical picture, and because Z_{2n-1} is in the algebra generated by Z_1, which allows us to perform the operation $\exp(-iZ_{2n-1}t) = \exp(-iZ_{L,n}t)$.

For quantum computation, we need to be able to perform at least one entangling two-qubit operation. We choose a controlled-Z operation, which can be performed by operating only on one physical qubit from each of the two logical qubits involved; to perform a controlled-Z between logical qubit n and m, we bring the physical qubits $(2n - 1)$ and $(2m - 1)$ to the control end, perform a controlled-Z between them, and bring them back. It is easy to check that again all unwanted phases cancel out. The controlled-Z could not be efficiently computed in the interplay with the many-body Hamiltonian H, because it cannot be generated by a quadratic Hamiltonian in the Jordan–Wigner picture. Therefore, this gate must be implemented on a time-scale t_g much faster than the natural evolution of the chain, i.e., $t_g \ll \min_j\{1/c_j\}$. We can soften this requirement by using control theory to generate $\exp(-iZ_1X_2t)$ by modulating $\beta_1(t)Y_1$ (this is a linear term in the Jordan–Wigner picture), and then using a fast Hadamard gate on the second site to obtain $\exp(-iZ_1Z_2t)$, which, together with $\exp(-iZ_1t)$ and $\exp(-iZ_2t)$, gives the controlled-Z gate. This leads to a remarkable conclusion: besides a fast Hadamard gate on the second qubit, all other controls required for quantum computation can be computed efficiently within the framework of optimal control.

The crucial question left open above, is how long does it actually take to implement the gates? In order to evaluate the efficiency, we have numerically simulated a range of chain lengths and studied the scaling of the logical swap operation time T with the (physical) chain length N. We set the coupling strength constant, namely $c_n = J$ $\forall$ n. To provide evidence of a polynomial scaling, we set the simulation time $T_N = N^2$ (all times are in units of $1/J$ and $\hbar = 1$) and verify for each N that we can find a specific $B_1{}^*(t)$ that performs the logical swap.

We quantify our success by calculating the error of the operation $\varepsilon = 1 - F$, where $F = (|\mathrm{tr}\, U^\dagger U_g|/N)^2$ is the gate fidelity between the time evolution U and the goal unitary U_g. This standard choice of fidelity is used for evaluating generic unitaries, and for our case it is well suited confirming that the swap gate $S_{kl} \otimes 1_{\mathrm{rest}}$ acts as the identity almost everywhere. However the normalisation factor $1/N^2$ could in principle wash out errors in the part of the gate that acts on qubits k and l only, resulting in the wrong scaling. Therefore, we checked the reduced gate fidelity (tracing out the rest of the system) on those qubits alone, finding that its fidelity remains above $1 - 10^{-4}$ for all N considered.

The function $B_1(t)$ is obtained using techniques from optimal control theory [32, 34]. Briefly, the procedure is as follows: (1) an initial guess is made for the function $B_1(t)$; (2) we run the optimal control algorithm to generate a new $B_1(t)$ which decreases the error of our operation; (3) steps 1 and 2 are iterated until the final error reaches a preselected threshold ε. In practice, it suffices to choose a threshold which is of the same order of magnitude as the error introduced by the Hadamard gate.

If the algorithm converges for each N and the corresponding T_N, giving the optimal pulse sequence $B_1{}^*(t)$, then we can assert that the scaling of the operation time is at least as good as $T_N = N^2$, up to a given precision. Simulating chain lengths up to $N = 40$, we find that $T_N = N^2$ can be achieved. We stress here that the chosen scaling law T_N may not necessarily describe the shortest time on which the physical swap gate can be performed. However, the dynamical Lie algebra of quasi-free fermions has a dimension of the order N^2, indicating that such scaling might be optimal.

2.7   Conclusions

We have seen that control theory provides a powerful framework for indirect control, and therefore for potential control schemes of large many-body systems. We could furthermore show that almost all physical relevant Hamiltonians provide full control, and that at least in some cases efficient mappings from the gate model to quantum control are possible. Under which conditions this is true, and if—and how—such schemes can furthermore be made fault-tolerant in the presence of noise remains an active area of research. One thing that is clear, however, is that in order to apply such schemes, good knowledge about the system Hamiltonian H_0 is required. In the next part, we will consider how such knowledge can be obtained using similar indirect schemes.

3   Indirect Hamiltonian Tomography of Spin Networks

3.1   The Gateway Scheme of Hamiltonian Tomography

It has recently been studied how a priori knowledge on the system could reduce the complexity of QPT. A noteworthy example is the method developed on the basis of compressed sensing [35, 36], which is originally a scheme to make a best estimation for all elements of a sparse matrix despite limited amount of data. Assuming the sparsity under physically plausible settings has been also a key in other works on indirect Hamiltonian identification. The results on which we base the most of the following description exploited the polynomial dimensionality of a subspace we probe [22, 23]. That is, there is already an exponential reduction for the number of parameters to be determined. While this assumption puts a condition on the type of Hamiltonians, it was shown that a larger class of Hamiltonians (for 1D spin chains) could also be estimated through a gateway Di Carlo et al. [37]. We shall see below that this is a special case of the generic estimation of quadratic Hamiltonians, which might describe the dynamics of either bosons or fermions on not only 1D chains but also more general networks.

Suppose that we have a network consisting of N spin-1/2 particles, such as the one in Fig. 3. Our aim is to estimate all the non-zero coupling strengths between spins and the intensities of the local magnetic fields. The assumptions we make are as follows:

1. The topology of the network is known. That is, information on the graph $G = (V, E)$ corresponding to the network is available, where nodes V of the graph correspond to spins and edges E connect spins that are interacting with each other.
2. The type of the interaction between spins, such as the Heisenberg, XX, etc., is a priori known.

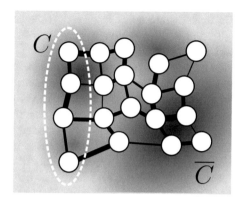

Fig. 3 *All* coupling strengths (*solid lines*) and local magnetic fields (background) of a 2-dimensional network $G = (V, E)$ of spins (*white circles*) can be estimated *indirectly* by quantum state tomography on a gateway C (enclosed by the *dashed red line*). The coupling strengths and field intensities are represented by the width of lines and the density of the background colour, respectively

3. The inhomogeneous magnetic field is applied in the z-direction.
4. The values of coupling strengths are all real and their signs are known.

Assumptions 1 and 2 are the key for reducing the complexity of the problem. In many experimental situations, these information are available due to the conditions for fabrication, albeit a number of exceptions. In the following, we describe the estimation scheme assuming Hamiltonians that have the following form:

$$H = \sum_{(m,n) \in E} c_{mn}(X_m X_n + Y_m Y_n + \Delta Z_m Z_n) + \sum_{n \in V} b_n Z_n, \tag{18}$$

for simplicity. Here, X_m, Y_m, and Z_m are the standard Pauli operators for spin-1/2, c_{mn} are the coupling strengths between the mth and nth spins, b_n are the intensity of local magnetic field at the site of nth spin, and Δ is an anisotropy factor that is common for all interacting pairs.

The Hamiltonians of the type of Eq. (18) have a nice property, $[H, \sum_n Z_n] = 0$, i.e., the total magnetisation is preserved under the dynamics generated by H. Thus the whole 2^N-dimensional Hilbert space is decomposed into the direct sum of subspaces, each of which corresponds to a specific number of total magnetisation. For the purpose of Hamiltonian tomography, analysing the dynamics in the single excitation sector $\mathcal{H}_1$, which has only a single up spin $|\uparrow\rangle$ among N spins, turns out to be sufficient. We will write a single excitation state as $|\mathbf{n}\rangle \in \mathcal{H}_1$ when only the spin $n \in V$ is in $|\uparrow\rangle$ with all others in $|\downarrow\rangle$, and $|\mathbf{0}\rangle = |\downarrow \ldots \downarrow\rangle$. In Sect. 3.5, we will treat more general cases, i.e., Hamiltonians that do not conserve the total magnetisation, such as the generic XX- or Ising-type Hamiltonians.

The task of Hamiltonian tomography is to estimate c_{mn} and b_n under the limited access to a small gateway $C \subset V$ only. Naturally, the challenge here is to obtain information about the inaccessible spins in $\overline{C} \equiv V \backslash C$, which could be a large majority of V. The question is, however, how small can C be such that we can (in principle) still learn all the couplings and fields in V?

This can be answered by using the *infecting* property, which has been introduced in Sect. 2.3 for a given graph G and a subset $C \subset V$ of nodes. The main theorem about hamiltonian identification under a limited access can be presented in terms of the infection property as follows. That is, *if C infects V, then all c_{mn} and b_n can be obtained by acting on C only*. Therefore, C can be interpreted as an upper bound on the smallest number of spins we need to access for the purpose of Hamiltonian tomography, i.e., given by the cardinality $|C|$ of the smallest set C that infects V. To prove this statement, let us assume that C infects V and that all eigenvalues E_j $(j = 1, \ldots, |V|)$ in $\mathcal{H}_1$ are known. Furthermore, assume that for all orthonormal eigenstates $|E_j\rangle$ in $\mathcal{H}_1$ the coefficients $\langle n|E_j\rangle$ are known for all $n \in C$. We show how these information lead to the full Hamiltonian identification, and then in Sect. 3.2 show how these necessary data, $E_j(\forall j)$ in $\mathcal{H}_1$ and $\langle n|E_j\rangle$ for all $j \in 1, \ldots, |V|$ and all $n \in C$, can be obtained by simple state tomography experiments.

Observe that the coupling strengths between spins *within C* are easily obtained because of the relation $c_{mn} = \langle m|H|n\rangle = \sum E_k \langle m|E_k\rangle\langle E_k|n\rangle$, where we defined $c_{mm} \equiv \langle m|H|m\rangle$ for the diagonal terms. Since C infects V there is a $k \in C$ and a $l \in \overline{C} \equiv V \backslash C$ such that l is the only neighbour of k outside of C, i.e.

$$\langle n|H|k\rangle = 0 \quad \forall n \in \overline{C} \backslash \{l\}. \tag{19}$$

For an example see Fig. 1. Using the eigenequation, we obtain for all j

$$E_j|E_j\rangle = H|E_j\rangle = \sum_{m \in C} \langle m|E_j\rangle H|m\rangle + \sum_{n \in V \backslash C} \langle n|E_j\rangle H|n\rangle.$$

Multiplying with $\langle k|$ and using Eq. (19) we obtain

$$E_j\langle k|E_j\rangle - \sum_{m \in C} c_{km}\langle m|E_j\rangle = c_{kl}\langle l|E_j\rangle. \tag{20}$$

By assumption, the left-hand side (LHS) is known for all j. This means that up to an unknown constant c_{kl} the expansion of $|l\rangle$ in the basis $|E_j\rangle$ is known. Through normalisation of $|l\rangle$ we then obtain c_{kl}^2 thus c_{kl} (by using the assumed knowledge on its sign) and hence $\langle l|E_j\rangle$. Redefining $C \Rightarrow C \cup \{k\}$, it follows by induction that all c_{mn} are known. Finally, we have

$$c_{mm} = \langle m|H|m\rangle = E_0 - \Delta \sum_{n \in N(m)} c_{mn} + 2b_m, \tag{21}$$

where $N(m)$ stands for the (directly connected) neighbourhood of m, and

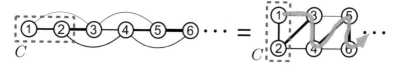

Fig. 4 An example of graphs for non-nearest neighbour interactions. The graph for next-nearest interaction (*left*) can be infected by C as it is easily seen after deforming (*right*)

$$E_0 = \frac{1}{2}\Delta \sum_{(m,n)\in V} c_{mn} - \sum_{n\in V} b_n \qquad (22)$$

is the energy of the ground state $|\mathbf{0}\rangle$. Summing Eq. (21) over all $m \in V$ and using Eq. (22), we can have the value of $\sum_{n\in V} b_n$, thus that of E_0 as well, since all other parameters are already known. Then we obtain the strength of each local magnetic field, b_m, from Eq. (21).

An interesting application of the above scheme is a one-dimensional(1D) spin chain with non-nearest neighbour interactions [38]. If spins interact with the next-nearest neighbours in addition to the nearest ones, the whole graph can be infected by setting the two end spins as C, as shown in Fig. 4. Similarly, if spins interact with up to rth nearest neighbours, all coupling strengths can be estimated by including the r spins at the chain end, from the first to the rth, in C.

3.2 Data Acquisition

In order to perform the above estimation procedure, we need to know the energy eigenvalues E_j in $\mathcal{H}_1$ and the coefficients $\langle \mathbf{n}|E_j\rangle$ for all $n \in C$ by controlling/measuring the spins in C. Suppose the spin 1 is in C. To start, we initialise the system as $|\mathbf{0}\rangle$ and apply a fast $\pi/2$-pulse on the spin 1 to make $\frac{1}{\sqrt{2}}(|\mathbf{0}\rangle + |\mathbf{1}\rangle)$. This can be done efficiently by acting on the spin 1 only; the basic idea is that by measuring the spin 1, and flipping it quickly every time when it was found in $|\uparrow\rangle$, the state of the network becomes $|\mathbf{0}\rangle$ within a polynomial time with respect to the network size $N = |V|$. The reason for this is twofold: the excitation-preserving property of the Hamiltonian guarantees that an up-spin cannot be observed more than N times and the propagation time of up-spins in the network is polynomial in N [39]. Then, we perform quantum state tomography on the spin $n \in C$ after a time lapse t. By repeating the preparation and measurements on spin n, we obtain the following matrix elements of the time evolution operator as a function of t:

$$e^{iE_0t}\langle\mathbf{n}|U(t)|\mathbf{1}\rangle = \sum_j \langle\mathbf{n}|E_j\rangle\langle E_j|\mathbf{1}\rangle e^{-i(E_j-E_0)t}. \tag{23}$$

If we take $n=1$ and Fourier transform Eq. (23) we can get information on the energy spectrum in $\mathcal{H}_1$. Up to an unknown constant E_0, which turns out to be irrelevant, we learn the values of all E_j from the peak positions. The height of the jth peak gives us the value of $|\langle\mathbf{1}|E_j\rangle|^2$ for *all* eigenstates. Thanks to the arbitrariness of the global phase, we can set $\langle\mathbf{1}|E_j\rangle > 0$. Hence observing the *decay/revival* of an excitation at $n=1$ we can learn some E_j and all the $\langle\mathbf{1}|E_j\rangle$.

In order to determine $\langle\mathbf{n}|E_j\rangle$ for other $n\in C$, we prepare a state at 1 and measure at n. Namely, setting $n(\neq 1)$ in Eq. (23) allows us to extract the coefficient $\langle\mathbf{n}|E_j\rangle$ correctly, including their relative phase with respect to $\langle\mathbf{1}|E_j\rangle$. Continuing this analysis over all sites in C, we get all information necessary for the Hamiltonian tomography. It could be problematic if there were eigenstates in $\mathcal{H}_1$ that have no overlap with *any* $n\in C$, i.e., $\langle\mathbf{n}|E_j\rangle = 0$. Fortunately, such eigenstates do not exist, as shown in [28]. Therefore we can conclude that all eigenvalues in the $\mathcal{H}_1$ can be obtained. Although tomography cannot determine the extra phase shift E_0, it does not affect the estimation procedure (it is straightforward to check that it cancels out in the above estimation).

Note that in order for the information about $\langle\mathbf{n}|E_j\rangle$ ($n\in C$) to be attained there should be no degeneracies in the spectrum of Eq. (23). For example, suppose there are two orthogonal states $|E_k^{(1)}\rangle$ and $|E_k^{(2)}\rangle$, both of which are the eigenstates of H corresponding to the same eigenvalue E_k. The height of the peak at E_k in the Fourier transform of $\langle\mathbf{1}|U(t)|\mathbf{1}\rangle$ would be $|\langle\mathbf{1}|E_k^{(1)}\rangle|^2 + |\langle\mathbf{1}|E_k^{(2)}\rangle|^2$. There is no means to estimate the value of each term from this sum, let alone the values of $\langle\mathbf{n}|E_k^{(1)}\rangle$ and $\langle\mathbf{n}|E_k^{(2)}\rangle$. Also even if there are no degeneracies, thus if E_j are all distinct, the peaks need to be sharp enough to be resolved. The issues on degeneracies and resolving peaks are discussed in the following Sects. 3.3 and 3.3.

3.3   Degeneracy

What if there were degenerate energy levels in the single excitation subspace $\mathcal{H}_1$? While 1D spin chains have no degeneracies [40], there could be in general spin networks. Of course "exact degeneracy" is highly unlikely; however, approximate degeneracy could make the scheme less efficient. In this section, we show that there *always* exists an operator B_C, which represents extra fields applied on C, such that it lifts all degeneracies of H in $\mathcal{H}_1$. Because C is only a small subset, the existence of such an operator is not a trivial problem at all. In the following, we demonstrate the existence of such a B_C by explicitly constructing it, assuming the full knowledge about H. Without the full knowledge of H (as is the case in the estimation scenario), we could only guess a B_C and have it right probabilistically. Nevertheless, as it is clear from the discussion below, the parameter space for B_C that does not lift all the degeneracies has only a finite volume. Thus even choosing B_C randomly can make the probability of lifting the degeneracies to converge exponentially fast to one.

Once all degeneracies are lifted, we can estimate the full Hamiltonian $H + \lambda B_C \otimes I_{\bar{C}}$ and subtracting the known part $\lambda B_C \otimes I_{\bar{C}}$ completes our identification task. Here, λ is a parameter for the strength of the fields. Although the extra fields on C do not necessarily have to be a small perturbation, let us consider a small λ to see the effect of λB_C on the energy levels, making use of the perturbation theory.

Let us denote the eigenvalues of H as E_k and the eigenstates as $|E_k^d\rangle$, where $d = 1, \ldots, D(k)$ is a label for the $D(k)$-fold degenerate states. Let us first look at one specific eigenspace $\{|E_k^d\rangle, d = 1, \ldots, D(k)\}$ corresponding to an eigenvalue E_k. Since the eigenstates considered here are in $\mathcal{H}_1$, we can always decompose them as

$$|E_k^d\rangle_{C\bar{C}} = |\phi_k^d\rangle_C \otimes |0\rangle_{\bar{C}} + |0\rangle_C \otimes |\psi_k^d\rangle_{\bar{C}} ,$$

where the unnormalised states $|\phi_k^d\rangle_C$ and $|\psi_k^d\rangle_{\bar{C}}$ are in the single excitation subspace on C and $\bar{C}$, respectively. The state $|\phi_k^d\rangle_C$ $(\forall d)$ cannot be null, i.e., $|\phi_k^d\rangle_C \neq 0$, because if there was an eigenstate in the form of $|0\rangle_C \otimes |\psi_k^d\rangle_{\bar{C}}$ then applying H repeatedly on it will necessarily introduce an excitation to the region C, in contradiction to being an eigenstate [28]. Furthermore, the set $\{|\phi_k^d\rangle_C, d = 1, \ldots, D(k)\}$ must be linearly independent: for, if there were complex numbers α_{kd} such that $\sum_d \alpha_{kd} |\phi_k^d\rangle_C = 0$, then a state in this eigenspace $\sum_d \alpha_{kd} |E_k^d\rangle_{C\bar{C}} = \sum_d \alpha_{kd} |0\rangle_C \otimes |\psi_k^d\rangle_{\bar{C}}$ would be an eigenstate with no excitation in C, again contradicting the above statement. This leads to an interesting observation that the degeneracy of each eigenspace can be maximally $|C|$-fold, because there can be only $|C|$ linearly independent vectors at most in $\mathcal{H}_1$ on C. Thus, the minimal infecting set of a graph, a topological property, is related to some bounds on possible degeneracies, a somewhat algebraic property of the Hamiltonian.

Now suppose that $\lambda_k B_{kC}$ is a perturbation that we will construct so that it lifts all the degeneracies for an energy eigenvalue E_k. Assuming $B_{kC}|0\rangle_C = 0$ turns out to be sufficient for our purpose. The energy shifts due to B_{kC} in the first order are given as the eigenvalues of the perturbation matrix $_{C\bar{C}}\langle E_k^d | B_{kC} \otimes I_{\bar{C}} | E_k^{d'}\rangle_{C\bar{C}} = {}_C\langle \phi_k^d | B_{kC} | \phi_k^{d'}\rangle_C$. We want the shifts to be different from each other to lift the degeneracy. To this end, recall that $\{|\phi_k^d\rangle_{\bar{C}}\}$ are linearly independent, which means that there is a similarity transform S_k (not necessarily unitary, but invertible) such that the vectors $|\chi_k^d\rangle_C \equiv S_k^{-1}|\phi_k^d\rangle_C$ are orthonormal. The perturbation matrix can then be written as $_C\langle \chi_k^d | S_k^\dagger B_{kC} S_k | \chi_k^{d'}\rangle_C$. If we set $S_k^\dagger B_{kC} S_k = \sum_d \varepsilon_{kd} |\chi_k^d\rangle_C \langle \chi_k^d |$, the Hermitian operator

$$B_{kC} \equiv \sum_d \varepsilon_{kd} \left(S_k^\dagger\right)^{-1} |\chi_k^d\rangle_C \langle \chi_k^d | S_k^{-1} \tag{24}$$

gives us energy shifts ε_{kd}. Therefore, as long as we choose mutually different ε_{kd}, the degeneracy in this eigenspace is lifted by B_{kC}. This happens for an arbitrarily small perturbation λ_k. So we choose λ_k such that the lifting is large while *no new degeneracies* are created, i.e. $||\lambda_k B_{kC}|| \neq \Delta E_{ij}$, where $\Delta E_{ij} = E_i - E_j$ are the energy gaps of H.

There may be some remaining degenerate eigenspaces of the perturbed Hamiltonian $H' = H + \lambda_k B_{kC}$. Fortunately, since B_{kC} conserves the number of excitations [see Eq. (24)], we can still consider only $\mathcal{H}_1$ and repeat the above procedure to find operators $B_{k'C}$ to lift degeneracy in each eigenspace spanned by $|E_{k'}^d\rangle$. Eventually we can form a total perturbation $B_C = \sum_k B_{kC}$ that lifts *all* degeneracies in $\mathcal{H}_1$. By perturbation theory a ball of finite volume around B_C has the same property. In practice, we expect that almost all operators will lift the degeneracy, with a good candidate being a simple homogeneous magnetic field on C. This is confirmed by numerical simulations [23].

3.4 Efficiency

The efficiency of the coupling estimation can be studied using standard properties of the Fourier transform (see [41] for an introduction). In experiments, the function $\langle n|U(t)|m\rangle (m, n \in C)$ is sampled for discrete times t_k, rather than for continuous time t, with an interval $\Delta t = t_{k+1} - t_k$. Therefore an important cost parameter is the total number of measured points, being proportional to the sampling frequency, $f = 1/\Delta t$. The minimal sampling frequency is given by the celebrated Nyquist–Shannon sampling theorem as $2f_{min} = E_{max}$, where E_{max} is the maximal eigenvalue of H in the first excitation sector.

Due to decoherence and dissipation, the other important parameter is the total time length $T (= \max(t_k))$ over which the functions need to be sampled to obtain a good resolution. This is given by the classical uncertainty principle that states that the frequency resolution is proportional to $1/T$. Hence the minimal time duration over which we should sample scales as $T_{min} = 1/(\Delta E)_{min}$, where $(\Delta E)_{min}$ is the minimal gap between the eigenvalues of the Hamiltonian. Also, in order for all peaks in the Fourier transform to be resolved, the height of the peaks, which are given by $|\langle n|E_j\rangle\langle E_j|m\rangle|$, should be high enough. That is, all energy eigenstates need to be well delocalised, otherwise most of $\langle E_j|m\rangle$ would have almost zero modulus.

Although a coherence time that is as long as T_{min} has been assumed so far to make the scheme work by letting the signal propagate back and forth many times, the gateway scheme is also applicable to systems with short coherence times by modifying it. For example, as shown in [42], instead of measuring the spin state in the accessible area, we may be able to measure in the energy eigenbasis $|E_n\rangle$, and then the Hamiltonian can be estimated. Such a global measurement is actually easier in some cases than measuring the state of a single component. With this modification to the scheme, however, the graph condition for the accessible area C needs to be slightly changed; it should be expanded, depending on the graph structure.

Another potential concern is the (Anderson) localisation. The localisation of excitation (or spin-up) will take place, if there is too much disorder in the coupling strengths (see, for example, [43]). Then couplings far away from the controlled region C can no longer be probed. In turn, this suggests a way of obtaining information on localisation lengths indirectly. That we cannot "see" beyond the localisation length would not be a serious problem as our primary purpose is to identify a quantum system we can control.

When localisation is negligible, the numerical algorithm to obtain the coupling strengths from the Fourier transform is very stable [40]. The reason is that the couplings are obtained from a linear system of equations, so errors in the quantum-state tomography or effects of noise degrade the estimation only linearly.

Let us also look at the scaling of the problem with the number of spins. Typically the dispersion relation in one-dimensional systems of length N is $\cos kN$, which means that the minimal energy difference scales as $(\Delta E)_{\min} \sim N^{-2}$ and thus the total time interval should be chosen as $T_{\min} \sim N^2$. This agrees well with our numerical results tested up to $N = 100$. For each sampling point a quantum-state tomography of a signal of an average height of N^{-1} needs to be performed. Since the error of tomography scales inverse proportionally to the square root of the number of measurements, roughly N^2 measurements are required for each tomography.

3.5 Quadratic Hamiltonians

So far, we have focused on the Hamiltonians that preserve the total magnetisation. Nevertheless, it is possible to generalise the above argument to a more general class. They are those that are quadratic in terms of annihilation and creation operators, that is

$$H = \sum_{m,n \in E} A_{mn} a_m^\dagger a_n + \frac{1}{2} \left(B_{mn} a_m^\dagger a_n^\dagger + B_{mn}^* a_n a_m \right), \tag{25}$$

which does not preserve the number of quasi-particles $\sum a_n^\dagger a_n$. Here, E is again the set of interacting nodes as in Eq. (18). For H to be Hermitian we must have $A = A^\dagger$ and $B^T = -\varepsilon B$, where $\varepsilon = 1$ for fermions and $\varepsilon = -1$ for bosons, depending on the particle statistics described by a and $a^\dagger$. For one-dimensional spin chains, the operators a and $a^\dagger$ are defined with the standard spin (Pauli) operators through the Jordan–Wigner transformation [44, 45],

$$a_n^\dagger a_n = \sigma_n^+ \prod_{m<n} Z_m, \text{ and } a_n^\dagger = \left(\prod_{m<n} Z_m \right) \sigma_n^-, \tag{26}$$

where $\sigma_n^{\pm} = (X_n \pm iY_n)/2$. The operators hereby defined, a_n and $a_n^{\dagger}$, satisfy the canonical anti-commutation relations for fermions, i.e., $\{a_m, a_n\} = 0$ and $\{a_m, a_n^{\dagger}\} = \delta_{mn}$. A 1D XX-type Hamiltonian

$$H = \sum_{m=1}^{N-1} c_m[(1+\gamma)X_m X_{m+1} + (1-\gamma)Y_m Y_{m+1}] + \sum_{m=1}^{N} b_m Z_m \qquad (27)$$

with anisotropy factor $\gamma \in [0, 1]$ can be rewritten in the form of Eq. (25) through the Jordan–Wigner transformation, and the matrices A and B will look like

$$A = \begin{pmatrix} -2b_1 & c_1 & & \\ c_1 & -2b_2 & c_2 & \\ & c_2 & -2b_3 & \\ & & & \ddots \end{pmatrix}, \ and \ B = \begin{pmatrix} 0 & \gamma c_1 & & \\ -\gamma c_1 & 0 & \gamma c_2 & \\ & -\gamma c_2 & 0 & \\ & & & \ddots \end{pmatrix}.$$

A physically important example of quadratic Hamiltonians is the Ising chain of spins with transverse magnetic fields, which is expressed by Eq. (27) with $\gamma = 1$ and is relevant for systems, such as superconducting qubits [9] and NMR. Note also that once the Hamiltonian of a given system is described in quadratic form, the operators a and $a^{\dagger}$ can represent not only fermions, but also bosons by requiring them to obey the bosonic commutation relations, $[a_m, a_n] = 0$ and $[a_m, a_n^{\dagger}] = \delta_{mn}$. In the following, we shall consider the problem of Hamiltonian tomography of Eq. (25) for 1D chains for simplicity, although the generalisation to more complex graphs is possible.

Since the Hamiltonian Eq. (25) does not preserve the number of particles, initialising the chain to be $|0 \ldots 0\rangle$ just by accessing the end node appears to be impossible. Nevertheless, this difficulty can be circumvented by making use of the property of such Hamiltonians. The quadratic Hamiltonian above can be diagonalised as $H = \sum_k E_k b_k^{\dagger} b_k + \text{const.}$ by transforming $\alpha = (a_1, \ldots, a_N, a_1^{\dagger}, \ldots, a_N^{\dagger})^t$ into $\beta = (b_1, \ldots, b_N, b_1^{\dagger}, \ldots, b_N^{\dagger})^t$ as $\beta = T\alpha$, so that operators b and $b^{\dagger}$ still satisfy the canonical (anti-)commutation relations. So, the quasi-particles described by b and $b^{\dagger}$ behave as free particles that almost do not interact with each other.

The "initialisation" works then as follows. Suppose we can initialise the chain to be in a fixed, but not necessarily known, state ρ_0. Though ρ_0 can be any state, a realistically plausible one might be a thermal state. We prepare two different states ψ_1 and ψ_2 locally at the end site after initialising the chain to be ρ_0. For each initial state we observe the time evolution at the same end site to get a reduced density matrix $\rho(t | \psi_i)$ $(i = 1, 2)$ as a function of time. Because the evolution of internal state of the chain is independent of that of the state at the chain end and vice versa (thanks to the insensitivity between quasi-particles), we can extract the pure response of the chain due to the difference between ψ_1 and ψ_2, by comparing $\rho(t | \psi_1)$ and $\rho(t | \psi_2)$.

The Hamiltonian of Eq. (25) can be rewritten as

$$H = \frac{1}{2}\alpha^\dagger M\alpha,$$

where M is a $2N \times 2N$ matrix

$$M \equiv \begin{pmatrix} A & B \\ -\varepsilon B^* & -\varepsilon A^* \end{pmatrix}, \tag{28}$$

with $\varepsilon = 1$ for fermions and $\varepsilon = -1$ for bosons. As in the previous case of the magnetisation-preserving Hamiltonians, we assume that all coupling strengths are real and their signs are known. Also the factor $\gamma = B_{n,n+1}/A_{n,n+1}$ (anisotropy) is assumed to be constant and known.

Now that we can take it for granted that this $2N \times 2N$ matrix M is symmetric and its entries are all real, a key observation is to reinterpret M as a Hamiltonian that describes the hopping of excitations over a graph of $2N$ nodes [24]. That is, the "Hamiltonian" M preserves the number of excitations in the $2N$-"spin" network, therefore we can apply the scheme discussed in previous sections. Of course, the state on which the Hamiltonian M acts is not a physical spin network, instead it is a fictitious state represented by a $2N \times 1$ vector $(a_1, \ldots, a_1^\dagger, \ldots)^T$. So the eigenvectors of M are something different from physical state vectors.

The graph for a 1D spin chain of Eq. (27) is shown in Fig. 5. Accessing the spin 1 in the real chain corresponds to accessing the nodes 1 and $N + 1$, since what we obtain from the measurement (and Fourier transform) are the values of E_j, $\langle 1|E_j \rangle$, and $\langle N + 1|E_j \rangle$ [24]. Here the state $|\mathbf{n}\rangle$ stands for the localised state on the fictitious $2N$-node graph.

Let us take an Ising chain of N spins with transverse magnetic fields, i.e., $\gamma = 1$ in Eq. (27), as a specific example to demonstrate how the estimation goes. To make use of the symmetry the graph in Fig. 5 possesses, let us define

$$|n^\pm\rangle := \frac{1}{\sqrt{2}}(|\mathbf{n}\rangle + |\mathbf{N} + n\rangle).$$

We already have the information about $\langle 1^\pm|E_j \rangle$, as well as E_j, from the measurement on the spin 1. The estimation procedure proceeds as in Sect. 3.1, namely by looking at $\langle 1^+|M|E_j \rangle$ we have

$$E_j\langle 1^+|E_j \rangle = -2b_1\langle 1^-|E_j \rangle,$$

whose LHS is known, thus b_1 can be obtained through the normalisation condition for $\langle 1^-|E_j \rangle$. Similarly, evaluating $\langle 1^-|M|E_j \rangle$ gives

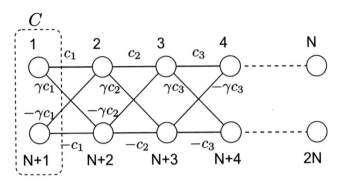

Fig. 5 A graph corresponding to the matrix M with A and B of Eq. (28) and $\varepsilon = 1$ (fermionic). For bosonic systems, there will be additional edges connecting nodes m ($1 \leq m \leq N$) and $N + m$, because B is symmetric, rather than antisymmetric. For both fermionic and bosonic cases, there are edges extruding and returning to the same node, corresponding to the diagonal elements of A, which are not shown here to illustrate the principal structure of the graph

$$E_j \langle 1^- | E_j \rangle = 2c_1 \langle 2^+ | E_j \rangle - 2b_1 \langle 1^+ | E_j \rangle,$$

from which c_1 and $\langle 2^+ | E_j \rangle$ can be known. Also, from $E_j \langle 2^+ | E_j \rangle = 2c_1 \langle 1^- | E_j \rangle - 2b_2$ $\langle 2^- | E_j \rangle$ we have b_2 and $\langle 2^- | E_j \rangle$, therefore we have obtained all parameters up to the second spin, so effectively expanded the accessible area to two spins. Then, this procedure can go on one by one till we reach the other end of the chain, i.e., the Nth spin, identifying all the parameters in the matrix M.

A remark on the initialisation follows. It was shown in [37] that, in the case of 1D XX chains of spins-1/2, the estimation of Hamiltonian parameters is possible without initialising the chain state. The smart trick there was that the spin 1 was initialised so that the average value of the z-component of spin, i.e., $\langle Z_1 \rangle$, was made zero at $t = 0$. The rationale behind it stems from the Jordan–Wigner transform. Since $a_n = \sigma_n^+ \prod_{m<n} Z_m$, if we set $\langle Z_1 \rangle = 0$, the averages of all a_n and $a_n^\dagger$ ($n > 1$) at $t = 0$ become zero. Their time evolution is expressed as (in the form of the vector α)

$$\alpha_n(t) = \sum_{m,k} e^{-iE_k t} T_{nk}^{-1} \left(T^{-1} \right)_{km}^\dagger \alpha_m(0), \tag{29}$$

from which we can see that, in the Jordan–Wigner picture, the initial state of spins from the second to the Nth gives no effect on the measurement result of the first spin. Here, T is a matrix that transforms α into $\beta = T\alpha$ as mentioned above to diagonalise the Hamiltonian. Hence the above initialisation of the first spin is equivalent to that of the whole chain in the Jordan–Wigner (fermionic) picture, and thus corresponds to a special case of our description on initialisation.

3.6 Conclusions

We have seen that despite a severe restriction on our accessibility a large quantum system can be controlled and its Hamiltonian can be identified. As a matter of fact, it is unrealistic for any existing control scheme to have a full access to the system, i.e., a full modulability for the $d^2 - 1$ parameters for independent Hamiltonians with d being the system dimensionality. In the case of methods based on electron/nuclear spin resonance, for instance, all we modulate is the external magnetic field and we do not have a full control over all inter-spin couplings. Therefore, a guiding theory of quantum control is needed to systematically understand and design feasible control schemes under a limited access. The results we have reviewed in this chapter are an example towards the more generic theory, already showing how powerful a restricted access can be. Although the limitation for the control in laboratories would vary, the same or modified methods as what we have seen here will be of help in making a shortcut towards the realisation of the full quantum control.

References

1. L.M.K. Vandersypen, I.L. Chuang, Rev. Mod. Phys. **76**, 1037 (2005)
2. L.M.K. Vandersypen, M. Steffen, G. Breyta, C.S. Yannoni, M.H. Sherwood, I.L. Chuang, Nature **414**, 883 (2001)
3. R. Laflamme, E. Knill, D.G. Cory, E.M. Fortunato, T.F. Havel, C. Miquel, R. Martinez, C.J. Negrevergne, G. Ortiz, M.A. Pravia, Y. Sharf, S. Sinha, R. Somma, L. Viola, Los Alamos Sci. **27**, 226 (2002)
4. J.J.L. Morton, A.M. Tyryshkin, A. Ardavan, K. Porfyrakis, S.A. Lyon, G.A.D. Briggs, Phys. Rev. A **71**, 012332 (2005)
5. J. Petta, A. Johnson, J. Taylor, E. Laird, A. Yacoby, M. Lukin, C. Marcus, M.P. Hanson, A. Gossard, Science **309**, 2180 (2005)
6. F.H.L. Koppens, C. Buizert, K.J. Tielrooij, I.T. Vink, K.C. Nowack, T. Meunier, L.P. Kouwenhoven, L.M.K. Vandersypen, Nature **442**, 766 (2006)
7. T. Hayashi, T. Fujisawa, H.D. Cheong, Y.H. Jeong, Y. Hirayama, Phys. Rev. Lett. **91**, 226804 (2003)
8. Y. Nakamura, Y.A. Pashkin, J.S. Tsai, Nature **398**, 786 (1999)
9. Y. Makhlin, G. Schön, A. Shnirman, Rev. Mod. Phys. **73**, 357 (2001)
10. D. Vion, A. Aassime, A. Cottet, P. Joyez, H. Pothier, C. Urbina, D. Esteve, M.H. Devoret, Science **296**, 886 (2002)
11. F. Jelezko, T. Gaebel, I. Popa, A. Domhan, A. Gruber, J. Wrachtrup, Phys. Rev. Lett. **93**, 130501 (2004)
12. R.J. Epstein, F.M. Mendoza, Y.K. Kato, D.D. Awschalom, Nat. Phys. **94**, 1 (2005)
13. M. Neeley, M. Ansmann, R.C. Bialczak, M. Hofheinz, N. Katz, E. Lucero, H.W. A. O'Connell, A.N. Cleland, J.M. Martinis, Nat. Phys. **4**, 523 (2008)
14. K. Yuasa, K. Okano, H. Nakazato, S. Kashiwada, K. Yoh, Phys. Rev. B **79**, 075318 (2009)
15. K. Sato, S. Nakazawa, S. Nishida, R. Rahimi, T. Yoshino, Y. Morita, K. Toyota, D. Shiomi, M. Kitagawa, T. Takui, *EPR of Free Radicals in Solids II* (Springer, Dordrecht, 2012)
16. K. Kraus, *States, Effects, and Operations* (Springer, New York, 1983)
17. S. Schirmer, D. Oi, S. Devitt, Inst. Phys. Conf. Ser. **107**, 012011 (2008)

18. S.J. Devitt, J.H. Cole, L.C.L. Hollenberg, Phys. Rev. A **73**, 052317 (2006)
19. K.C. Young, M. Sarovar, R. Kosut, K.B. Whaley, Phys. Rev. A **79**, 062301 (2009)
20. D. Burgarth, S. Bose, C. Bruder, V. Giovannetti, Phys. Rev. A **79**, 060305(R) (2009)
21. D. Burgarth, K. Maruyama, M. Murphy, S. Montangero, T. Calarco, F. Nori, M.B. Plenio, Phys. Rev. A **81**, 040303(R) (2010)
22. D. Burgarth, K. Maruyama, F. Nori, Phys. Rev. A **79**, 020305(R) (2009)
23. D. Burgarth, K. Maruyama, New J. Phys. **11**, 103019 (2009)
24. D. Burgarth, K. Maruyama, F. Nori, New J. Phys. **13**, 013019 (2011)
25. S. Lloyd, A.J. Landahl, J.J.E. Slotine, Phys. Rev. A **69**, 012305 (2004)
26. F. Albertini, D. D'Alessandro, Linear Algebra Appl. **350**, 213 (2002)
27. S.G. Schirmer, H. Fu, A.I. Solomon, Phys. Rev. A **63**, 063410 (2001)
28. D. Burgarth, V. Giovannetti, Phys. Rev. Lett. **99**, 100501 (2007)
29. S. Severini, J. Phys. A Math. Gen. **41**, 482002 (2008)
30. N. Alon, A propagation process on Cayley graphs (2008). Preprint. http://www.cs.tau.ac.il/~nogaa/PDFS/pn.pdf
31. F. Barioli, W. Barrett, S.M. Fallat, H.T. Hall, L. Hogben, B. Shader, P. van den Driessche, H. van der Holst, Linear Algebra Appl. **433**, 101 (2010)
32. N. Khaneja, R. Brockett, S.J. Glaser, Phys. Rev. A **63**, 032308 (2001)
33. A. Kay, P.J. Pemberton-Ross, Phys. Rev. A **81**, 010301(R) (2010)
34. D. D'Alessandro, *Introduction to Quantum Control and Dynamics* (Taylor and Francis, Boca Raton, 2008)
35. D. Gross, Y.K. Liu, S.T. Flammia, S. Becker, J. Eisert, Phys. Rev. Lett. **105**, 150401 (2010)
36. A. Shabani, M. Mohseni, S. Lloyd, R.L. Kosut, H.A. Rabitz, Phys. Rev. A **84**, 012107 (2011)
37. C.D. Franco, M. Paternostro, M.S. Kim, Phys. Rev. Lett. **102**, 187203 (2009)
38. P. Cappellaro, C. Ramanathan, D.G. Cory, Simulations of information transport in spin chains (2007). arXiv:0706.0342
39. D. Burgarth, V. Giovannetti, in *Proceedings*, 2007, ed. by M. Ericsson, S. Montangero (Pisa, Edizioni della Normale, 2008). arXiv:0710.0302
40. G.M.L. Gladwell, *Inverse Problems in Vibration* (Kluwer, Dordrecht, 2004)
41. R.N. Bracewell, *The Fourier Transform and Its Application* (McGraw-Hill, Princeton, 1999)
42. K. Maruyama, D. Burgarth, A. Ishizaki, T. Takui, K.B. Whaley, Quantum. Inf. Comput. **12**, 0763 (2012)
43. C.K. Burrell, T.J. Osborne, Phys. Rev. Lett. **99**, 167201 (2007)
44. P. Jordan, E. Wigner, Z. Phys. **47**, 631 (1928)
45. E. Lieb, T. Schultz, D. Mattis, Ann. Phys. **16**, 406 (1961)

NMR Quantum Information Processing

**Dawei Lu, Aharon Brodutch, Jihyun Park, Hemant Katiyar,
Tomas Jochym-O'Connor, and Raymond Laflamme**

Abstract Quantum computing exploits fundamentally new models of computation based on quantum mechanical properties instead of classical physics, and it is believed that quantum computers are able to dramatically improve computational power for particular tasks. At present, nuclear magnetic resonance (NMR) has been one of the most successful platforms amongst all current implementations. It has demonstrated universal controls on the largest number of qubits, and many advanced techniques developed in NMR have been adopted to other quantum systems successfully. In this review, we show how NMR quantum processors can satisfy the general requirements of a quantum computer, and describe advanced techniques developed towards this target. Additionally, we review some recent NMR quantum processor experiments. These experiments include benchmarking protocols, quantum error correction, demonstrations of algorithms exploiting quantum properties, exploring the foundations of quantum mechanics, and quantum simulations. Finally we summarize the concepts and comment on future prospects.

Keywords Nuclear magnetic resonance • Quantum information processing • Quantum computing • Quantum simulation

1 Introduction

With each passing year, computers are used to solve more problems, faster and more efficiently. Nevertheless it seems that many problems are, and will remain, unsolvable by computers based on standard technologies. Three gigantic obstacles,

D. Lu (✉) • A. Brodutch • J. Park • H. Katiyar • T. Jochym-O'Connor
Department of Physics and Astronomy, Institute for Quantum Computing
and University of Waterloo, Waterloo, ON, Canada, N2L 3G1
e-mail: dawei.lu.qip@gmail.com

R. Laflamme
Department of Physics and Astronomy, Institute for Quantum Computing
and University of Waterloo, Waterloo, ON, Canada, N2L 3G1

Perimeter Institute for Theoretical Physics, Waterloo, ON, Canada, N2L 2Y5

Canadian Institute for Advanced Research, Toronto, ON, Canada, M5G 1Z8

© Springer New York 2016
T. Takui et al. (eds.), *Electron Spin Resonance (ESR) Based Quantum Computing*,
Biological Magnetic Resonance 31, DOI 10.1007/978-1-4939-3658-8_7

on the road leading to future computers, cannot be circumvented by classical means. (A) *Microscopic quantum effects*: Moore's law [1] states that the number of transistors in a dense integrated circuit doubles approximately every 18 months. At this rate in a few years, we will have to store each of bit information at the atomic scale, and microscopic quantum effects will play a dominant role. (B) *Dissipation*: All processes in classical computers are irreversible and dissipative. The energy for implementing a single logical gate is an order of magnitude larger than the Laudaur energy [2], which is the minimal cost consumed by the erasure of single bit information. This leads to problems of heating and energy consumption that grow with the number of operations per unit time. (C) *Computational complexity*: Some problems are simply intractable on a classical computer. For instance, storing the state of 71 spins demands 2.4×10^{21} bits, approximately the content of all information currently stored by mankind [3]! These limitations require us to seek out radically new technologies for processing and storing information. While the first two problems may be temporarily circumvented by switching to new platforms that implement classical algorithms, there is no doubt that quantum effects must be dealt with in the near future. Moreover, quantum algorithms are currently the only known way to transverse the obstacle of computational complexity for an important class of problems that include quantum simulations.

Quantum information processors [4] exploit fundamentally new models of computation based on quantum mechanical properties instead of classical physics. While there is no fixed physical platform or the underlying information processing model, most of the known candidates must, almost by definition, deal with quantum effects. Moreover, most known models are in principle reversible, and minimize the erasure of information and thermal dissipation [5]. Most importantly, there is a good reason to believe that quantum computers can solve some problems exponentially faster than a classical computer [4]. For example, fifty quantum bits (qubits) are sufficient to simulate the dynamical behaviour of fifty spins.

Although fascinating and stimulating, the enthusiasm for building large-scale quantum computers [6, 7] is partly challenged by the substantial practical difficulty in controlling quantum systems. At present, a number of physical systems can be used to implement small-scale quantum processors. These include [6] trapped ions and neutral atoms, superconducting circuits, spin-based magnetic resonance, impurity spins in solids, photons and others. Amongst all current implementations, nuclear magnetic resonance (NMR) [8, 9] has been one of the most successful platforms: having demonstrated universal controls on the largest number of qubits. Meanwhile, many advanced techniques developed in NMR have been adapted to other quantum systems successfully. Therefore, despite the huge difficulties in initialization and scalability, NMR remains indispensable in quantum computing as it continues to provide new ideas, new methods and new techniques, as well as implement quantum computing tasks in this interdisciplinary field.

In Sect. 2 below, we present the basics of quantum information processing (QIP) and the implementation of NMR quantum processors. We show how these processors can satisfy the general requirements of a quantum computer, and describe advanced techniques developed towards this target. In Sect. 3, we review some recent NMR quantum processor experiments. These experiments include benchmarking protocols, quantum error correction, demonstrations of algorithms exploiting quantum properties, exploring the foundations of quantum mechanics, and quantum simulations. Finally in Sect. 4, we summarize the concepts and comment on future prospects.

2 NMR Basics

As of 2015, there are many different proposals for quantum computing architectures and it is unclear which architecture will result in a quantum computer. While the computational model is well defined, the underlying physical implementations are still unknown. There are however, five well-accepted physical requirements [10] that must be satisfied by any potential candidate. The so-called DiVincenzo criteria are: (1) a scalable physical system with well characterized qubits; (2) the ability to initialize the state of the qubits to a simple fiducial state, such as $|000\ldots\rangle$; (3) a universal set of quantum gates; (4) a qubit-specific measurement capability; (5) long relevant decoherence times, much longer than the gate operation time. In this section, we describe how NMR completely or partially satisfies the requirements one by one, and interpret the relevant techniques exploited for each aspect. All concepts, unless specified, refer to liquid-state NMR which is more comprehensible.

2.1 Well-Defined Qubits

A two-level quantum system which is analogous to a spin-1/2 particle can encode a qubit. The two levels, usually labeled $|0\rangle$ and $|1\rangle$, are the equivalent of $\sigma_z +1$ and -1 eigenstates, respectively. These are often referred to as the computational basis states. Spin-1/2 systems, such as ^{1}H, ^{13}C and ^{19}F nuclear spins, are natural qubits, and are thus used in vast majority of NMR quantum computation experiments.[1] When a nuclear spin is placed in a static magnetic field B_0 along z direction, the dynamical evolution will be dominated by the internal Hamiltonian (set $\hbar = 1$)

$$H_\omega = -(1 - \sigma)\gamma B_0 I_z = -\frac{1}{2}\omega_0 \begin{bmatrix} 1 & 0 \\ 0 & -1 \end{bmatrix}, \tag{1}$$

where γ is the nuclear gyromagnetic ratio, σ is the chemical shift arising from the partial shielding of B_0 by the electron cloud surrounding the nuclear spin, and $\omega_0 = (1 - \sigma)\gamma B_0$ is the Larmor precession frequency. I_z is the angular momentum

---

[1] For simplicity, we only consider spin ½ systems in this chapter.

operator related to Pauli matrix σ_z as $\sigma_z = 2I_z$, and so on for I_x and I_y. The energy difference between the computational basis states $|0\rangle$ and $|1\rangle$ is the Zeeman splitting ω_0.

For multiple-spin systems, heteronuclear spins are easily distinguished due to the distinct γ and thus very different ω_0 in the magnitude of hundreds of MHz, while homonuclear spins are often individually addressed by the distinct σ due to different local environments. Furthermore, the qubit-qubit interactions are the natural mediated spin-spin interactions called Hamiltonian J-coupling terms. The dipole-dipole interactions are averaged out due to rapid tumbling in liquid solution. The Hamiltonian is

$$H_J = \sum 2\pi J_{ij}\left(I_x^i I_x^j + I_y^i I_y^j + I_z^i I_z^j\right) \approx \sum 2\pi J_{ij} I_z^i I_z^j. \tag{2}$$

The approximation is valid when the weak coupling approximation $\Delta\omega_0 \gg 2\pi|J_{ij}|$ is satisfied, which is always the case for heteronuclear spins and moderately distinct homonuclear spins.

Therefore, the total internal Hamiltonian for an n-spin system is

$$H_{\text{int}} = -\sum \omega_0^i I_z^i + \sum 2\pi J_{ij} I_z^i I_z^j, \tag{3}$$

which forms a well-defined multi-qubit system used in most NMR quantum computing experiments.

2.2 Initialization

Initialization is a process to prepare the system in a known state such as the ground state $|00\ldots\rangle$, which is generally a pure state. The Boltzmann distribution requires extremely low temperature, about tens of mK at 1 GHz, to prepare such state in liquid-state NMR. To avoid working at such low temperatures, a pseudo-pure state (PPS) [11, 12] is used in almost all NMR experiments.

An n-qubit PPS is described as

$$\rho_{\text{PPS}} = \frac{1-\varepsilon}{2^n}\widehat{I} + \varepsilon|00\ldots\rangle\langle 00\ldots|, \tag{4}$$

where $\widehat{I}$ denotes the identity matrix and $\varepsilon \sim 10^{-5}$ is the polarization. In NMR, the identity term is invariant under unital operations; these include pulses, free Hamiltonian evolution, and T_2 decoherence. Moreover, the identity does not contribute to measured signal as we will see later. Thus the dynamical behaviour of the PPS is the same as that of a pure state. The creation of PPS from thermal equilibrium inevitably involves non-unitary transformations since the eigenvalues of the PPS and thermal equilibrium state are different. Several approaches such as temporal averaging [13], spatial averaging [11], logical labeling [12], and cat-state [14] have been proposed to date. However, none of these methods are scalable due to exponential signal decay as a function of the number of qubits [15]. There are scalable methods for preparing qubits in a PPS. One such method, algorithmic cooling, is presented in detail in Chap. 8.

2.3 Universal Gates

Physically, a quantum algorithm is a dynamical process taking the initial state to a final state. One of the breakthroughs of quantum computing was the realization that it is possible to efficiently break this dynamical process into a finite set of elementary gates such as the set that includes finite single-qubit rotations and the controlled-NOT (CNOT) gate [4]. In NMR, we can apply external radiofrequency (RF) pulses in the transversal x–y plane to realize single-qubit rotations. The external Hamiltonian for a single qubit in the lab frame is written as

$$H_{\text{ext}} = -\gamma B_1 \left[\cos \left(\omega_{\text{rf}} t + \varphi \right) I_x - \sin \left(\omega_{\text{rf}} t + \varphi \right) I_y \right], \tag{5}$$

where B_1 is the amplitude of the RF pulse, ω_{rf} is the frequency, and φ is the phase. For simplicity, we often set $\omega_{\text{rf}} = \omega_0$ and work in the rotating frame at frequency ω_{rf}, where the internal Hamiltonian vanishes and the external one remains stationary. Using the propagator in the rotating frame

$$U = e^{i \gamma B_1 \left(\cos \varphi I_x - \sin \varphi I_y \right) t} \tag{6}$$

and choosing appropriate B_1, φ and pulse width t, one can approximate arbitrary angle rotations around any axis in the x–y plane. Using Bloch's theorem, we can decompose single-qubit unitary into rotations around two fixed axes

$$e^{i\alpha} R_x(\beta) R_y(\gamma) R_x(\delta). \tag{7}$$

A CNOT gate is a unitary gate which has two input qubits usually called control and target. The gate flips the target when the control is in the $|1\rangle$ state, and does nothing if the control is in the $|0\rangle$ state. In NMR pulse notation, the gate can be written as

$$U_{\text{CNOT}} = \sqrt{i} R_z^1(\pi/2) R_z^2(-\pi/2) R_x^2(\pi/2) U(1/2J) R_y^2(\pi/2), \tag{8}$$

where $U(1/2J) = \exp\left(-i\pi I_z^1 I_z^2\right)$ indicates the J-coupling evolution for time $t = 1/2J$. The undesired terms in the internal Hamiltonian can be removed via refocusing techniques by inserting π pulses in appropriate positions during the evolution. Note that this refocusing scheme is inefficient to design when the size of system increases. Alternatively, the sequence compiler technique which can track the off-resonance and coupling effects followed with correcting the phase and coupling errors is scalable and particularly powerful [16].

In principle, any quantum circuit can be implemented by RF pulses and internal Hamiltonian evolutions. In practice however, the requirement for ultra-high precision is hard to implement. Conventional composite pulses are accurate in small-size systems but hard to scale due to relaxation during the relatively long duration. To overcome this problem, optimized pulse engineering techniques inspired by optimal control theory for NMR quantum computing have been developed in recent years. Here we primarily focus on the GRadient Ascent Pulse Engineering (GRAPE) techniques [17].

2.3.1 Pulse Engineering Based on GRAPE Algorithm

Given some theoretical unitary evolution U_{th}, the aim of a pulse engineering algorithm is to find an experimental pulse sequence U_{exp} which, together with the free evolution, produces the desired unitary up to some error. The distance between the theoretical and experimental pulse is given by the Hilbert-Schmidt fidelity

$$\Phi = \left| \text{tr}\left(U_{th} U_{exp}^{\dagger} \right) \right|^2 / 4^n. \tag{9}$$

In NMR, the experimental unitary is an N step digitized pulse where unitary operator for the mth step is

$$U_m = e^{-i\left[H_{int} + \sum u_k(m) H_{ext} \right] \Delta t}, \tag{10}$$

where $u_k(m)$, the controllable RF fields, remains constant at each step. The optimization process starts with a guess for the optimal sequence. At each subsequent iteration, we alter $u_k(m)$ according to the gradient

$$u_k(m) \rightarrow u_k(m) + \epsilon \frac{\Delta \Phi}{\Delta u_k(m)}. \tag{11}$$

After a number of iterations, the fidelity Φ will reach a local maximum, and will usually provide a high-fidelity GRAPE pulse to implement U_{th}.

The GRAPE optimization method is much faster than conventional numerical optimization methods. It is robust to RF inhomogeneities and drift of chemical shifts, as well as friendly to the spectrometer due to its smoothness. The major drawback of GRAPE technique is the inefficiency with respect to the system size. However, separating the entire system into small subsystems may moderately reduce the complexity [16]. Another drawback is possible discrepancies between the designed pulse and implemented pulse. A feedback system called pulse fixing can be employed to correct these systematic imperfections.

2.3.2 Pulse Fixing

Non-linearities in pulse generation and amplification, and bandwidth constraints of the probe-resonant circuit, prohibit a perfect match between the designed pulse and real one. The solution is measuring the control field at the sample and closing a feedback loop which can iteratively adjust the control pules so that the real field at the sample matches the designed one. First, a pickup coil is used to measure the fields in the vicinity of the sample, and the data is fed back to compare with the target pulse. Then a new pulse attempting to compensate the imperfection is generated based on the measurement result, and sent back to the pulse generator. A good match between design and experiment is typically reached after 8–10 loops.

2.4 Measurement

The measurement in NMR is accomplished with the aid of an RF coil positioned at the sample. This apparatus can detect the transversal magnetization of the ensemble, and transform the time-domain signals into frequency-domain NMR spectra via Fourier transform. The detection coil is very weak coupled to the nuclear spins, and does not contribute much to decoherence. However, due to the interactions with the heat bath and inhomogeneity of the static field, the nuclear spins still decohere, leading to free induction decay (FID) of the time-domain signal. The weak measurement process cannot extract much information from a single spin and is not projective. Nonetheless, the ensemble averaged measurement provided by bulk identical spins can, for some purposes, provide more information than a projective measurement.

The FID measurement allows us to extract the expectation values of the readout operators in the x–y plane in a single experiment. Pauli observables outside the x–y plane can be rotated into the x–y plane first and then measured in the allowed basis. In this way, full quantum state tomography [18, 19] is achievable in NMR to determine all elements of the density matrix describing the quantum state.

2.5 Decoherence

Decoherence remains a fundamental concern in quantum computation as it leads to the loss of quantum information. It is traditionally parameterized by the energy relaxation rate T_1 and the phase randomization rate T_2. T_1 originates from couplings between the spins and the lattice, which are usually tens of seconds in an elaborate liquid sample. T_2 originates from spin-spin interactions such as the unaccounted terms in the internal Hamiltonian. For NMR quantum computing, the timescale T_2^* which involves the effect of inhomogeneous fields is often more important than the intrinsic T_2 time. Characteristic T_2^* ranges from tens of milliseconds to several seconds, compared to the two-qubit gate time about several milliseconds. For simple quantum tasks, it is sufficient as hundreds of gates can be finished before T_2^* has elapsed. However, for complex algorithms, other ideas have to be employed to counteract the decoherence and preserve the information. Here we introduce how to use RF selection technique to improve T_2^*.

2.5.1 RF Selection

In NMR, the RF inhomogeneity can be mostly eliminated by running an RF selection sequence. This is a sequence of pulses followed by a gradient field that removes polarization on all but a small part of the sample. The part which is left polarized is restricted to a more homogeneous field strength. We have used the RF selection sequence as

$$R_x(\pi/2)[R_{-x}(\pi)]^{64}[R_{\theta_i}(\pi)R_{-\theta_i}(\pi)]^{64}R_y(\pi/2) + \text{Gradient}, \tag{12}$$

where the sum over θ_i should be $\pi/8$ and the number of loops can be varied according to the requirement of homogeneity. The RF selection sequence is applied prior to computation sequences in the experiment, and the signals produced by the inhomogeneous portion of the sample are discarded after the gradient pulse. RF selection improves the timescale T_2^* significantly at the cost of signal loss. For instance, raising the homogeneity to $\pm 2\%$ will result in around 12% residual signal.

3 Recent Experiments

3.1 Benchmarking

Characterizing the level of coherent control is important in evaluating quantum devices. It allows for a comparison between different devices, and indicates the prospects of these devices with respect to the fault-tolerant quantum computing [20]. The traditional approach for characterizing any quantum process is known as quantum process tomography [21, 22], which has been realized in up to 3-qubit systems in experiment [23–28]. However an arbitrary process on a n-qubit system has $O(2^{4n})$ free parameters. So, while quantum process tomography fully characterizes the process, it requires exponential number of experiments, making it impractical even for moderately large systems. For most practical purposes however, we do not need to determine the value of all free parameters experimentally. For quantum error correction, a few parameters related to the level of noise are required. Several useful techniques such as twirling [29–31], randomized benchmarking [32–34], and Monte Carlo estimations [35, 36] can be used to characterize a given quantum process. In the following, we describe an experimental realization of the twirling process.

Twirling is the process of conjugating a quantum process by random (Harr-distributed) unitaries. The quantum process is then reduced to a depolarizing channel with a single parameter to describe the strength of the noise. The twirling procedure provides a way to estimate the average fidelity of an identity operation with a few experiments depending only on the desired accuracy. It can be extended to characterize the noise of various unitary operations such as those in the Clifford group.[2] It is however, not useful for separating preparation and measurement errors. Randomized benchmarking is the generalization of twirling by applying a sequence of Clifford gates and measuring the fidelity decay as the function of an increasing number of gates. The decay rate is independent of the preparation and readout errors up to an additional normalization, but the shortcoming is it cannot provide the information for a particular quantum process. Monte Carlo estimations have the same scaling as the twirling protocol in the case of Clifford gates, but are not as natural as twirling if the probability of a given weighted error is required.

In this section, we focus on the twirling and randomized benchmarking protocols, and describe the relevant NMR experiments [29, 31, 34, 37] briefly. We show that reliable coherent control has been achieved in NMR quantum computing up to seven qubits.

3.1.1 Characterization of a Quantum Memory

Ideally, qubits in a quantum memory do not evolve dynamically, i.e., the dynamical evolution is the identity. The original twirling protocol, proposed by Emerson et al. [29], considers noisy quantum memories, where the quantum process is a faulty identity Λ. The average fidelity of this process is defined as

$$\overline{F}(\Lambda) = \int d\mu(\psi)\langle\psi|\Lambda(|\psi\rangle\langle\psi|)|\psi\rangle, \tag{13}$$

where $d\mu(\psi)$ is the unitary invariant distribution of pure states known as Fubini-Study measure [32]. It is equivalent to average over random unitaries distributed according to the Harr measure $d\mu(V)$ [32].

$$\overline{F}(\Lambda) = \int d\mu(V)\langle\psi|V^\dagger\Lambda V(|\psi\rangle\langle\psi|)|\psi\rangle, \tag{14}$$

---

[2] The Clifford group is the group of unitary operations that leave take Pauli operators to Pauli operators.

Formally, the continuous integral of Eq. (14) can be replaced by a finite sum over a unitary 2-design [30] such as the Clifford group C.

$$\overline{F}(\Lambda) = \frac{1}{|C|} \sum_{C_i \in C} \langle \psi | C_i^\dagger \Lambda C_i (|\psi\rangle\langle\psi|) |\psi\rangle. \tag{15}$$

It is possible to show [29] that the average fidelity above can be derived from an experiment where instead of conjugating by elements of the Clifford group C we conjugate over the single-qubit Clifford group C_1 applied to each qubit individually together with a permutation. In this way, Λ is symmetrized to a Pauli channel instead of a depolarizing channel; however, the task of noise characterization is simplified to the finding probability of no error Pr(0) in this channel.

$$\overline{F}(\Lambda) = \frac{2^n \text{Pr}(0) + 1}{2^n + 1}, \tag{16}$$

where n is number of qubits.

To measure the probability of no error Pr(0), we can probe the Pauli channel with the input state $|00\ldots0\rangle$, followed by a projective measurement in the n-bit string basis. For an ensemble system such as NMR, we can use n distinct input states $\rho_w = Z_w I_{n-w}$, where w is the Pauli weight defined as the number of nonidentity factors in the Pauli operator. This is followed by a random permutation operation π_n and a random 1-qubit Clifford. The average of the output states returns the scaled parameter of the input. Figure 1 shows the circuit for both cases.

To estimate Pr(0) to precision δ, it is enough to perform $\log(2n/\delta^2)$ experiments [29] such that each experiment requires random conjugation by a 1-qubit Clifford and permutation.

The NMR experiments to demonstrate the above protocol were implemented on both a 2-qubit liquid sample chloroform $CHCl_3$ and 3-qubit single-crystal sample Malonic acid $C_3H_4O_4$. To evaluate the level of quantum memories, C48 pulse sequence [38] was utilized to suppress the evolution of the internal Hamiltonian. Two experiments including one cycle of a C48 sequence with 10 μs pulse spacing and two cycles C48 with 5 μs pulse spacing were performed to characterize the

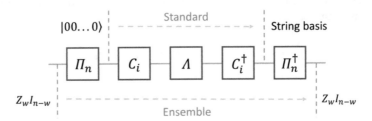

Fig. 1 Quantum circuit to implement the twirling protocol for the purpose of quantum memories. The standard one requires one input state $|00\ldots0\rangle$ and conjugation by C_i, whereas the ensemble one requires n distinct input states and an additional permutation π_n

unknown residual noise. The results show that the probabilities of one-, two-, and three-body noise terms all decrease substantially by using the latter sequence. For instance, Pr(0) increases from 0.44 for the one-cycle case to 0.84 for the two-cycle case.

3.1.2 Characterization of Clifford Gates

Moussa et al. proposed [31] a slight modification of the original twirling protocol, to efficiently estimate the average fidelity of a Clifford gate, by inserting an identity process in the original twirling protocol. If a noisy quantum operation $U_N = U \circ \Lambda$ can be represented by a noisy process Λ followed by the application of the target unitary U, an identity process written as $U^\dagger U$ can be inserted between $C_i^\dagger$ and Λ in Eq. (15). Thus, the average fidelity of a noisy identity Λ transforms to the average fidelity of a noisy unitary gate U_N

$$\overline{F}(\Lambda) = \frac{1}{|C|} \sum_{C_i \in C} \langle \psi | C_i^\dagger U^\dagger \circ U_N \circ C_i(|\psi\rangle\langle\psi|) | \psi \rangle. \tag{17}$$

This is further simplified by combining the pieces following U_N into a new measurement $M_{\text{new}} = UC_iMC_i^\dagger U^\dagger$. Note that for an ensemble system, the permutation operations π_n need to be applied accordingly, see Fig. 2. In general, this new measurement is difficult to implement as U is usually impossible to realize in experiment. However, if U is an element of the Clifford group and the original measurement M is a Pauli measurement (always the case in NMR), M_{new} can be calculated efficiently. The remaining steps are the same as the characterization of quantum memories described in the original twirling protocol.

Despite the limitation of the protocol to characterize only Clifford gates, the modified twirling protocol is still significant since Clifford gates construct the elementary units in the vast majority of fault-tolerant quantum computations based on stabilizer codes, where universality is granted by magic state preparations [39]. In addition, the evolution of states under Clifford gates can be tracked efficiently, as mentioned above.

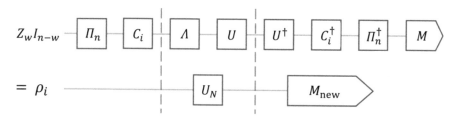

Fig. 2 Quantum circuit for modified twirling protocol to certify noisy Clifford gates. An identity process $U^\dagger U$ is inserted to generate the aim U_N. $\rho_i = C_i\pi_n(Z_wI_{n-w})\pi_n^\dagger C_i^\dagger$ is a random Pauli state and $M_{new} = UC_i\pi_nM\pi_n^\dagger C_i^\dagger U^\dagger$ is an efficiently pre-computed Pauli operator if U is a Clifford gate

The first experiment for certifying Clifford gates was implemented by a 3-qubit single-crystal sample Malonic acid $C_3H_4O_4$ in NMR. The aim was to certify the encoding operation of the phase variant of the 3-qubit quantum error correcting code [40]. This can be decomposed into two CNOT gates and three single qubit Hadamard gates. A GRAPE pulse [17] with the length 1.5 ms was designed to implement this encoding operation, and was rectified by pulse fixing in experiment. The estimation of the average fidelity before and after the rectification is 86.3 % and 97.3 %, respectively. After factoring out the preparation and measurement errors, the average fidelity of the rectified implementation was improved to be over 99 %.

Another experiment of certifying a 7-qubit Clifford gate in NMR was carried out recently [37]. The sample was Dichlorocyclobutanone and the seven carbons formed a 7-qubit quantum processor. The target Clifford gate was chosen as the one to generate the maximal coherence from single coherence with the aid of a few local gates. A 80 ms GRAPE pulse was obtained to realize this operation with a theoretical fidelity over 99 %, followed with the rectification by pulse fixing in experiment. 1656 Pauli input states were randomly sampled out of the entire Pauli group, which consists of 16,383 elements, to achieve a 99 % confidence level. The average fidelity of this Clifford gate is 55.1 %, which is reasonable because high-weight Pauli states are extremely fragile to the effect of decoherence. To assess the gate imperfections, the decoherence effect was simulated under the assumption that it could be factored out. The average fidelity with the elimination of decoherence increased to 87.5 %. As the Clifford gate involved about six two-qubit gates and twelve single-qubit gates, the average error per gate was estimated about 0.7 %, attributed to the imperfections in designing and implementing the GRAPE pulse. The NMR spectra observed after applying this Clifford gate were used as further evidence of the level of control.

3.1.3 Randomized Benchmarking of Single- and Multi-qubit Control

The twirling protocol requires a lower error rate in preparation and measurement than the quantum gate being certified, and cannot identify errors that are due to preparation and measurement. As a result, randomized benchmarking was developed as a modification of the twirling protocol that enables the estimation of error rates per gate for a particular quantum system, independent of the preparation and measurement errors.

The idea is similar to the one used for characterizing a single Clifford gate, but replacing the single Clifford gate with a sequence of one- and two-qubit Clifford gates, that are uniformly sampled from the Clifford group. The outcome is the fidelity decay as a function of the number of Clifford gates in the sequence. Assuming that the errors are independent of the gates, the preparation and measurement errors provide only an additional normalization to the fidelity decay curve. Note that the sequence must be constructed by Clifford gates, to enable the output state tracking and reversal gate designing.

Both single- and three-qubit experiments have been performed in NMR [34]. For the single-qubit experiment, the sample was unlabeled chloroform. The Clifford gates were randomly chosen from $\pi/2$ and π rotations around x, y, or z axis, and applied sequentially for utmost 190 times. Traditional Gaussian pulses, BB1 composite pulses, and GRAPE pulses were all tested, with the average fidelity 2.1×10^{-4}, 1.3×10^{-4}, and 1.8×10^{-4}, respectively. The results were initially somewhat surprising as the optimized GRAPE pulses could not surpass the performance of the BB1 pulses. The explanation is that GRAPE pulses are more sensitive to implementation imperfections such as finite bandwidth effects.

3-qubit experiments were performed using ^{13}C-labeled trissilane-acetylene, and the Clifford group generating set was chosen to be the Hadamard, PHP† (a Hadamard conjugated by a phase gate) and nearest-neighbour CNOT gates. The sequence was constructed by randomly choosing the gates from the above group, with 2/3 probability to implement the single-qubit gates and 1/3 probability to implement the two-qubit CNOT gates. All the operations were optimized by 99.95 % fidelity GRAPE pulses. Starting from a fixed initial state ZII, the theoretical output could be tracked and recovered to return to ZII in the end. By comparing the signal loss as a function of number of gates and fitting the exponential fidelity decay, the average error per gate is about 4.7×10^{-3}, which is an order of magnitude higher than the expected error 4.4×10^{-4} obtained from the GRAPE imperfection and decoherence. This implies there are still unknown factors which have yet to be handled in the pulse design.

3.2 Error Correction and Topological Quantum Computing

To build a reliable and efficient QIP device, a quantum system should be resilient to errors caused by unwanted environmental interaction and by imperfect quantum control. The progressive development of quantum error correction codes (QECC) and fault-tolerant methods in the past two decades have been central to determining the feasibility of implementing a quantum computer. The threshold theorem proves that implementing a robust quantum computer is possible in principle, provided that the error correction schemes can be implemented physically above certain accuracy [41–43]. Using error correction methods, a quantum computer can tolerate faults below a given threshold that depends on the error correction scheme used. Despite many outstanding achievements in the theoretical field, implementing such schemes in physical experiments remains a significant challenge, in large due to the requirement for a relatively large number of qubits. NMR was one of the early platforms used to take up the challenge of demonstrating fault tolerance in real experiments. In this section, we outline some of the fundamentals of fault tolerance and review some experimental implementations of QECC in NMR.

The basic ideas behind quantum error correction schemes [4, 44] are similar to those used in classical error correction methods, which exploit the idea of

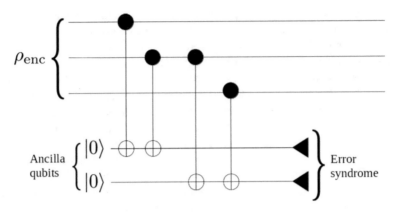

Fig. 3 To detect the error in the encoded state, the ancilla qubits are used to obtain information about the error. Subsequently, the error syndromes can be used to detect and identify the errors. With this knowledge, we can recover the state by applying appropriate recovery operation to the erroneous state

redundancy. Suppose the information carried in a classical bit is copied (encoded) onto two other bits. The *logical* bit is now the encoded three *physical* bits. For simplicity, let us assume we are interested only in storing the information. During the storage time, bit flipping errors can occur, and the errors need to be corrected. For this purpose, we need to check repeatedly whether the three bits are all in the same state. Whenever a discrepancy occurs, we can use a majority vote to bring all three bits to the same states. The method assumes that the probability of two erroneous bits is much lower than the probability of a single erroneous bit.

Extending the classical scheme to the quantum case requires some care. First of all, we need to avoid direct measurement on an encoded state to prevent a quantum superposition from collapsing. As shown in Fig. 3, this can be done by adding ancilla qubits to the circuit and applying appropriate gates to obtain sufficient information about the error without learning the state of the logical qubit. Subsequently, the ancilla qubits can be measured to obtain an error syndrome, which ideally contains the relevant information about which qubit is affected by what kind of error. Secondly, a quantum encoding scheme can exists without violating the 'no cloning principle' of quantum states. The quantum encoding step repeats the state only on a computational basis, which is different from copying a state (i.e., $\alpha|0\rangle + \beta|1\rangle \overset{\text{encoding}}{\to} \alpha|000\rangle + \beta|111\rangle.$, not $(\alpha|0\rangle + \beta|1\rangle)^{\otimes 3}$).

Any decoherence phenomenon can be decomposed into two types of errors: X and Z. Here, X and Z are Pauli matrices. X (or bit flip) errors flip the spin states, from $|0\rangle$ to $|1\rangle$ and vice versa, whereas Z (or phase flip) errors have the effect

$$\frac{1}{\sqrt{2}}[|0\rangle + |1\rangle] \underset{Z}{\Leftrightarrow} \frac{1}{\sqrt{2}}[|0\rangle - |1\rangle]. \tag{18}$$

In an NMR system, Z errors are similar to the T_2 decoherence effect, while T_1 is in the class of X errors although it is not symmetric. Depending on circumstances, a code might focus on correcting one of the two types. Since the two types are closely related, a code that corrects one type can be easily modified to fix the other type. To correct for both types of errors, a larger code might be necessary. For example, Shor's nine qubit code [45] is a code based on two 3-qubit codes, one for X errors and one for Z errors.

Several early QECC, such as the three-qubit phase error correcting code and five qubit error correcting code, were first implemented using an NMR QIP device [44, 46, 47]. The three-qubit phase error and five-qubit error correction codes correct a single qubit phase error and an arbitrary single qubit error, respectively [48]. These implementations demonstrated the benefits of quantum error correction, showing that error correction indeed protects the quantum information even in the presence of gate imperfections. Ideally, to protect quantum information from decoherence, the error corrections should be applied repeatedly. This requires resetting ancilla qubits to a pure state after each error correction state such that they can be reused for the next round. To achieve this, the time it takes to reset ancilla qubits should be considerably shorter than the duration of a desired circuit. In NMR, the natural reset time is T_1. Consequently, the lifetime of the circuit is comparable to the time it takes to reset the ancilla qubits. Moreover, even if the T_1 values of ancilla qubits are an order of magnitude shorter, these qubits will reset to a thermal equilibrium state (in NMR systems) instead of the desired pure state. Therefore, existing NMR implementations are limited to a single round of correction. A single round includes encoding, decoherence, decoding, and error correction steps. The solution to this problem is an active area of research. Methods such as algorithmic cooling can be used to increase the number of rounds [49].

Recently, Zhang et al. [50] realized the implementation of logical gates (Identity, Not, and Hadamard) on encoded qubits to demonstrate the use of quantum error correcting codes in an information processing task. The previous demonstration of single round of the five-qubit error correction code [44] was extended by applying a logical gate after the encoding step. To realize this additional step, they used a dipolar coupled system which reduced the duration of the experiment by the order of magnitude compared to Ref. [44], which was about 300 ms. To implement each gate, each of the five physical qubits was subjected to I, X, Z, and XZ errors (16 possible errors). Comparing the averaged fidelities of the 16 outgoing states with and without the error correction, they showed that the gates perform better when error correction is applied. The improvement in terms of average fidelity was 0.0837, 0.0528, and 0.0196, for Identity, Not, and Hadamard gates, respectively.

To perform fault-tolerant quantum computing, it is important that errors do not propagate badly. It is critical to ensure that when qubits interact, errors from one qubit do not propagate uncontrollably to the rest of the system. One way to do so is to compute and correct errors transversally [51, 52]. For example, consider

Fig. 4 A bad propagation of errors. An error in the control qubit propagates to the target qubit as well

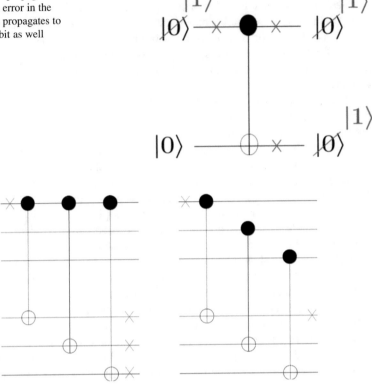

Fig. 5 Two different ways to implement a CNOT gate between the two three-qubit codes: the example on the left is an example of a bad implementation of a CNOT gate between the two three-qubit codes. An error on the first qubit of the first block can propagate to all the qubits in the second block. On the contrary, the right example propagate to at most one error on the bottom encoded qubit and thus remains correctable

applying a CNOT gate between two logical qubits (see Fig. 4), a bit flip error on the control qubit will propagate to the target qubit.[3]

In an error correction model, different methods to implement the logical gates can lead to different models for error propagation. For example, there are two ways to apply a CNOT between two logical qubits, encoded using the three-qubit code, $\alpha|0\rangle + \beta|1\rangle \rightarrow \alpha|000\rangle + \beta|111\rangle$ (see Fig. 5). In the first case, an error occurs on the first qubit of the first block. This error will propagate to all the qubits in the second block, causing a logical error which is not correctable. By implementing a CNOT gate as shown in the second case, we can avoid this bad propagation of errors. One error on the logical control qubit will propagate to at-most one error in the logical

---

[3] In general, a protected space does not necessarily encode a single qubit, and single qubit gates are often not transversal.

target qubit. Each can be corrected individually. This second case is an example of a transversal CNOT gate.

By applying the gates transversally between the encoded blocks, we can ensure errors propagate in a controllable manner. Unfortunately, for any given code, it is not possible to implement a universal set of gates transversally [53]. One way to overcome this problem in constructing a universal fault-tolerant quantum computer is to use special states known as magic states along with the transversal gates [54–57]. These special states can be used together with transversal gates to perform an operation which is otherwise not transversal. Other proposed techniques include concatenation of two different codes [58], transversal gates with the addition of gauge fixing [59], as well as code conversion [60]. However, magic state preparation is currently one of the most well-studied techniques. One method of special interest is the transversal Clifford plus the use of the T-type magic state used to implement the remaining gate in the universal gate set [39].

Preparation of a high fidelity magic state may be critical for universal fault-tolerant quantum computation. *Magic state distillation* is a method to prepare a number of high fidelity magic states from the larger number of low fidelity magic states. Souza et al. [61] demonstrated magic state distillation for the first time using NMR. They showed that they have sufficient control to distill five imperfect magic states into a single higher fidelity magic state. The higher fidelity target T-type magic state

$$\rho_M = \left[I + (\sigma_x + \sigma_y + \sigma_z)/\sqrt{3} \right]/2 \qquad (19)$$

was prepared from the five copies of imperfect states

$$\rho = \left[I + p(\sigma_x + \sigma_y + \sigma_z)/\sqrt{3} \right]/2 \qquad (20)$$

where $p = \sin \alpha$, $\alpha \in [\pi, 3/2\pi]$. To quantify how close the imperfect state is from the target magic state, they measured the m-polarization defined as $p_m = 2\mathrm{Tr}(\rho_M \rho)$. They showed that the m-polarization increases after performing the magic state distillation based on the five qubit error correction code, if the input m-polarization (m-polarization averaged over the five imperfect states) is large enough ($> \sim 0.65$).

3.2.1 Topological Quantum Computing Using Anyons

If the quantum error correction method introduced above is an algorithmic way to protect quantum information, topological quantum computation is the work towards realizing a physical medium that is naturally resilient to decoherence. Anyons, exotic quasi-particles, can be used to realize such a medium. In anyonic topological codes, the computation is encoded in a degenerate ground state of a two-dimensional system that supports anyons [62].

Due to their fault-tolerant nature, anyonic systems have been gaining much attention lately for their prospects in building quantum memories and topological quantum error correction architectures [62, 63]. Currently, most of the contributions to the field have been theoretical, due to the difficulty in building the relevant topological systems. Here we will briefly discuss the past and future contributions of NMR to the field of experimental topological quantum computation. To lead to this discussion, we will first introduce anyons and their properties. For simplicity, we will treat anyons as fundamental particles, although a more correct term would be quasi-particles, excitations that behave like particles. After discussing the basic properties, we will discuss how fault-tolerant quantum computation can be achieved with anyons in a general setting, and we shall conclude the topic with an explanation of a specific anyonic error correction scheme which has been demonstrated in NMR.

Anyons are particles that can be created in a two-dimensional system, such as a spin lattice system [64]. They have a unique property which distinguishes them from other fundamental particles such as bosons or fermions. This property, known as fractional statistics, plays a key role in Topological Quantum Computing (TQC). Unlike bosons and fermions, anyons behave in a non-trivial way under particle exchange.

This operation of exchanging the positions of particles is referred to as a 'braiding operation' [62] in general. Here, we will focus on an operation where we exchange the positions of two particles twice. Intuitively, we would expect the system to come back to its original state as in the case of bosons and fermions. However, if we exchange the positions of two anyons twice, the wavefunction can either obtain a phase factor, ranging from 0 to 2π (abelian anyon), or evolve according to a unitary matrix (non-abelian anyon).

This interesting phenomenon is the result of different topologies that can be manifested in the two-dimensional case. Exchanging the positions of two particles twice is equivalent to moving one particle around the other as shown in Fig. 6. Such a braiding path can always be contracted to a point for a three-dimensional case, whereas the braiding path confined on a plane (a two-dimensional case) cannot be contracted to a point (for more detailed explanation, refer to Fig. 7). This may result in anyons with non-trivial statistics.

Although we cannot build a truly two-dimensional system [62, 63], we can physically realize an effective two-dimensional system. Therefore, anyons do not

Fig. 6 The operation that exchanges the particles twice is equivalent to circulating one particle around the other. The effect of this operation in two dimensions depends on the topology

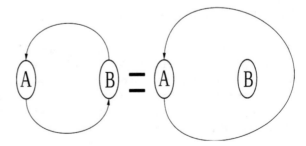

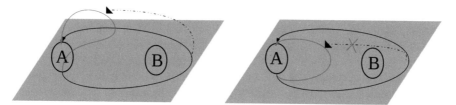

Fig. 7 The topological difference of the braiding path between the three-dimensional (*left*) and the two-dimensional (*right*) cases (circles with A and B represent particles): the braiding path (*black*), can be smoothly deformed to the *red* path for the three dimensional case (imagine the situation where we are pulling one end of the *black* loop, and we also have freedom to move this loop *up* and *down*). Similarly, this red loop can be further deformed to a point, which is effectively doing nothing on the system. However, in a two-dimensional case, since the *black* loop is confined in a plane, we cannot continuously deform the path to the *red* one (unless we make a cut). Here, again, imagine pulling one end of the *black* loop, but without the freedom of moving the loop *up* and *down*. The loop gets stuck because of the particle B

appear as fundamental particles, but as quasi-particles, usually localized defects or excitations of quantum systems.

The quantum states of anyons can be used for QIP. By creating and moving anyons around, we can encode our information in the anyonic state space. As long as the quasi-particles are stable, the information stays safe. Gate operations can be implemented by braiding anyons. In this way, we ensure that the state evolves exactly, since the statistics constitute a unique particle property. This property is exact and path independent. It does not matter which paths we use to braid the anyons, as long as the topology of the paths are the same. In other words, the path depends only on its global (topological) property, not a local property. This feature provides flexibility when implementing a braiding operation, since there is no need to form a precise loop and small wiggles in the path have no effect.

To use anyons for quantum computing, we should first come up with a consistent mathematical model which describes the braiding and fusion statistics of different types of anyons [62, 65]. Working out a mathematical model with appropriate braiding and fusion statistics to implement a desired circuit is non-trivial. Moreover, having a mathematical anyonic model which can perform universal set of quantum gates using only topological operations, i.e., the Fibonacci anyonic (non-abelian) model [62], does not necessarily mean we can realize the model experimentally. In fact, although there has been experimental demonstration of existence of abelian anyons [66], the experimental evidence of non-abelian anyons is still not conclusive, despite extensive ongoing progress [67].

While TQC is fascinating, there is a lot of interest in using anyons for only part of the design, for example in quantum memories and QECC. Since many of these ideas rely on exploiting abelian anyons, they can be physically realized with near future technology.

One well-known topological quantum error correction scheme is the quantum double model [62, 63]. In this model, quantum information is encoded into a collective state of interacting spins on a two-dimensional surface. This encoding scheme takes the spatial relationship between the qubits into account, unlike conventional QECC. These topological systems have certain important properties. First of all, the Hamiltonian of these systems possesses a finite energy gap between degenerate ground states and the excited states. Information encoded in the ground state is therefore protected by this energy gap, since a jump from the ground state to the excited state has an associated energy cost. Also, the information is encoded in a non-local way, for example, not only in one particular spin but rather in the state of the entire system. Hence, local errors cannot alter the information. Most importantly, any local errors (excitations) are realized as the creation of a pair of anyons. This is the critical underlying feature which gives rise to the properties mentioned above. Thus, the errors can be corrected by annihilating the anyons, connecting the two through a topologically trivial loop which is contractible to a point. Some gate operations can be realized by moving anyons through topologically non-trivial loops. Such encoding schemes have several desirable features: high feasibility, requiring only nearest-neighbor interaction; robustness to local perturbations; and access to topological operations.

Since the underlying Hamiltonian that supports anyons is not the natural Hamiltonian of a molecule in a magnetic field, anyonic systems are not directly implementable in an NMR system. However, there has been an experimental demonstration of the toric code [63], an example of quantum double models. Feng et al. [68] took a state preparation approach. Instead of realizing the Hamiltonian of the toric code, they prepared its ground state, which is a highly entangled state. This approach cannot realize all the properties of the toric code, notably the protection of the ground states by the energy gap. However, it can be used to study the properties of the codespace (the grounds state) that are independent of the Hamiltonian. Particularly, how those properties behave under non-ideal noise and whether we have sufficient control to realize the braiding operations on the codespace with current technology. With the state preparation approach, Feng et al. [68] simulated a small instance (six-qubit system) of the toric code [69] and demonstrated operations equivalent to the creation, manipulation, and braiding operations of anyons in the toric code system. The experiment showed that we have a sufficient control to realize such operations. Similar experiments were also performed in quantum optics [70, 71]. Extending such experiments, we can also explore the path independence property of anyonic braiding operations with NMR. Such small-system experiments of NMR QIP make small steps towards experimental TQC.

3.3 DQC1

While liquid-state NMR was the first test bed for QIP, objections about the 'quantumness' of this platform were raised early on due to the amount of noise in the system. One objection [72] was that liquid-state NMR systems at room temperature could not produce entanglement—Schrodinger's "characteristic trait of quantum mechanics" [73]—and are therefore not quantum in the real sense of the

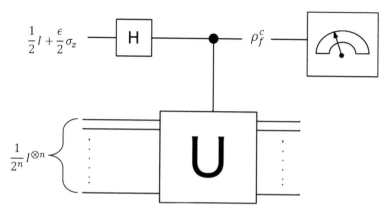

Fig. 8 The DQC1 circuit for evaluating the normalized trace of a unitary matrix with 2^n diagonal elements. The output state shown by Eq. (23) on the control qubit is measured to estimate the normalized trace of U. This task is believed to be computationally hard for a classical computer

word. To challenge that idea, Knill and Laflamme [74, 75] came up with an algorithm which is specifically tailored to NMR systems. The algorithm called *Deterministic quantum computing with 1 qubit* (DQC1) was designed for a processor that has highly mixed input states, intermediate unitary operations, and ensemble readout. The input state has n spins in the maximally mixed state and one pseudo-pure spin.

For simplicity, we describe a specific version of the DQC1 algorithm for estimating the normalized trace of a $2^n \times 2^n$ unitary matrix. This task is expected to be hard to compute (i.e., it scales exponentially with n) due to the exponential number of elements in the sum.[4] Consider the circuit in Fig. 8; the input is the $n + 1$ qubit state,

$$\frac{1}{2^{n+1}} \left[2\epsilon |0\rangle\langle 0| + (1 - \epsilon)I \right] \otimes I^{\otimes n}. \tag{21}$$

We call the first (pseudo-pure) qubit the *control* and the other n maximally mixed qubits the *target*. The output is

$$\frac{1}{2^{n+1}} \left[2\epsilon |0\rangle\langle 0| \otimes I^{\otimes n} \right]$$

$$+ \frac{1 - \epsilon}{2^{n+1}} \left[|1\rangle\langle 1| \otimes U_n I^{\otimes n} U_n^\dagger + |1\rangle\langle 0| \otimes U_n I^{\otimes n} + |0\rangle\langle 1| \otimes I^{\otimes n} U_n^\dagger \right]. \tag{22}$$

---

[4] The argument regarding the number of elements to be summed is somewhat simplistic, since we only require an estimate. Nevertheless, there is good reason to expect the computation scale exponentially with n [78].

Tracing out the target, we get the final state for the control,

$$\rho_f^c = \frac{1}{2}I + \frac{1}{2^{n+1}}\text{Re}[\text{Tr}(U_n)]\sigma_x + \frac{1}{2^{n+1}}\text{Im}[\text{Tr}(U_n)]\sigma_y. \qquad (23)$$

The readout $\langle\sigma_x\rangle$ and $\langle\sigma_y\rangle$ is natural for NMR. We assume that U has an efficient description in terms of a quantum circuit so that the algorithm is relatively easy to implement.

To prepare the initial state, it is possible to use the thermal state and depolarize the n target qubits. One way to achieve this is to rotate them into the x–y plane and then apply a gradient to the magnetic field. The gradient randomizes the phase and the target system is left in a maximally mixed state.

The DQC1 computational complexity class is the class of problems that can be solved efficiently using the DQC1 model. This class is unchanged even if we allow a constant k pseudo-pure qubits (DQC-k), instead of a single pseudo-pure qubit. To show that a processor has the computing power to solve problems in this class, it is sufficient to show that it can solve a single problem which is complete for this class.[5] The first experimental implementation of a complete problem for DQC1 was an algorithm for approximating the Jones polynomial at the fifth root of unity [76, 77], which is a problem derived from knot theory. Details of the problem are given in Ref. [77]; for our purposes, it is sufficient to note that the algorithm is a special case of the algorithm in Fig. 8. The unitary gate U_n is the braid representation of the relevant knot, and the Jones polynomial at the fifth root of unity is approximated using the weighted trace of U_n, a block diagonal matrix in the computational basis. The exact structure of the relevant matrices U_n (as n grows) makes the problem complete for DQC1.

The algorithm requires two pseudo-pure qubits, so the target system is prepared in the state

$$\frac{1}{2^n}\left[2\epsilon'|00\rangle\langle00| + (1-\epsilon')I\right] \otimes I^{\otimes n-1}. \qquad (24)$$

As noted above, this does not change the complexity class. The matrix U_n is block diagonal and the pseudo-pure qubit on the target system is rotated so that the final result is a weighed sum of the trace of the two blocks. The experiment [76] was performed on trans-chrotonic acid, a 4-qubit molecule prepared in an initial state of two pseudo-pure qubits and two maximally mixed qubits. The aim was to distinguish between six distinct Jones polynomials corresponding to braid representations encoded in the two blocks of the 8×8 unitary matrix.

Decoherence was a major source of noise in the experiment. To compensate, the reference spectrum was measured using a similar experiment with the identity instead of the controlled unitary. The other sources of error were gate fidelities;

---

[5] Strictly speaking, it should also be scalable.

these were maximized using GRAPE [17]. The algorithm was implemented for 18 different braids that had to be divided into six different groups corresponding to the six distinct values of the Jones polynomials. The results gave a 91 % success rate at distinguishing different values.

While this experiment demonstrates good control, it is not clear how far it is possible to scale the number of qubits with similar gate fidelities. The issue of noise in DQC1 is problematic, since there is no known error correction procedure within this scheme. It is not yet known at which point this approximation algorithm fails due to errors.

The DQC1 model undermines the claim that entanglement is the essence from which quantum computer derive their power. It is known that for any bipartite cut, the DQC1 algorithm can generate only a small amount of entanglement [78]. Perhaps more importantly, in the trace estimation algorithm, the control is never entangled with the target. Since entanglement seems to play a major role in pure state QIP, it was suggested [74, 78] that a more general form of quantum correlation called quantum discord [79, 80] plays a similar role to in DQC1. Studies on the relation between quantum discord and quantum computing were extended to other measures with some success [79]. One issue with these quantities is that they are usually hard to calculate. However, a DQC1 algorithm can be used for calculating one quantum correlation measure called the geometric discord [81]. An experiment for measuring the geometric discord in DQC1 was also implemented in NMR using similar methods to the experiment for estimating the Jones polynomial [81].

3.4 Foundation

One of the first suggested uses for quantum computers was to test the foundations of quantum mechanics [82]. One may say that fault-tolerant quantum computers will be the ultimate test of the theory, but for the time being simpler experiments have been carried out on small quantum processors. In NMR, such tests are sometimes problematic due to the major downsides of ensemble QIP: the noise and the lack of projective measurements. Nevertheless, a number of experiments related to foundations have been carried out on NMR processors. In the following, we describe two experiments, a state-independent test of contextuality that avoids the need for pure states and a weak measurement protocol that overcomes the inability to perform projective measurements.

3.4.1 Quantum Measurement and the Von Neumann Scheme

Both of the protocols below rely on a particular implementation of the von Neumann measurement scheme. For a Pauli observable $\sigma_{\hat{n}}$ and a spin $\frac{1}{2}$ system S initially in the state $\alpha|\uparrow\rangle + \beta|\downarrow\rangle$ (written in the eigenbasis of $\sigma_{\hat{n}}$), a projective measurement has the following properties: (a) The outcome is ± 1 with probability given by the Born rule $P(+1) = |\alpha|^2$, $P(-1) = |\beta|^2$ and (b) the state of S after the measurement is the corresponding eigenstate of $\sigma_{\hat{n}}$.

In the von Neumann scheme, the measurement result is recorded on an ancillary system called the meter, in our case a spin ½ initially prepared in the $|0\rangle$ state. The measurement is a unitary interaction between the meter and the system such that, after the interaction, the state is $\alpha|\uparrow\rangle|0\rangle + \beta|\downarrow\rangle|1\rangle$. We can then say that a meter readout of $|0\rangle$ corresponds to $a+1$ or $\uparrow$ result and $|1\rangle$ corresponds to $a-1$ or $\downarrow$ result. In NMR, the meter can interact with single quantum system and then we take the average of this meter.

3.4.2 Testing Contextuality

One difference between quantum and classical systems is that measurements are inherently probabilistic and disturbing. Since the early days of quantum theory there were suggestions that the probabilistic nature of the theory is due to an incomplete description and that an underlying ontological hidden variable can be used to make the theory deterministic. Theoretical results give bounds often called no-go theorems regarding the possibility of an underlying hidden variable theory, the most famous of these is Bell's theorem [83] regarding local realism. Another theorem often attributed to Bell is the Kochen-Specker theorem regarding contextuality [84]. Simply stated, the theorem shows that a hidden variable theory cannot give probabilities to measurement results independently of the context of these measurements.

Contextuality inequalities involve degenerate observables and must therefore apply to systems with at least three Hilbert space dimensions. They usually involve specific states that violate the inequality, usually pure states. Cabello [85] came up with a simple inequality which is state independent and therefore more natural for NMR. The inequality involves measurements on two spins. There are nine observables (the entries in Table 1) and six correlation measurements (the rows and columns of Table 1). Each measurement is a correlation measurement of the

Table 1 The six measurements and nine observables for the test of contextuality

	c_1	c_2	c_3	
r_1	IZ	ZI	ZZ	+1
r_2	XI	IX	XX	+1
r_3	XZ	ZX	YY	+1
	+1	+1	−1	

For any quantum states, the measurements yield the same deterministic result. However, if one tries to assign a deterministic value to each of the nine observables, the table cannot be completed. A simple analysis shows that if one assigns values to each observable, the measurements obey an inequality $\beta = r_1 + r_2 + r_3 + c_1 + c_2 - c_3 \leq 4$; however, for any quantum state we get $\beta = 6$

product of three commuting (or co-measurable) observables O_1, O_2, O_3 (e.g., R_1 = IZ · ZI · ZZ). Now let us assume that quantum mechanics is an incomplete theory and that there is a more complete description of nature (a hidden variable) such that we know that the outcomes of independent measurements of these observables should be o_1, o_2, o_3. Since the observables commute, we know that the result of a measurement of the product $O_1O_2O_3$ must give the outcome $o_1o_2o_3$. Looking at Table 1, we can see that these products (for each row or column) are proportional to the identity, so regardless of the state they should give +1 for all row measurement and the two column measurements c_1, c_2 and −1 for the final column c_3. Adding these up, we get $\beta = r_1 + r_2 + r_3 + c_1 + c_2 - c_3 = 6$. However, if we try to give values to each measurement (i.e., each observable in the table), we cannot possibly reach the value of 6. The upper bound is 4. So, the inequality reads $\beta = r_1 + r_2 + r_3 + c_1 + c_2 - c_3 \leq 4$ for all non-contextual hidden variable theories.

An experimental test of these inequalities requires six correlation measurements (the rows and columns of Table 1). In NMR, these correspond to different experimental setups. Each measurement is a set of three unitary interactions with a single meter spin. Each single interaction corresponds to the von Neumann scheme presented above; however, since the spin ½ meter is modular i.e., two π rotations are equivalent to no rotation, the meter only records the correlations. $A + 1$ result on the meter corresponds to an even number of +1 results for the three observables and $a - 1$ result corresponds to an odd number. The readout is an ensemble average. Since the experiment can be done with any initial system state, including the maximally mixed state, the model requires only that the meter spin is pseudo-pure. It is therefore within the class DQC1 (see Sect. 3.3).

The experiment [86] was performed using a macroscopic single crystal of malonic acid with ~3 % of the molecules triply abled with ^{13}C. The gates were generated using GRAPE with an average fidelity of 99.8 % and time of 1.5 ms. Following the six experiments, a value of $\beta = 5.2 \pm 0.1$ was obtained, giving a violation of more than 25 % with respect to the maximal classical value. Deviations from the predicted value, $\beta = 6$, can be explained by taking decoherence into account.

3.4.3 Weak Measurements

Weak measurements are performed by taking the standard von Neumann measurement and making the interaction very weak. The result of such a measurement is a *shift* of the meter's wave function by a value proportional to the expectation value of the system S. An interesting phenomenon occurs if after the weak measurement, S is measured in a different basis. In this case the shift is proportional to a weak value $\langle \phi | \sigma_{\hat{n}} | \psi \rangle / \langle \phi | \psi \rangle$, where $|\psi\rangle$ is the preparation, $|\phi\rangle$ is the post-selection (i.e., the state corresponding to the result of the final measurement) and $\sigma_{\hat{n}}$ is the weakly measured observable. For non-trivial post-selection, the weak value can be complex and arbitrarily large.

The challenge in NMR is post-selection. Since there are no projective measurements, it is impossible to post-select those molecules that gave the desired result for the final measurement. However, by using the von Neumann procedure for post-selecting, and furthermore getting rid of the systems that fail post-selection by adding noise, it is possible to perform the full weak measurement [87].

Large and complex weak values are a signature of non-trivial post-selection. In an experiment [87], the final signal is diminished by $|\langle \phi | \psi \rangle|$ due to the noise added in the post-selection step. This makes very large weak values hard to observe. However, complex weak values are not difficult to observe as long as $|\langle \phi | \psi \rangle|$ is not too small. In addition, decoherence causes the calculated weak values to be slightly lower than the ideal result, this is more apparent as $|\langle \phi | \psi \rangle|$ grows. Overall, in the experiment weak values of 2.3 (compared with a maximal eigenvalue of 1) as well as complex weak values of magnitude 1 were observed with good precision. Attempts to observe larger weak values did not reach the theoretical predictions due to decoherence and relatively strong coupling that had to be used to counter the small signal.

3.5   Quantum Simulation

Simulating a generic quantum system is believed to be a hard problem for a classical computer. Due to the exponential size of the Hilbert space as a function of subsystems a simulation may require an exponential number of parameters that need to be stored and updated. In 1982 Feynman suggested that a controllable quantum system can be used to simulate other quantum systems [88]. Feynman's idea was one of the motivating forces for quantum computing. However, in many cases, quantum simulators are easier to construct than universal quantum computers. In the past decades, progress has been made in making the first steps in using one quantum system to simulate another one [89]. In the following, we outline a few quantum simulation experiments done in NMR.

3.5.1   Digital Quantum Simulation of the Statistical Mechanics of a Frustrated Magnet [90]

The straightforward approach to simulate the evolution of a quantum system is by directly implementing a similar Hamiltonian on a different system. This method often called *analog* [91] requires the design of a very specific physical system that can simulate a very specific set of Hamiltonians. In *digital* quantum simulations, the initial state is represented by qubits and the time evolution is approximated by applying a sequence of short-time unitary gates [92]. The digital simulators are more general and usually require better control, often to the level of universal quantum computers.

To study the ground state of an Ising Hamiltonian, it is possible to use an adiabatic (analogue) method; however, this method requires that the energy gap between the ground state and first excited state is large enough to avoid excitations.

In general it is very hard to determine energy gap efficiently [93]. In the digital simulation [86], the ground state is prepared using a quantum circuit which is composed efficiently from the Hamiltonian.

An Ising Hamiltonian for 3 spin ½ particles is given by [94]

$$H = J(Z_1Z_2 + Z_2Z_3 + Z_1Z_3) + h(Z_1 + Z_2 + Z_3), \tag{25}$$

where Z_i is the Pauli-Z matrix for the spin i. For $J > 0$, the coupling is anti-ferromagnetic, and the spins tend to align in opposite direction to minimize energy. On the other hand, h has the effect of aligning spins in same direction. These two opposite forces result in a frustrated ground states and a very rich phase diagram.

At $h = 0$, there are six possible configuration of ground state possible i.e., the ground state is sixfold degenerate, so the entropy of the system can be non-zero even at $T \rightarrow 0$. Now if by changing h a little bit in either positive or negative direction, three of the six configurations are preferred. By increasing h further such that it becomes the dominant factor in the Hamiltonian, all the spins will align in the same direction and the ground state will be non-degenerate at $h = -2J$ and $2J$, see Fig. 9. The purpose of the simulation was to study the magnetization, $Z_1 + Z_2$

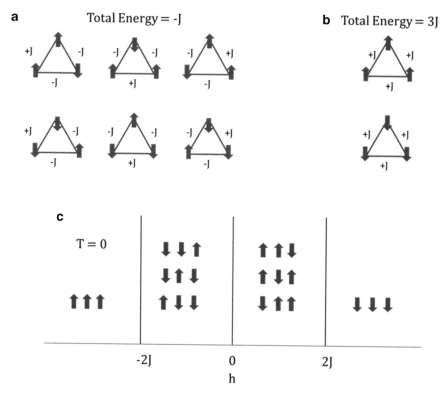

Fig. 9 (**a**) The six possible configuration for the ground state of Ising spin chain with a magnetic field $h = 0$, (**b**) the configuration at $h = \pm 2J$, and (**c**) The configurations preferred as a function of h

$+ Z_3$ and entropy equals to $\text{Tr}(\rho \log \rho)$, where ρ is the density matrix of Ising spin chain of the three spin system as a function of h.

The total magnetization as a function of h is a step function. For $h < -2J$ the spins all the spins will point upwards, giving maximum magnetization in upward direction. For $-2J < h < 0$, the tendency to align anti-parallel due to the first part of the Hamiltonian makes one out of three spins to point downwards, similarly, for $0 < h < 2J$, two of three spins face downwards and for $h > 2J$, all of them point downwards. For $h = 0$, all six combinations are equally likely, the system has zero net magnetization.

As for entropy, in the region $h < -2J$ and $h < 2J$ all the spins are aligned in the same direction the entropy is minimal, similarly in $-2J < h < 2J$ (excluding the point $h = 0$) the ground state is threefold degenerate and the entropy is higher. The maximum entropy being at $h = 0$. Two more points with higher entropy are $h = -2J$ and $h = 2J$.

In the experiment ^{13}C-labeled trans-crotonic acid was used as the four qubit processor. Three carbons were used to simulate the three spin chain while the fourth one was used to measure the expectation value of various Pauli operators at the end of the protocol and reconstruct the density matrix. This way of reading off elements from the fourth carbon's spectra was useful due to its well resolved spectra compared to the other three. The starting state was a coherent encoding of the thermal states [95, 96]. Different unitary evolutions corresponded to variation in the Hamiltonian parameters. These were decomposed into single-qubit gates and 2-qubit evolutions so that the variation in the Hamiltonian parameters required only phase shift in the applied RF pulses. This method exploits the ability to manipulate phases in the RF pulses to high precision (resolution of 10^4 per rad). Since entropy is a non-linear function of the state, small errors in the density matrix result in higher errors in the calculated entropy.

3.5.2 Quantum Simulation of Entanglement in Many Body Systems [79]

At zero temperature all the thermal fluctuations resulting in phase transition cease, but as seen in the previous experiment, quantum fluctuation can still occur. These quantum fluctuations give rise to quantum phase transitions (QPTs), under specific conditions. These conditions can be tuned by controlling a parameter in the Hamiltonian of the system, for example, the magnetic field. The result of these quantum fluctuations is an abrupt change in the ground state wave function [97]. It is not always possible to keep track of the ground state wave function to see when the QPT has occurred, but one can use different properties which are easier to track. One quantity that plays a role is entanglement; however, measuring entanglement in a many-body system is a challenging task [98, 99]. In Ref. [79], the ground state of an XXZ spin chain [100] was simulated and the geometric entanglement (GE) was measured to study QPTs.

The GE of a pure state $|\Phi\rangle$ is given by the expression [101, 102]:

$$E|\Phi\rangle = -\log_2\Lambda_{\max}^2, \quad \text{with} \quad \Lambda_{\max} = \max_{\psi}|\langle\Psi|\Phi\rangle| \qquad (26)$$

Where maximization is over all pure product states. $\Lambda_{\max}$ can be interpreted as the distance from the closest product state $|\Psi\rangle$ which is equivalent to the probability to end up in this state after performing the optimal local projective measurement on every spin. Experimentally GE can be obtained by an iterative method, which converges very quickly to its maximal value as a function of number of iterations.

The iterative method is: choose a random local measurement basis and pick one direction for each spin. Vary the basis of the ith spin, to find the measurement that yields the largest measurement probability. Next, move on to the next, $(i+1)$th spin and perform the same procedure. Repeat the procedure by sweeping back and forth until the global maximum is reached.

The XXZ spin chain is described by the Hamiltonian

$$H_{XXZ} = \sum_{i=1}^{N}(X_iX_{i+1} + Y_iY_{i+1} + \gamma Z_iZ_{i+1}), \qquad (27)$$

Where X_i, Y_i, and Z_i denote the Pauli matrices acting on ith spin, γ is a control parameter and the boundary condition are periodic i.e., $N+1 \equiv 1$. The XXZ chain can be solved exactly [100] and its ground states have a rich phase diagram. For $\gamma < -1$, the ground state is in a ferromagnetic Ising phase. At $\gamma = -1$, first-order phase transition occurs and from $-1 < \gamma \leq 1$ the ground state is in a gapless phase. Again at $\gamma = 1$ there is an ∞ order phase transition and for $\gamma > 1$ the ground state is in the anti-ferromagnetic phase [103].

The calculation of ground state energy shows discontinuity at $\gamma = -1$, whereas it is analytic across $\gamma = 1$ and so is any correlation function. As a consequence measures based on correlation functions are insensitive to the ∞ order transition. GE on contrast shows a jump at $\gamma = -1$ and a cusp (i.e., the derivative is discontinuous) at $\gamma = -1$, making it a better measure to study QPTs [104].

In principle, the closest product state is not known and the iterative method described above provides an efficient method to find the maximum overlap and hence the GE. The advantage of measuring GE was that both first and ∞ order quantum phase transition were detected, with the transition points being when either GE or its first-order derivative is discontinuous. On the other hand, all the traditional statistical-physical methods for QPTs, such as correlation functions and low-lying excitation spectra, will be continuous at the ∞ order phase transition, since the ground state energy is continuous.

The experiment was performed using the four carbons in crotonic acid dissolved in acetone-d6. Various ground states could be prepared by only varying single spin rotations and the quantum gates were prepared using the GRAPE algorithm [17]. For $\gamma < -1$, the experimental value of Λ_i^2 was measured to be 0.92, 0.048, and 0.019 compared to theoretical values of 1, 1/16, and 0 respectively. A polynomial fit of Λ_2^2 and Λ_3^2 shows that they intersect at $\gamma = 0.92$ compared with the theoretical value, $\gamma = 1$. To account for this discrepancy an inverse decay parameter was added to experimental data. The new experimental value decay into account gives an intersection of Λ_2^2 and Λ_3^2 at $\gamma = 1.02$.

3.5.3   Quantum Data Bus in Dipolar Coupled Nuclear Spin Qubits [105]

In both (quantum and classical) forms of computation and communication, one important task is to transfer an arbitrary state from one (qu)bit to another. Many quantum state transfer (QST) protocols exists [106–109] such as applying a SWAP gate between the qubits. The SWAP gate can be applied by evolving the qubits of interest under the dipolar coupling, but experimentally it is difficult when the spins cannot be addressed individually, for example, in large-size solid state systems. In Ref. [105] a QST protocol was implemented by exploiting a scheme of applying gates iteratively to only two qubits at one end of the qubit chain, irrespective of the size of the chain. Each iteration transfers part of the information from the point of origin to the desired location in the chain, and with fidelity of transfer reaching unity with more number of iteration performed. Dipolar couplings of a liquid crystal sample were used. These are much stronger than the scalar couplings, making gate time significantly shorter [110]. The benefit of this scheme is that one does not need a global control of the spin, or individual control of all the spins in the chain. Two individually addressable qubits are sufficient to perform this protocol.

The aim is to transfer an arbitrary state $\alpha|0\rangle + \beta|1\rangle$ from j to N in a N-spin system. The Hamiltonian for the spins up to $N - 1$ is given by

$$H = \frac{1}{2}\pi \sum_{(j,k=1;k>j)}^{(N-1)} D_{jk}\left(2\sigma_z^j\sigma_z^k - \sigma_x^j\sigma_x^k - \sigma_y^j\sigma_y^k\right) \tag{28}$$

where $\sigma_{x,y,z}^j$ represents the Pauli matrices with j representing the spin on which it acts. Evolving the N-1 spins under this Hamiltonian for time τ gives $U_\tau = e^{-i\tau H}$

$$\text{with} \quad U_\tau|0\rangle = e^{i\theta}|0\rangle \ ; \qquad U_\tau|j\rangle = \sum_{k=1}^{N-1} a_k|k\rangle \tag{29}$$

where $|0\rangle$ and $|j\rangle$ represent all spin pointing up and all spins up except the spin j pointing down, respectively. The bold characters indicate multiple spin state. Now the main iterative gate is carefully chosen such that after n iterations the following transformations occur $(\alpha|0\rangle + \beta + |j\rangle) \rightarrow \alpha e^{in\theta}|0\rangle + \beta|N\rangle$, where $e^{in\theta}$ is a known phase induced by the gate U_τ. Since the process is unitary we can invert it to transfers arbitrary state from position N to j. Hence one can prepare an arbitrary state at any location of the spin chain by having control on only two spins of the chain. Another useful extension of this method is to be able to prepare an entangled state between any two locations of the spin chain. This can be easily achieved by slightly changing the way in which the iterative gate is calculated.

The experiments were performed on a 4 spin chain provided by the four protons of the orthochlorobromobenzene (C6H4ClBr) dissolved in a liquid crystal solvent ZLI-1132. We transferred σ_x, σ_y, and σ_z from spin 1 to spin 4 on the four spin system we have, the experimental fidelities were 0.654 ± 0.046, 0.660 ± 0.052, and 0.693 ± 0.037 respectively after 100 iterations. The next part of experiment involved entangled state where spin 1 and 4 are entangled. The experimental fidelity was calculated as 0.77. The major sources of imperfections are attributed to the inhomogeneities of the magnetic field, imperfect implementation of the GRAPE pulses, and to the decoherence.

4 Conclusion and Perspective

Liquid-state NMR, one of the first proposals for quantum processors [11, 12], has clearly demonstrated major steps towards the realization of ideas and concepts of quantum information science in the laboratory. However, NMR is an unlikely candidate for a quantum computer due to the lack of scalability in practice. Despite impressive control, the ratio of gate time to decoherence is still too small as the sizes of systems grow to more than a dozen qubits. One way to address this limitation is to extend liquid-state NMR to solid-state NMR, where various dynamical nuclear polarization techniques can be employed and the speed of gate operations can be increased via much larger dipolar couplings. Another way to achieve scalability is to involve electrons as actuators in electron spin resonance (ESR) systems [111], to achieve indirect control of nuclear spins in a much faster approach [112].

Even if other platforms will be used to implement an eventual quantum computer, NMR still plays a leading role in progressing towards this goal. The experiments and techniques reviewed in this chapter should convince the reader that most quantum computing schemes within seven qubits or less are reasonably straightforward to implement in NMR. The control demonstrated in NMR exceeds the capabilities of any other system used today. The advanced techniques developed in NMR quantum computation, such as GRAPE pulses and pulse fixing, have been extended to many other systems successfully to realize high-fidelity control. The lessons learned in the history of NMR quantum computation have and continue to be indispensable in the development of experimental quantum computation.

Acknowledgement We thank Rolf Horn for helpful comments and discussions. This work is supported by Industry Canada, NSERC and CIFAR.

References

1. G. Moore, Electronics **38**, 114 (1965)
2. R. Landauer, IBM J. Res. Dev. **5**, 183 (1961)
3. M. Hilbert, P. López, Science **332**, 60 (2011)
4. M.A. Nielsen, I.L. Chuang, *Quantum Computation and Quantum Information: 10th Anniversary Edition* (2011), p. 702
5. C.H. Bennett, IBM J. Res. Dev. **17**, 525 (1973)
6. T.D. Ladd, F. Jelezko, R. Laflamme, Y. Nakamura, C. Monroe, J.L. O'Brien, Nature **464**, 45 (2010)
7. I. Buluta, S. Ashhab, F. Nori, Rep. Prog. Phys. **74**, 104401 (2011)
8. L.M.K. Vandersypen, Rev. Mod. Phys. **76**, 1037 (2005)
9. J.A. Jones, Prog. Nucl. Magn. Reson. Spectrosc. **59**, 91 (2011)
10. D.P. DiVincenzo, Fortschritte Der Phys. **48**, 771 (2000)
11. D.G. Cory, A.F. Fahmy, T.F. Havel, Proc. Natl. Acad. Sci. **94**, 1634 (1997)
12. N.A. Gershenfeld, I.L. Chuang, Science **275**, 350 (1997)
13. E. Knill, I. Chuang, R. Laflamme, Phys. Rev. A **57**, 3348 (1998)
14. E. Knill, R. Laflamme, R. Martinez, C. Tseng, Nature **404**, 21 (2000)
15. W.S. Warren, Science **277**, 1688 (1997)
16. C.A. Ryan, C. Negrevergne, M. Laforest, E. Knill, R. Laflamme, Phys. Rev. A **78**, 12328 (2008)
17. N. Khaneja, T. Reiss, C. Kehlet, T. Schulte-Herbrüggen, S.J. Glaser, J. Magn. Reson. **172**, 296 (2005)
18. I.L. Chuang, L.M.K. Vandersypen, X. Zhou, D.W. Leung, S. Lloyd, Nature **393**, 143 (1998)
19. I.L. Chuang, N. Gershenfeld, M. Kubinec, Phys. Rev. Lett. **80**, 3408 (1998)
20. J. Preskill, Proc. R. Soc. A Math. Phys. Eng. Sci. **454**, 385 (1998)
21. I.L. Chuang, M.A. Nielsen, J. Mod. Opt. **44**, 2455 (1997)
22. J. Poyatos, J. Cirac, P. Zoller, Phys. Rev. Lett. **78**, 390 (1997)
23. R.C. Bialczak, M. Ansmann, M. Hofheinz, E. Lucero, M. Neeley, A.D. O'Connell, D. Sank, H. Wang, J. Wenner, M. Steffen, A.N. Cleland, J.M. Martinis, Nat. Phys. **6**, 409 (2010)
24. A. Childs, I. Chuang, D. Leung, Phys. Rev. A **64**, 012314 (2001)
25. Y.S. Weinstein, T.F. Havel, J. Emerson, N. Boulant, M. Saraceno, S. Lloyd, D.G. Cory, J. Chem. Phys. **121**, 6117 (2004)
26. J. O'Brien, G. Pryde, A. Gilchrist, D. James, N. Langford, T. Ralph, A. White, Phys. Rev. Lett. **93**, 080502 (2004)
27. M. Riebe, K. Kim, P. Schindler, T. Monz, P. Schmidt, T. Körber, W. Hänsel, H. Häffner, C. Roos, R. Blatt, Phys. Rev. Lett. **97**, 220407 (2006)
28. J. Chow, J. Gambetta, L. Tornberg, J. Koch, L. Bishop, A. Houck, B. Johnson, L. Frunzio, S. Girvin, R. Schoelkopf, Phys. Rev. Lett. **102**, 090502 (2009)
29. J. Emerson, M. Silva, O. Moussa, C. Ryan, M. Laforest, J. Baugh, D.G. Cory, R. Laflamme, Science **317**, 1893 (2007)
30. C. Dankert, R. Cleve, J. Emerson, E. Livine, Phys. Rev. A **80**, 012304 (2009)
31. O. Moussa, M.P. da Silva, C.A. Ryan, R. Laflamme, Phys. Rev. Lett. **109**, 070504 (2012)
32. J. Emerson, R. Alicki, K. Życzkowski, J. Opt. B Quantum Semiclassical Opt. **7**, S347 (2005)
33. E. Knill, D. Leibfried, R. Reichle, J. Britton, R. Blakestad, J. Jost, C. Langer, R. Ozeri, S. Seidelin, D. Wineland, Phys. Rev. A **77**, 012307 (2008)
34. C.A. Ryan, M. Laforest, R. Laflamme, New J. Phys. **11**, 013034 (2009)
35. S.T. Flammia, Y.-K. Liu, Phys. Rev. Lett. **106**, 230501 (2011)
36. M.P. da Silva, O. Landon-Cardinal, D. Poulin, Phys. Rev. Lett. **107**, 210404 (2011)
37. D. Lu, H. Li, D. Trottier, J. Li, A. Brodutch, A. P. Krismanich, A. Ghavami, G. I. Dmitrienko, G. Long, J. Baugh, R. Laflamme, Phys. Rev. Lett. **114**, 140505 (2015)
38. D.G. Cory, J.B. Miller, A.N. Garroway, J. Magn. Reson. **90**, 205 (1990)
39. S. Bravyi, A. Kitaev, Phys. Rev. A **71**, 022316 (2005)

40. S.L. Braunstein, arXiv:quant-ph/9603024v1 (1996)
41. J. Preskill, Proc. R. Soc. A **454**, 385 (1998)
42. D. Aharonov, M. Ben-Or, in Proceedings of the 29th Annual ACM Symposium on Theory of Computing, El Paso, 1997 (ACM, New York, 1997), p. 176
43. E. Knill, R. Laflamme, W. Zurek, Science **279**, 342 (1998)
44. E. Knill, R. Laflamme, R. Martinez, C. Negrevergne, Phys. Rev. Lett. **86**, 5811 (2001)
45. P.W. Shor, Phys. Rev. A **52**, R2493(R) (1995)
46. D.G. Cory, M.D. Price, W. Maas, E. Knill, R. Laflamme, W.H. Zurek, T.F. Havel, S.S. Somaroo, Phys. Rev. Lett. **81**, 2152 (1998)
47. J. Zhang, D. Gangloff, O. Moussa, R. Laflamme, Phys. Rev. A **84**, 034303 (2011)
48. R. Laflamme, C. Miquel, J.P. Paz, W.H. Zurek, Phys. Rev. Lett. **77**, 198 (1996)
49. M. Ben-Or, D. Gottesman, R. Gan, arXiv:1301.1995 (2013)
50. J. Zhang, R. Laflamme, D. Suter, Phys. Rev. Lett. **109**, 100503 (2012)
51. D. Gottesman, arXiv:quant-ph/0507174 (2005)
52. E. Knill, Nature **434**, 39 (2005)
53. B. Eastin, E. Knill, Phys. Rev. Lett. **102**, 110502 (2009)
54. E.T. Campbell, D.E. Browne, Phys. Rev. Lett. **104**, 030503 (2010)
55. E.T. Campbell, D.E. Browne, in *Lecture Notes in Computer Science (including Subser. Lect. Notes Artif. Intell. Lect. Notes Bioinformatics)* (2009), pp. 20–32
56. W. Van Dam, M. Howard, Phys. Rev. Lett. **103**, 170504 (2009)
57. M. Howard, J. Wallman, V. Veitch, J. Emerson, Nature **509**, 351 (2014)
58. T. Jochym-O'Connor, R. Laflamme, Phys. Rev. Lett. **112**, 010505 (2014)
59. A. Paetznick, B.W. Reichardt, Phys. Rev. Lett. **111**, 090505 (2013)
60. J. Anderson, G. Duclos-Cianci, D. Poulin, Phys. Rev. Lett. **113**, 080501 (2014)
61. A.M. Souza, J. Zhang, C.A. Ryan, R. Laflamme, Nat. Commun. **2**, 169 (2011)
62. J.K. Pachos, *Introduction to Topological Quantum Computation* (Cambridge University Press, Cambridge, 2012)
63. A.Y. Kitaev, Ann. Phys. (N. Y). **303**, 2 (2003)
64. F. Wilczek, Phys. Rev. Lett. **49**, 957 (1982)
65. A. Kitaev, Ann. Phys. (N. Y). **321**, 2 (2006)
66. F. Camino, W. Zhou, V. Goldman, Phys. Rev. B **72**, 155313 (2005)
67. R.L. Willett, C. Nayak, K. Shtengel, L.N. Pfeiffer, K.W. West, Phys. Rev. Lett. **111**, 186401 (2013)
68. G. Feng, G. Long, R. Laflamme, Phys. Rev. A **88**, 022305 (2013)
69. Y. Han, R. Raussendorf, L. Duan, Phys. Rev. Lett. **98**, 150404 (2007)
70. C.Y. Lu, W.B. Gao, O. Gühne, X.Q. Zhou, Z.B. Chen, J.W. Pan, Phys. Rev. Lett. **102**, 030502 (2009)
71. J.K. Pachos, W. Wieczorek, C. Schmid, N. Kiesel, R. Pohlner, H. Weinfurter, New J. Phys. **11**, 083010 (2009)
72. S.L. Braunstein, C.M. Caves, R. Jozsa, N. Linden, S. Popescu, R. Schack, Phys. Rev. Lett. **83**, 1054 (1999)
73. E. Schrödinger, Die Naturwissenschaften **23**, 823 (1935)
74. E. Knill, R. Laflamme, Phys. Rev. Lett. **81**, 5672 (1998)
75. R. Laflamme, D.G. Cory, C. Negrevergne, L. Viola, arXiv:quant-ph/0110029 (2001)
76. G. Passante, O. Moussa, C.A. Ryan, R. Laflamme, Phys. Rev. Lett. **103**, 250501 (2009)
77. G. Passante, *Ph.D. Thesis*, University of Waterloo (2012)
78. A. Datta, S. Flammia, C. Caves, Phys. Rev. A **72**, 042316 (2005)
79. K. Modi, A. Brodutch, H. Cable, T. Paterek, V. Vedral, Rev. Mod. Phys. **84**, 1655 (2012)
80. H. Ollivier, W.H. Zurek, Phys. Rev. Lett. **88**, 017901 (2001)
81. B. Dakić, V. Vedral, Č. Brukner, Phys. Rev. Lett. **105**, 190502 (2010)
82. D. Deutsch, Proc. R. Soc. London A **400**, 97 (1985)
83. J.S. Bell, Physics **1**, 195 (1964)
84. S. Kochen, E.P. Specker, J. Math. Mech. **17**, 59 (1967)

85. A. Cabello, Phys. Rev. Lett. **101**, 210401 (2008)
86. O. Moussa, C.A. Ryan, D.G. Cory, R. Laflamme, Phys. Rev. Lett. **104**, 160501 (2010)
87. D. Lu, A. Brodutch, J. Li, H. Li, R. Laflamme, New J. Phys. **16**, 53015 (2014)
88. R. Feynman, Int. J. Theor. Phys. **21**, 467 (1982)
89. I.M. Georgescu, S. Ashhab, F. Nori, Rev. Mod. Phys. **86**, 153 (2014)
90. J. Zhang, M.-H. Yung, R. Laflamme, A. Aspuru-Guzik, J. Baugh, Nat. Commun. **3**, 880 (2012)
91. I. Buluta, F. Nori, Science **326**, 108 (2009)
92. I. Kassal, J.D. Whitfield, A. Perdomo-Ortiz, M.-H. Yung, A. Aspuru-Guzik, Annu. Rev. Phys. Chem. **62**, 185 (2011)
93. B. Altshuler, H. Krovi, J. Roland, Proc. Natl. Acad. Sci. U. S. A. **107**, 12446 (2010)
94. G.H. Wannier, Phys. Rev. **79**, 357 (1950)
95. M.-H. Yung, D. Nagaj, J.D. Whitfield, A. Aspuru-Guzik, Phys. Rev. A **82**, 060302 (2010)
96. D. Lidar, O. Biham, Phys. Rev. E **56**, 3661 (1997)
97. S. Sachdev, *Quantum Phase Transitions*, 2nd Edition (Cambridge University Press, Cambridge, 2011), p. 517
98. O. Gühne, G. Tóth, Phys. Rep. **474**, 1 (2009)
99. L. Amico, A. Osterloh, V. Vedral, Rev. Mod. Phys. **80**, 517 (2008)
100. V.E. Korepin, N.M. Bogoliubov, A.G. Izergin, *Quantum Inverse Scattering Method and Correlation Functions* (Cambridge University Press, Cambridge, 1997)
101. T.-C. Wei, P. Goldbart, Phys. Rev. A **68**, 042307 (2003)
102. T.-C. Wei, D. Das, S. Mukhopadyay, S. Vishveshwara, P. Goldbart, Phys. Rev. A **71**, 060305 (2005)
103. J.M. Kosterlitz, D.J. Thouless, J. Phys. C: Solid State Phys. **6**, 1181 (2002)
104. R. Orús, T.-C. Wei, Phys. Rev. B **82**, 155120 (2010)
105. J. Zhang, M. Ditty, D. Burgarth, C.A. Ryan, C.M. Chandrashekar, M. Laforest, O. Moussa, J. Baugh, R. Laflamme, Phys. Rev. A **80**, 12316 (2009)
106. S. Bose, Phys. Rev. Lett. **91**, 207901 (2003)
107. P. Cappellaro, C. Ramanathan, D. Cory, Phys. Rev. Lett. **99**, 250506 (2007)
108. M. Christandl, N. Datta, A. Ekert, A. Landahl, Phys. Rev. Lett. **92**, 187902 (2004)
109. E.B. Fel'dman, A.I. Zenchuk, Phys. Lett. A **373**, 1719 (2009)
110. T. Mahesh, D. Suter, Phys. Rev. A **74**, 062312 (2006)
111. M. Mehring, J. Mende, W. Scherer, Phys. Rev. Lett. **90**, 153001 (2003)
112. Y. Zhang, C.A. Ryan, R. Laflamme, J. Baugh, Phys. Rev. Lett. **107**, 170503 (2011)

Heat Bath Algorithmic Cooling with Spins: Review and Prospects

Daniel K. Park, Nayeli A. Rodriguez-Briones, Guanru Feng, Robabeh Rahimi, Jonathan Baugh, and Raymond Laflamme

Abstract Application of multiple rounds of Quantum Error Correction (QEC) is an essential milestone towards the construction of scalable quantum information processing devices. The requirements for multiple rounds QEC are high control fidelity and the ability to extract entropy from ancilla qubits. Nuclear Magnetic Resonance (NMR) based quantum devices have demonstrated high control fidelity with up to 12 qubits. On the other hand, the major challenge in the NMR QEC experiment is to efficiently supply ancilla qubits in highly pure states at the beginning of each round of QEC. Purification of spin qubits can be accomplished through Heat Bath Algorithmic Cooling (HBAC). It is an efficient method for extracting entropy from qubits that interact with a heat bath, allowing cooling below the bath temperature. For practical HBAC, hyperfine coupled electron-nuclear spin systems are more promising than conventional NMR quantum processors, since electron spin polarization is about 10^3 times greater than that of a proton under the same experimental conditions. We provide an overview on both

D.K. Park (✉)
Natural Science Research Institute, KAIST, Daejon, South Korea, 34141

Institute for Quantum Computing, University of Waterloo, Waterloo, ON, Canada, N2L 3G1

Department of Physics and Astronomy, University of Waterloo, Waterloo, ON, Canada, N2L 3G1
e-mail: kdpspin@gmail.com

N.A. Rodriguez-Briones • G. Feng
Institute for Quantum Computing, University of Waterloo, Waterloo, ON, Canada, N2L 3G1

Department of Physics and Astronomy, University of Waterloo, Waterloo, ON, Canada, N2L 3G1

R. Rahimi
Science and Research Branch Azad University, Tehran, Iran

Institute for Quantum Computing, University of Waterloo, Waterloo, ON, Canada, N2L 3G1

Department of Physics and Astronomy, University of Waterloo, Waterloo, ON, Canada, N2L 3G1

© Springer New York 2016
T. Takui et al. (eds.), *Electron Spin Resonance (ESR) Based Quantum Computing*, Biological Magnetic Resonance 31, DOI 10.1007/978-1-4939-3658-8_8

theoretical and experimental aspects of HBAC focusing on spin and magnetic resonance based systems, and discuss the prospects of exploiting electron-nuclear hyperfine coupled systems for the realization of HBAC and multiple-round QEC.

Keywords Electron spin resonance • Electron nuclear double resonance • Quantum information processing • Heat bath algorithmic cooling

1   Introduction

Quantum Information Processing (QIP) has the potential to perform exponentially faster computation and revolutionize current technology by harnessing the systems governed by the laws of quantum mechanics. To reach this goal, we need to be able to control imperfections and imprecision occurring when theoretical ideas are implemented in the physical world. Quantum Error Correction (QEC) is a theory that aims to bridge this. The first steps towards developing experimental QEC have been taken, but there is still more to be done. Application of multiple rounds of QEC is an essential milestone towards the construction of scalable QIP devices, but experimental realizations of it are still in their infancy. The requirements for multiple round QEC are high control fidelity and the ability to extract entropy from ancilla qubits. Nuclear Magnetic Resonance (NMR)-based quantum devices have demonstrated high control fidelity with up to 12 qubits [1]. Hence, these devices are excellent test beds that can be explored in the lab today for the ideas of quantum control and QEC. More details on NMR QIP can be found in [2, 3]. The major challenge in the NMR QEC experiment is to efficiently supply ancilla qubits in highly pure states at the beginning of each round of QEC. This challenging requirement was recently alleviated by Criger et al. in [4]. They showed that QEC could still suppress the error rate using mixed ancilla qubits as long as the

J. Baugh
Institute for Quantum Computing, University of Waterloo, Waterloo, ON,
Canada, N2L 3G1

Department of Physics and Astronomy, University of Waterloo, Waterloo, ON,
Canada, N2L 3G1

Department of Chemistry, University of Waterloo, Waterloo, ON, Canada, N2L 3G1

R. Laflamme
Institute for Quantum Computing, University of Waterloo, Waterloo, ON,
Canada, N2L 3G1

Department of Physics and Astronomy, University of Waterloo, Waterloo, ON,
Canada, N2L 3G1

Perimeter Institute for Theoretical Physics, Waterloo, ON, Canada, N2J 2W9

Canadian Institute for Advanced Research, Toronto, ON, Canada, M5G 1Z8 polarization or purity of the ancilla qubits is above certain threshold value. Purifying qubits in NMR can be obtained through Heat Bath Algorithmic Cooling (HBAC). It is an efficient method for extracting entropy from qubits that interact with a heat bath, allowing cooling below the bath temperature. In a nutshell, HBAC recurrently applies two steps: Given n number of system qubits each with polarization ϵ_0, cool $n - m$ qubits by compressing entropy into m qubits. The polarization of m qubits is exchanged with the heat bath polarization ϵ_b. By repeating these steps, $n - m$ qubits can attain a final polarization ϵ_f that is greater than ϵ_b. There is an asymptotic limit for ϵ_f that depends on n and ϵ_b. Proof-of-principle experiments for 3-qubit HBAC have been performed in a solid state NMR (SSNMR) system, demonstrating sufficient level of control to execute multiple rounds of HBAC. However, under typical experimental conditions, nuclear spin polarization at thermal equilibrium is very small, and therefore precise control over tens of nuclear spin qubits is required for reaching polarization of order unity on one qubit. For practical HBAC and QEC, hyperfine-coupled electron-nuclear spin systems are more promising than conventional NMR Quantum Computing (QC), since electron spin polarization is about 10^3 times greater than that of a proton under the same experimental conditions. This is due to the higher gyromagnetic ratio of the electron spin. Another consequence is that the electron spin relaxation rate is typically about 10^3 faster than that of nuclear spins. Faster spin relaxation and higher polarization makes the electron an excellent heat bath for cooling nuclear spins.

In this review, we provide an overview on both theoretical and experimental aspects of HBAC focusing on spin and magnetic resonance-based systems. The chapter is organized as follows. The challenge of preparing nearly pure ancilla qubits in conventional NMR system is discussed in Sect. 2. Section 3 discusses the theory of HBAC in detail. Section 4 reviews SSNMR experiments that demonstrated sufficient control fidelity for realizing HBAC and motivates the use of electron spins by explaining the shortcomings of NMR QC. Section 5 introduces electron-nuclear spin ensemble QC and the prospects of implementing HBAC in this type of system.

2 State Preparation Challenge in Ensemble Quantum Computation

NMR QIP is one example of ensemble quantum computation models, where an ensemble of identical quantum systems is manipulated in parallel, and the only measurable quantities are expectation values of certain observables. That is, there is no access to projective measurement. In this section, we review concepts related to spin polarization and present the challenge of preparing nearly pure spin qubits.

2.1 Polarization

For a spin at temperature T, the occupancy of a state with energy E is calculated by the Gibbs distribution $n(E) = e^{-E/k_B T}/Z$, where k_B is the Boltzmann constant and Z is the partition function. The polarization ϵ is defined as the population difference between two energy levels normalized by the total number of spins. When the Zeeman energy dominates the energy splitting, the polarization of a spin-1/2 system can be expressed as

$$\epsilon = n(E_0) - n(E_1) = \tanh\left(\frac{\Delta E}{2k_B T}\right) = \tanh\left(\frac{\hbar \gamma B_0}{2k_B T}\right), \tag{1}$$

where ΔE is the energy difference between the two levels, γ is the gyromagnetic ratio, and B_0 is the strength of the external magnetic field. Equation (1) establishes the relationship between polarization and gyromagnetic ratio, magnetic field strength, and temperature.

2.2 Pseudo-Pure State

The density matrix describing a spin ensemble at thermal equilibrium can be written in the eigenbasis of σ_z, corresponding to the direction of the applied static magnetic field, as

$$\rho = \frac{1}{2}\begin{bmatrix} 1+\epsilon & 0 \\ 0 & 1-\epsilon \end{bmatrix} = \frac{1}{2}(\mathbb{I} + \epsilon\sigma_z), \tag{2}$$

where $\mathbb{I}$ is the unit matrix and σ_z is the Pauli operator. For n spin qubits, the thermal equilibrium state can be transformed to a pseudo-pure state through non-unitary processes using standard NMR techniques of temporal or spatial averaging [5, 6]:

$$\rho_{pps}^n = (1-\alpha)\mathbb{I}_n + \alpha|\psi\rangle\langle\psi|, \tag{3}$$

$$\alpha = \frac{(1+\epsilon)^n - 1}{2^n - 1}, \tag{4}$$

where $|\psi\rangle\langle\psi|$ is a pure state, $\mathbb{I}_n$ is $2^n \times 2^n$ normalized unit matrix, and α quantifies the purity of the state. A typical NMR experiment operates at $B_0 \approx 7$ T and room temperature in which nuclear spin polarizations are extremely small ($\epsilon \approx 10^{-5}$ for proton). Moreover, in the absence of methods like algorithmic cooling which can compress entropy, the signal of a pseudo-pure state decreases exponentially in the number of qubits.

2.3 NMR QEC with Mixed Ancilla Qubits

In [4], Criger et al. showed that even if ancilla qubits are not pure, augmented QEC can still suppress the error rate as long as the polarization of ancilla qubits exceeds certain values which depend on the error correction code. For example, in the conventional 3-qubit QEC code for phase flip error, one can imagine that two ancilla qubits in the NMR experiment are in mixed states with polarizations ϵ_1 and ϵ_2, respectively. The probability amplitude of the lowest energy state of the two qubit has to be greater than 0.5 in order for the augmented QEC to suppress the error rate and improve the fidelity of a state exposed to the noisy channel, i.e., $(1 + \epsilon_1)(1 + \epsilon_2)/4 > 0.5$. If $\epsilon_1 = \epsilon_2 = \epsilon$, then $\epsilon > \sqrt{2} - 1 \approx 0.41$ must be satisfied. This is far above what can be achieved in a reasonable NMR setup. One can imagine having a SSNMR setup in which the experiment can be carried out at low temperature. However, in order to meet the polarization requirement given above, the temperature must be below $17\,\text{mK}$ for ^1H at a field of 7 T. As the temperature is lowered, the nuclear T_1 relaxation time is increased and therefore the wait time for thermal state initialization can become impractically long.

In the following sections, we present the main ideas and experimental realizations of HBAC, which is a promising tool for preparing nearly pure spin qubits in experiments that are feasible with today's technology.

3 Theory of Algorithmic Cooling

Purification of quantum states is essential for realizing fault tolerant quantum information processors. The procedure is needed not only for initializing the physical system for many algorithms, but also to dynamically supply fresh pure ancilla qubits for error correction. For quantum computation models that rely on ensemble of identical systems such as NMR or Electron Spin Resonance (ESR) QC, acquisition of nearly pure quantum states in a scalable manner is extremely challenging [7]. A potential solution is algorithmic cooling (AC), a protocol which purifies qubits by removing entropy from subset of them, while increasing the entropy of the rest [8, 9]. An explicit way to implement this idea in quantum computations was given by Schulman et al. [10]. They showed that it is possible to reach polarization of order unity using only a number of qubits which is polynomial in the initial polarization. However, their method was limited by the Shannon bound, which imposes a constraint on the entropy compression step in closed systems.

This idea was further improved by adding contact with a heat bath to pump entropy out of the system and transfer it into the heat bath [11], a process known as Heat Bath Algorithmic Cooling (HBAC). Based on this new idea, many practical cooling algorithms have been designed [12–16]. In short, HBAC purifies qubits by

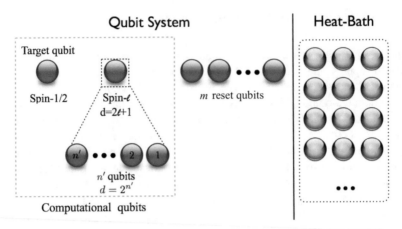

Fig. 1 Heat bath algorithmic cooling can cool the target spin-1/2 by compressing entropy into d-dimensional spin-l (equivalent to a string of $n' = \log_2 d$ qubits if l is a half integer), and exchanging the entropy of spin-l with that of the reset qubits that are in contact with a cold heat bath. The target spin-1/2 and the spin-l are referred to as the computational qubits

applying alternating rounds of entropy compression and pumping out entropy from the system of interest to a thermal bath. Theoretical details are explained below.

As an example, we consider a system consisting of a string of qubits: one target qubit (a spin-1/2) which is to be cooled, a spin-l system which aids in the entropy compression, and m reset qubits that can be brought into thermal contact with the heat bath. When l is a half integer, having spin-l is equivalent to having $n' = \log_2 d$ qubits, where d is the dimension of the Hilbert space of spin-l. The spin-1/2 and the spin-l are referred to as computational qubits (Fig. 1).

The idea of the first step of HBAC is to redistribute the entropy among the string of qubits by applying an entropy compression operation U. This is a unitary (reversible) process that extracts entropy from n computational qubits as much as possible and moves it to m reset qubits, resulting in the cooling of the computational qubits while warming the reset qubits (Fig. 2).

In the second step, m reset qubits are brought into thermal contact with a heat bath and reset to the cold bath temperature, resulting in the cooling of the total $n + m$ qubit system. This step is equivalent to tracing over the reset qubits and replacing them with qubits from the heat bath. The heat bath is assumed to be very large so that the action of qubit–bath interaction on the bath is negligible (Fig. 3).

The total effect of these two steps on a system with initial state ρ can be expressed as follows:

$$\rho \xrightarrow{C} \rho' = U\rho U^\dagger \tag{5}$$

Quantum Computer

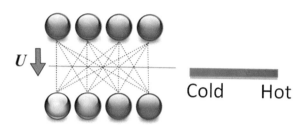

Fig. 2 Entropy compression step. A compression operation U raises the entropy on one side of the system, while lowering it on the other. In the figure, the *top part* represents the string of qubits before the compression. *Dotted lines* indicate redistribution of entropy among all qubits, resulting in the separation of cold and hot regions as shown in the *bottom part*

Fig. 3 The refresh step. The reset qubits are brought into thermal contact with a heat bath and the entropy of the qubit system is reduced. In the figure, two reset qubits are used as an example

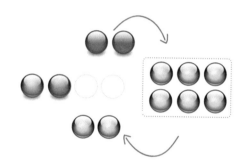

$$\rho' \xrightarrow{R} \rho'' = Tr_m\left(\rho'\right) \otimes \rho_{\epsilon_b}^{\otimes m} \tag{6}$$

where C and R stand for compression and reset, $Tr_m()$ is the partial trace operation over m reset qubits, and $\rho_{\epsilon_b} = \frac{1}{2}\begin{pmatrix} 1+\epsilon_b & 0 \\ 0 & 1-\epsilon_b \end{pmatrix}$ represents a qubit possessing the heat bath polarization ϵ_b.

These reversible compression and refreshing steps are iteratively applied until the target qubit reaches the desired temperature, or the cooling limit is reached. The physical requirements for reset and computational qubits are different. A reset qubit should strongly interact with the bath in order to rapidly relax and attain the bath temperature, and a computational qubit should have long relaxation time to remain polarized after being cooled through entropy compression.

In [13], Schulman et al. introduced the optimal (optimal in terms of entropy extraction per cooling step) algorithm for HBAC, the Partner Pairing Algorithm (PPA). The PPA is explained in detail in the following section.

3.1 Partner Pairing Algorithm

Consider a system with $n-1$ computational qubits and one reset qubit. Let ρ and ρ_{ϵ_b} be the density matrices of the n qubits and of the reset qubit after contact with the thermal bath, respectively. ρ can be partitioned into $2^{n-1} \times 2^{n-1}$ blocks M_{ij} by the basis states $\{|0\rangle, |1\rangle\}$ of the reset qubit:

$$
\rho = \begin{pmatrix}
\begin{bmatrix} \rho_{11} & \rho_{12} \\ \rho_{21} & \rho_{22} \end{bmatrix} & \begin{bmatrix} \rho_{13} & \rho_{14} \\ \rho_{23} & \rho_{24} \end{bmatrix} & \cdots & \\
\begin{bmatrix} \rho_{31} & \rho_{32} \\ \rho_{41} & \rho_{42} \end{bmatrix} & \begin{bmatrix} \rho_{33} & \rho_{34} \\ \rho_{43} & \rho_{44} \end{bmatrix} & & \\
\vdots & & \ddots & \vdots \\
& \cdots & & \begin{bmatrix} \rho_{2^n-1,\, 2^n-1} & \rho_{2^n-1,\, 2^n} \\ \rho_{2^n,\, 2^n-1} & \rho_{2^n,\, 2^n} \end{bmatrix}
\end{pmatrix} \qquad (7)
$$

$$
= \begin{pmatrix}
M_{11} & M_{12} & \cdots & \\
M_{21} & M_{22} & \ddots & \vdots \\
\vdots & & & \\
& \cdots & & M_{2^{n-1},\, 2^{n-1}}
\end{pmatrix}
$$

where M_{ij} is the ij-block of ρ (for example, $M_{11} = \begin{bmatrix} \rho_{11} & \rho_{12} \\ \rho_{21} & \rho_{22} \end{bmatrix}, M_{12} = \begin{bmatrix} \rho_{13} & \rho_{14} \\ \rho_{23} & \rho_{24} \end{bmatrix}$,

and etc.)

Refreshing the reset qubit (Eq. (6)) has the effect of changing every block M_{ij} to M'_{ij} as follows:

$$
M'_{ij} = \frac{Tr\left(M_{ij}\right)}{2} \begin{pmatrix} 1+\epsilon_b & 0 \\ 0 & 1-\epsilon_b \end{pmatrix}. \qquad (8)
$$

In the PPA, entropy compression operation permutes the diagonal elements of the density matrix of the system, rearranging them such that states in increasing lexicographic order have nonincreasing probability. For example, the probability amplitude of states starting with 0 (0...00, 0...01, etc.) is increased while that of states starting with 1 is decreased. This operation aims to increase the polarization of the first qubit. The compression can no longer improve the polarization of the first qubit once the states are already ordered as described above.

3.2 Illustrative Example: PPA for Three Qubits

We take a system of three qubits (one reset qubit and two computational qubits) as an example to illustrate the PPA. ρ_0 is the initial density matrix of the three qubit system and without loss of generality, ρ_0 is in a maximally mixed state, and the heat bath has polarization ϵ_b.

First, contact between the reset qubit and the heat bath is established. Then, the compression operator U permutes the probabilities of the basis states and sorts them in nonincreasing order:

$$d(\rho_0) = \frac{1}{8}\begin{bmatrix} 1 \\ 1 \\ 1 \\ 1 \\ 1 \\ 1 \\ 1 \\ 1 \end{bmatrix} \xrightarrow{R} d\left(\rho_0'\right) = \frac{1}{8}\begin{bmatrix} 1 + \varepsilon_b \\ 1 - \varepsilon_b \\ 1 + \varepsilon_b \\ 1 - \varepsilon_b \\ 1 + \varepsilon_b \\ 1 - \varepsilon_b \\ 1 + \varepsilon_b \\ 1 - \varepsilon_b \end{bmatrix} \xrightarrow{C} d\left(\rho_0''\right) = \frac{1}{8}\begin{bmatrix} 1 + \varepsilon_b \\ 1 + \varepsilon_b \\ 1 + \varepsilon_b \\ 1 + \varepsilon_b \\ 1 - \varepsilon_b \\ 1 - \varepsilon_b \\ 1 - \varepsilon_b \\ 1 - \varepsilon_b \end{bmatrix}, \qquad (9)$$

where $d(\rho)$ are the eigenvalues of ρ, and R and C stand for refresh and compression steps, respectively. This compression is equivalent to swapping the first computational qubit with the reset qubit. After this iteration, the polarization of the first qubit is increased from 0 to ϵ_b. Upon repeating above two steps again, we effectively swap the second computational qubit with the reset qubit that is at thermal equilibrium with the bath:

$$d(\rho_1) := d\left(\rho_0''\right) \xrightarrow{R} d\left(\rho_1'\right) = \frac{1}{8}\begin{bmatrix} (1+\varepsilon_b)^2 \\ 1 - \varepsilon_b^2 \\ (1+\varepsilon_b)^2 \\ 1 - \varepsilon_b^2 \\ 1 - \varepsilon_b^2 \\ (1-\varepsilon_b)^2 \\ 1 - \varepsilon_b^2 \\ (1-\varepsilon_b)^2 \end{bmatrix} \xrightarrow{C} d\left(\rho_1''\right) = \frac{1}{8}\begin{bmatrix} (1+\varepsilon_b)^2 \\ (1+\varepsilon_b)^2 \\ 1 - \varepsilon_b^2 \\ 1 - \varepsilon_b^2 \\ 1 - \varepsilon_b^2 \\ 1 - \varepsilon_b^2 \\ (1-\varepsilon_b)^2 \\ (1-\varepsilon_b)^2 \end{bmatrix}. \qquad (10)$$

In this iteration, the polarization of the first computational qubit remains the same, while the polarization of the second qubit is increased from 0 to ϵ_b. If the refresh and compression steps are repeated once more,

$$d(\rho_2) := d\left(\rho_1''\right) \xrightarrow{R} d\left(\rho_2'\right) = \frac{1}{8}\begin{bmatrix} (1+\varepsilon_b)^3 \\ (1+\varepsilon_b)^2(1-\varepsilon_b) \\ (1+\varepsilon_b)^2(1-\varepsilon_b) \\ (1+\varepsilon_b)(1-\varepsilon_b)^2 \\ (1+\varepsilon_b)^2(1-\varepsilon_b) \\ (1+\varepsilon_b)(1-\varepsilon_b)^2 \\ (1+\varepsilon_b)(1-\varepsilon_b)^2 \\ (1-\varepsilon_b) \end{bmatrix} \xrightarrow{C} d\left(\rho_2''\right) = \frac{1}{8}\begin{bmatrix} (1+\varepsilon_b)^3 \\ (1+\varepsilon_b)^2(1-\varepsilon_b) \\ (1+\varepsilon_b)^2(1-\varepsilon_b) \\ (1+\varepsilon_b)^2(1-\varepsilon_b) \\ (1+\varepsilon_b)(1-\varepsilon_b)^2 \\ (1+\varepsilon_b)(1-\varepsilon_b)^2 \\ (1+\varepsilon_b)(1-\varepsilon_b)^2 \\ (1-\varepsilon_b)^3 \end{bmatrix}.$$

$$(11)$$

In this iteration, the polarization of the first qubit increases to $1.5\epsilon_b - 0.5\epsilon_b^3$.

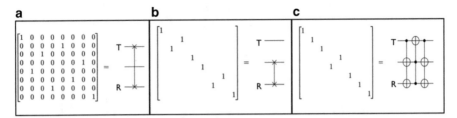

Fig. 4 Matrices and circuit symbols representing the unitary operations of the PPA on three qubits that are initially in a completely mixed state. In the circuit diagram, the top qubit is the target qubit (denoted T) and the bottom qubit is the reset qubit (denoted R). A swap operation is represented as two Xs located on the qubits that are exchanged connected by a *vertical line*. A controlled-not (CNOT) gate is denoted by a *dot* and an *open circle* connected by a *vertical line*. The *open circle* is on the target qubit of the CNOT operation, and the *dot* is on the controlled qubit. (**a**) In the first iteration, the compression gate swaps the target qubit and the reset qubit. (**b**) In the second iteration, the second qubit and the reset qubit are swapped. (**c**) The third iteration boosts the first qubit polarization to $1.5\epsilon_b - 0.5\epsilon_b^3$. From the second round of HBAC and on, entropy compressions are the repetition of the second and third gates of the first round

The gate representations of three entropy compression steps are shown in Fig. 4a, b, and c, respectively. Three iterations complete the first round of 3-qubit HBAC. In the next round, the required compression gates are alternating applications of the operations shown in Fig. 4b and c.

The evolution of the polarization of the first qubit under the PPA with $\epsilon_b \ll 1/2$ is shown in Fig. 5. The circuit asymptotically boosts the polarization on the first qubit up to twice the heat bath polarization; this limit is discussed in the next section.

An interesting question is to know what is the maximum achievable cooling using this method, and how many iterations of HBAC are necessary to obtain a certain polarization.

3.3 Cooling Limit

Through numerical simulations, Moussa [17] (see also [13]) observed that if $\epsilon_b \ll 1/2^{n-2}$, where n is the number of computational plus reset qubits, the maximum polarization the target qubit can have is $2^{n-2} \epsilon_b$. But when $\epsilon_b > 1/2^{n-2}$, a polarization close to one can be reached. Recently, the cooling limit of the PPA (starting with completely mixed qubits) was solved analytically: the maximum polarization of the target qubit can be expressed as a function of the number of computational and reset qubits and the heat bath polarization [18, 19]. This exact solution is consistent with the upper bound found by Schulman et al. [15]. The cooling limit corresponds to the stage at which it is not possible to continue extracting entropy from the system, i.e., when the state of the system is not changed by the compression and refresh steps. The system achieves this limit asymptotically, converging to a steady state. Starting from the completely mixed state, the

Target qubit polarization (3-qubit PPA)

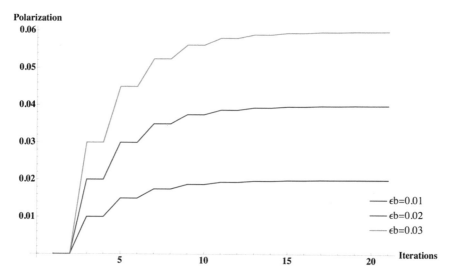

Fig. 5 Evolution of the target qubit polarization under the PPA method, using a system of 3 qubits, for three values of heat bath polarization ϵ_b. Each iteration consists of a reset and a compression procedure. Note the asymptotic polarization is $2\epsilon_b$, as expected for $\epsilon_b \ll 1/2$ in the case of three qubits

density matrix always remains in a diagonal form after each HBAC step. In general, the state of the computational qubits ρ_{comp} is therefore completely described by its diagonal elements: $d(\rho_{\text{comp}}) = (A_1^t, A_2^t \ldots, A_{2d}^t)$ after t iterations of HBAC (see Fig. 1 for the meaning of d).

The cooling limit is reached when there is no operation that can compress the entropy of the computational qubits, or equivalently, when the diagonal elements of the total state are already sorted. This limit occurs when the elements of ρ_{comp} satisfy the following condition (see Fig. 1 for the meaning of m):

$$A_i(1 - \epsilon_b)^m = A_{i+1}(1 + \epsilon_b)^m. \tag{12}$$

This condition together with normalization gives the exact solution of the steady state of the computational qubits, $\widetilde{\rho}_{\text{comp}}$:

$$d(\widetilde{\rho}_{\text{comp}}) = A_1(1, \ Q, \ Q^2, \ Q^3, \ \ldots, \ Q^{2d-1}), \tag{13}$$

where $A_1 = \frac{1-Q}{Q(1-Q^{2d})}$ and $Q = \left(\frac{1-\epsilon_b}{1+\epsilon_b}\right)^m$.

The maximum achievable polarization corresponds to the polarization of the state in the cooling limit. From the steady state, the maximum polarization of the target qubit is as follows:

$$\epsilon_{max} = \frac{(1+\epsilon_b)^{md} - (1-\epsilon_b)^{md}}{(1+\epsilon_b)^{md} + (1-\epsilon_b)^{md}}. \tag{14}$$

In the limit of low heat bath polarization, $\epsilon_b \ll 1/(md)$, the polarization of the steady state is proportional to md, in agreement with simulations. As the value of the heat bath polarization increases beyond md, the final polarization grows arbitrarily close to 1. The final polarization of the target qubit as a function of the heat bath polarization is shown in Fig. 6 for different numbers of qubits.

In order to see how quickly ϵ_{max} approaches 1, we introduce $\delta_{max} = 1 - \epsilon_{max}$. Using Eq. (14), δ_{max} can be expressed as:

$$\delta_{max} = \frac{2}{e^{md \ln\left(\frac{1+\epsilon_b}{1-\epsilon_b}\right)} + 1} = \frac{2}{e^{m2^{n'} \ln\left(\frac{1+\epsilon_b}{1-\epsilon_b}\right)} + 1}. \tag{15}$$

This expression shows that the maximum polarization reaches 1 exponentially in the size of the Hilbert space d (or doubly exponentially in n', the number of computational qubits excluding the target qubit).

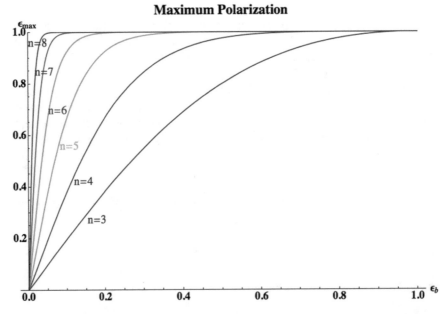

Maximum Polarization

Fig. 6 Maximum polarization achievable for the target qubit versus heat bath polarization ϵ_b and the number of qubits. The maximum polarization increases doubly exponentially in n', the number of computational qubits excluding the target qubit. This plot shows the results for $n = 3, 4, 5, 6, 7$, and 8, where n is the sum of computational qubits and one reset qubit (i.e., $n' = 1, 2, 3, 4, 5$, and 6)

4 Experimental Algorithmic Cooling with NMR QIP

Experimental realization of algorithmic cooling requires high fidelity control and the ability to reset qubits. Liquid State NMR (LSNMR) QIP has successfully demonstrated precise quantum control of up to 12 qubits, and hence it can provide sufficient quantum control for the experimental demonstration of algorithmic cooling. Nevertheless, the only way to reset qubits in LSNMR relies on spin-lattice relaxation, characterized by the time scale T_1. Reset qubits must have very short T_1 values compared to the computational qubits. One can imagine a molecule in which one nuclear spin has a very rapid T_1 and the reset to 99 % of the thermal polarization can be achieved by waiting $5T_1$. However, other spin qubits must have much slower T_1 process in order to maintain their polarizations during the reset step. Furthermore, the short T_1 on the reset qubit limits its T_2 and the fidelity of control. Despite these limitations, some preliminary steps towards full PPA have been experimentally realized in LSNMR by using protons (^{1}H nuclei) as reset qubits and ^{13}C nuclei as computational qubits [20, 21]. These experiments showed selective reset operations to polarize all three spin qubits close to the bath temperature. Nevertheless, the final compression step which polarizes a target qubit colder than the heat bath was not implemented. Meanwhile, Chang et al. implemented cooling solely by the final compression gate (Fig. 4c) on three fluorines in C_2F_3Br using LSNMR [22]. Full implementation of HBAC in LSNMR was accomplished much later in [23].

On the other hand, a network of dipolar coupled spins in SSNMR offers a reset step that does not require a relaxation process in the system of interest. A large number of dipolar coupled spins can be thought of as a spin bath, and other spins can be brought in thermal contact with the bath and reach thermal equilibrium at the spin bath temperature. Moreover, SSNMR experiments can be operated at low temperature, providing a higher bath polarization. In this section, we review the experimental demonstration of 3-qubit algorithmic cooling using a molecular single crystal.

4.1 Brief Review of Solid State NMR QC

SSNMR QIP makes use of the techniques developed in LSNMR QIP, and offers several advantages: the decoherence rates can be made slow using refocusing techniques, while spin-spin couplings much larger than in LSNMR can be exploited to realize faster quantum gates [24].

Features of the internal Hamiltonian of SSNMR that differ from LSNMR are the anisotropic chemical shift and dipole–dipole couplings between nuclei. The anisotropic chemical shift should be described by a tensor δ. In the secular approximation (at large dc magnetic field), the form of the dipole–dipole interaction Hamiltonian depends on whether the interacting spins belong to the same isotopic species or not and can be written as follows:

$$\text{Homonuclear:} \quad H_D^{ij} = d_{ij}\left(3\hat{I}_z^i\hat{I}_z^j - \hat{\boldsymbol{I}}^i \cdot \hat{\boldsymbol{I}}^j\right), \tag{16}$$

$$\text{Heteronuclear:} \quad H_D^{ij} = d_{ij}\left(2\hat{I}_z^i\hat{I}_z^j\right), \tag{17}$$

$$d_{ij} = -\hbar\frac{\mu_0}{4\pi}\frac{\gamma_i\gamma_j}{r_{ij}^3}\frac{3\cos^2\theta_{ij}-1}{2}, \tag{18}$$

where μ_0 is the permeability of free space, γ_i is the gyromagnetic ratio of spin i, r_{ij} is the distance between interacting spins, and θ_{ij} is the angle between the vector connecting the two spins and the external magnetic field. There are also J-couplings in SSNMR, which are usually an order of magnitude smaller than the dipole–dipole couplings, and for which the isotropic component cannot be distinguished from dipolar couplings. Nuclei with $S > 1/2$ interact with external electric field gradients, a phenomenon known as quadrupolar interaction. In this chapter, we limit our discussions to spin-$1/2$ systems, and hence quadrupolar interactions do not appear in the internal Hamiltonian.

Because of the orientation dependence of the internal Hamiltonian and the ensemble nature of NMR QIP, the solid sample should be a single crystal, where each unit cell contains only one molecule (or >1 magnetically equivalent molecules).

4.2 SSNMR Algorithmic Cooling Experiment

Experimental HBAC using SSNMR was first demonstrated by Baugh et al. in 2005 [25]. They implemented the PPA for three qubits using a single crystal of malonic acid $CH_2(COOH)_2$ (Fig. 7) as the quantum processor at $B_0 = 7.1$ T and room temperature.

In each unit cell of malonic acid, there are two molecules that are related by a center of symmetry and magnetically equivalent to each other ($P\bar{1}$ space group). The molecules in which all three carbons are isotopically labelled as ^{13}C (3-^{13}C) were used as quantum information processors, while the 100% abundant ^{1}H spins in the crystal were used as the heat bath. The concentration of 3-^{13}C molecules in the crystal was 3.2%. There were also about 1.1% molecules with one ^{13}C spin and about $(1.1\%)^2$ molecules with two ^{13}C spins due to natural abundance of ^{13}C spins, the latter being a small enough concentration to neglect. The small fraction of molecules with one ^{13}C produces detectable NMR signal, but these are inconsequential for QIP purposes. The structure of the molecule, spin Hamiltonian parameters used for the experiment that were obtained from spectral fitting, and ^{1}H-decoupled ^{13}C spectrum are shown in Fig. 7.

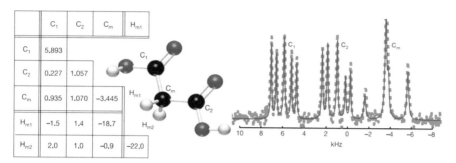

Fig. 7 From [25]. Characteristics of the dilute 3-^{13}C malonic acid spin system. On the right is the ^{1}H-decoupled ^{13}C spectrum. The *blue dashed line* is the experimental NMR spectrum, and the *red line* is the fit. The peaks are grouped into three multiplets which can be assigned to C_1, C_2, and C_m. In each multiplet, the central peak comes from the natural abundance of ^{13}C, and is inconsequential for QIP purposes. The table gives the parameters of the Hamiltonian. The diagonal values are chemical shifts and the off-diagonal values are dipolar couplings. All values are in kHz. Reprinted by permission from Macmillan Publisher Ltd: Nature 438, 470–473 (2005), copyright (2005)

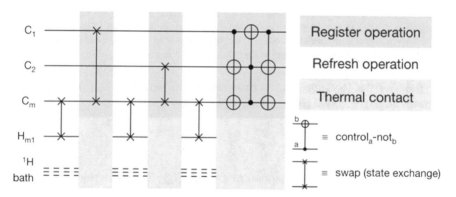

Fig. 8 The schematic circuit of the solid state NMR PPA experiment (reproduced from [25]). The circuit contains three iterations: three refresh steps and three reversible polarization compression steps, which are labelled as "register operation". Reprinted by permission from Macmillan Publisher Ltd: Nature 438, 470–473 (2005), copyright (2005)

The quantum circuit for 3-qubit PPA is shown in Fig. 8. The experiment was designed to increase the polarization of C_1, and C_m was the qubit interacting with the heat bath. As discussed in Sect. 3, the algorithm combines two steps: refreshing step and reversible polarization compression step. The refreshing step, illustrated in Fig. 8, is realized via the SWAP gate between C_m and H_{m1}. As shown in the spin Hamiltonian parameters in Fig. 7, the orientation of the crystal with respect to the magnetic field was chosen in such a way that only H_{m1} had a large coupling with C_m. The other heteronuclear couplings were negligibly small and all the homonuclear couplings were refocused during the refresh step.

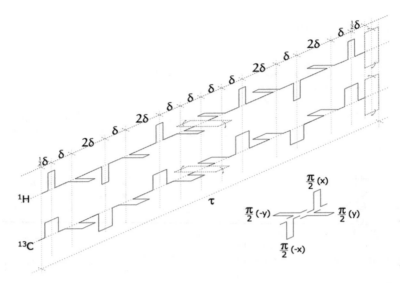

Fig. 9 From [17]. The "time-suspension" sequence of hard pulses for implementing the ^{1}H-^{13}C SWAP gate. Each rectangle corresponds to a $\pi/2$ rotation about a Bloch sphere axis ($\pm x$ or $\pm y$) denoted by the orientation of the rectangle, and δ is the shortest time delay between pulses. The sequence decouples homonuclear couplings, and transforms the heteronuclear Hamiltonian to an exchange Hamiltonian. The total time of the pulse sequence is $\tau = 3/(2d_{ij})$

The SWAP is implemented by "time-suspension" sequence [26] (Fig. 9) which induces effective spin-exchange Hamiltonian in the form

$$H_{eff}^{ij} = \frac{d_{ij}}{3} \left(\hat{I}^i \cdot \hat{I}^j \right), \tag{19}$$

where spin i and spin j correspond to C_m and H_{m1}. The evolution of duration $\tau = 3/(2d_{ij})$ under this spin-exchange Hamiltonian is equivalent to the SWAP.

Due to experimental imperfections, only about 83 % of the thermal ^{1}H polarization is transferred to C_m, which is referred to as the effective bath polarization. The final compression step was realized using strongly modulating pulses [27]. The pulse was designed to be robust to radio frequency (RF) field inhomogeneity. During the application of permutation gates, ^{1}H spins in the crystal were strongly decoupled from ^{13}C spins, and "spin-locked" by a transverse, phase-matched RF field, which preserved the ^{1}H polarization and allowed the H_{m1} to re-equilibrate with the hydrogen bath through spin diffusion mediated by hydrogen–hydrogen dipolar couplings. In the beginning of the experiment, all ^{13}C spins were initialized in completely mixed states by rotating the thermal polarization to a transverse Bloch sphere axis and dephasing it. After first five steps of the experiment as illustrated in Fig. 8, ideally the polarization of all three ^{13}C spins should equal to the bath polarization ϵ_B. Then in principle, the final gate boosts the polarization of C_1 to $1.5\epsilon_B$ to first order in ϵ_B. In the experiment, the final polarization of C_1 was

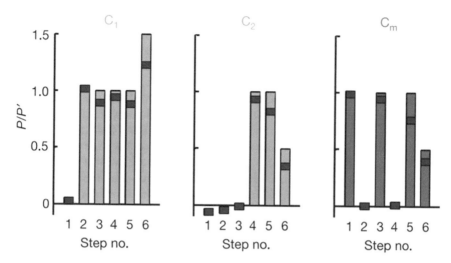

Fig. 10 From [25]. Theoretical and experimental qubit polarizations at each step for C_1, C_2, and C_m. Bars indicate ideal qubit polarizations; shaded bands are experimental values. The thickness of shaded bands indicates experimental uncertainty. Reprinted by permission from Macmillan Publisher Ltd: Nature 438, 470–473 (2005), copyright (2005)

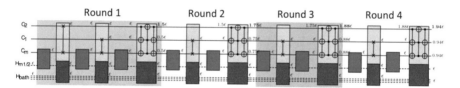

Fig. 11 The schematic circuit of the four-round PPA experiment, reproduced from [28]. Theoretical values of attainable polarizations are provided with respect to the heat bath polarization ϵ at each stage of the experiment. Reprinted figure with permission from C. A. Ryan, O. Moussa, J. Baugh, and R. Laflamme, Phys. Rev. Lett. 100, 140501 (2008). Copyright (2008) by the American Physical Society

1.22 ± 0.03 times the effective bath polarization. Major sources of error were a nonideal process of spin diffusion that prevented perfect refresh of C_m as shown in Fig. 10, and RF control imperfections. In spite of experimental errors, C_1 attained polarization higher than that of the heat bath.

In 2008, Ryan et al. experimentally demonstrated four rounds of algorithmic cooling that consist of nine iterations (Fig. 11) in the same experimental system (malonic acid) [28]. Perfect control without decoherence would theoretically result in improving one of the ^{13}C polarizations to $1.94\epsilon_B$ after four rounds of the PPA.

The experiment resembles the work in [25] in the sense that three ^{13}C spins were used as the computational qubits, and the abundant ^{1}H spins were used as the heat bath. But the refresh and the polarization compression steps were implemented differently. In the refresh step, the polarization was transferred from H_{m1} and H_{m2} at the same time. The orientation of the sample was chosen in such a way that both H_{m1} and H_{m2} have large dipolar couplings with C_m. Instead of applying a multi-pulse sequence to realize the refreshing step, cross polarization (CP) [29] which was found to be better in preserving the heat bath polarization was used. The permutation gates applied on ^{13}Cs were numerically optimized using the GRadient Ascent Pulse Engineering (GRAPE) algorithm [30]. The pulse design takes several error sources into considerations: distributions of the static magnetic field and the RF control field, and the finite bandwidth of the NMR probe resonant circuit. Also, the optimized pulses were corrected for nonlinearities in the pulse generation and transmission to the sample through a procedure that measures the RF pulse at the sample and corrects it via feedback. With all these tools, the level of control was improved and enabled four rounds of PPA. The polarization of each ^{13}C at the end of each round is shown in Fig. 12.

After four rounds of PPA, the polarization of C_2 reached $1.69\epsilon'_B$, where ϵ'_B is the polarization of C_m after the first reset. Experimental error was dominated by two factors—imperfection of ^{1}H decoupling and the network of dipolar coupled protons in the bath leading to a nonideal process of spin diffusion.

These experiments were significant milestones towards implementation of active error correction in solid state spin ensemble QIP. It demonstrated sufficient control fidelity to realize HBAC to prepare an ancilla qubit whose polarization is higher than the cold bath polarization. Now the control tools are available, and what

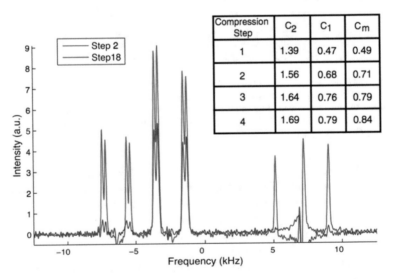

Compression Step	C_2	C_1	C_m
1	1.39	0.47	0.49
2	1.56	0.68	0.71
3	1.64	0.76	0.79
4	1.69	0.79	0.84

Fig. 12 From [28]. Table of the measured polarization (with respect to the initial refresh step) of each spin after each round of PPA. The spectra show a comparison of the first refresh step (swapped to C_2) and the final signal after four rounds of PPA. It shows clearly that the polarization of C_2 is boosted well beyond the bath polarization. Reprinted figure with permission from C.A. Ryan, O. Moussa, J. Baugh, and R. Laflamme, Phys. Rev. Lett. 100, 140501 (2008). Copyright (2008) by the American Physical Society

remains a challenge of experimental QEC is to identify a system that provides a heat bath that can be polarized to much higher values than the thermal nuclear bath.

4.3   Limitations to HBAC Using NMR

The SSNMR experiment discussed in this section successfully improved polarization of one nuclear spin beyond the heat bath polarization. Nevertheless, the ultimate goal of dynamical supply of nearly pure ancilla qubits for QEC is still far from reach. For example, the 3-qubit dephasing QEC code requires two ancilla qubits with polarizations of 0.41 at minimum (see Sect. 2.3). In order to achieve this polarization on one nuclear spin at room temperature and $B_0 \approx 7$ T, perfect quantum control on 17 coupled ^{1}H with no losses due to decoherence would be required. The condition can be relaxed if the heat bath temperature is colder. However, operating NMR HBAC at cryogenic temperatures is not an ideal solution for preparing cold heat bath since T_1 of nuclear spins become undesirably long at low temperature. This naturally leads to exploiting electron spin since the electron gyromagnetic ratio is much higher than that of nuclei which results in higher thermal equilibrium polarization and faster T_1 relaxation.

In the following section, we discuss implementation of HBAC using a combination of electron and nuclear spin resonance in hyperfine-coupled quantum processors.

5   HBAC with Hyperfine-Coupled Electron-Nuclear Spin Ensemble

The fundamentals of ESR QC are analogous to NMR QC, and many of the techniques used for manipulating nuclear spins can also be applied to control electrons. One obvious advantage is that higher gyromagnetic ratio of an electron γ_e (about 660 times greater than that of proton) leads to higher polarization. Decoherence and relaxation rates also scale with γ, and hence electron T_1 relaxation rate is about 3 orders of magnitude larger than that of nuclei. Thus, the electron spin is an excellent candidate for the reset qubit, and the reset can be done simply by waiting for a time about $5T_1$. Anisotropic hyperfine interaction is an advantage for designing nuclear quantum gates since it provides a control handle for fast manipulations of nuclear spins. However, in the case of HBAC, strong anisotropic hyperfine interaction can be a disadvantage because electron T_1 relaxation process induces nuclear polarization decay in the presence of anisotropic hyperfine interaction. If the interaction is strong, the loss of nuclear polarization while resetting the electron can be significant. Fortunately, one can choose the crystal orientation to reduce the anisotropic hyperfine coupling strength so that the nuclear spin decay induced by electron T_1 is small enough to allow cooling of a target spin species below bath temperature [31]. We discuss the spin Hamiltonian in more detail in the following section, and also discuss the crystal orientation selection for realistic implementations.

5.1   The Electron-Nuclear Spin Hamiltonian

The spin Hamiltonian for a 1 electron, k nuclear spin-1/2 system can be written as

$$H = \beta_e g_{\mu\nu} B_\mu \hat{S}_\nu + \sum_{n=1}^{k} \left(A_{\mu\nu}^n \hat{S}_\mu \hat{I}_\nu^n - \gamma_n \hat{I}_\mu^n B_\mu \right), \tag{20}$$

where $\hat{S}$ and $\hat{I}$ represent electron and nuclear spin operators, β_e is Bohr magneton, $\vec{B}$ is the external magnetic field, and γ_n is the gyromagnetic ratio for nuclear spin n. We set $\hbar = 1$ so that all Hamiltonians will appear in angular frequency units. The second rank tensors g and A^n are the electron g-tensor and the nth nuclear spin hyperfine coupling tensor, respectively. The nuclear dipole–dipole interaction is neglected since it is typically at least two orders of magnitude weaker than the hyperfine terms.

Pulsed ESR spectrometers are classified according to the frequency of the microwave source. Most commonly, ESR experiments are conducted at X-band (8–12 GHz) frequency, mainly due to the relatively low cost of microwave amplifiers and other components in this frequency range. In X-band ESR, the electron Zeeman interaction is the dominating term of the Hamiltonian. By convention, the coordinate system is chosen such that $\vec{B} = B_0 \hat{z}$, and the electron spin is quantized along that direction. When the magnitudes of nuclear Zeeman energy and the hyperfine interaction are comparable and much smaller than the electron Zeeman energy, the spin Hamiltonian is well approximated as

$$H = \omega_S \hat{S}_z + \sum_{n=1}^{k} \left[-\omega_I^n \hat{I}_z^n + \hat{S}_z \left(a_n \hat{I}_z^n + b_n \hat{I}_x^n \right) \right]. \tag{21}$$

Here, $\omega_S = \beta_e g_{zz} B_0$ and $\omega_I^n = \gamma_n B_0$ are electron and nuclear Larmor frequencies, respectively, and $a_n = A_{zz}^n$ and $b_n = \sqrt{\left(A_{zx}^n \right)^2 + \left(A_{zy}^n \right)^2}$.

There are two schemes for achieving universal control in electron nuclear systems. In the first scheme, the nuclear spins are directly manipulated by external RF pulses that are on resonance with NMR transition frequencies. This technique is known as Electron Nuclear Double Resonance (ENDOR) [32]. The second approach is to exploit the anisotropic hyperfine coupling and indirectly manipulate nuclear spins via microwave (MW) pulses acting on the electron. For brevity, we will name the latter approach Anisotropic Hyperfine Control (AHC). In the following section, we explain how to achieve universal control of electron-nuclear coupled systems through AHC in more detail.

5.2 Indirect Control via Anisotropic Hyperfine Coupling

The anisotropy of hyperfine coupling permits nuclear spin manipulation solely by irradiating MW pulses at electron spin transitions. The control universality of a 1 electron, N nuclear spin coupled system via anisotropic hyperfine interaction was proved in [33], and demonstrated experimentally in [34] for a single nuclear spin qubit gate and in [35] for a gate involving two nuclear spin qubits. The advantage of the indirect control technique is that it simplifies the instrumentation as additional RF excitations are not needed, and faster gate implementation relative to ENDOR can be achieved when the hyperfine coupling strength exceeds the Larmor frequency of the nucleus in a given external field. Here we use 1 electron, 1 nuclear spin system as an example to illustrate the idea. In the presence of $\vec{B} = B_0\hat{z}$ and the hyperfine interaction, the nuclear spin is quantized along the direction of an effective field

$$\vec{B}_n = \left(B_0 \pm \frac{a}{2\gamma_n}\right)\hat{z} \pm \frac{b}{2\gamma_n}\hat{x}, \tag{22}$$

and the $\pm$ sign depends on whether the electron spin is parallel (spin up) or antiparallel (spin down) to the external field. As a consequence, when $b \neq 0$, the direction of the nuclear spin quantization axis is dictated by the electron spin state. We introduce $\theta_\uparrow = \arctan\left(\frac{-b}{a+2\omega_I}\right)$ and $\theta_\downarrow = \arctan\left(\frac{-b}{a-2\omega_I}\right)$ to denote the angle of nuclear spin quantization axes from $\hat{z}$ axis, and $\Theta = (\theta_\uparrow - \theta_\downarrow)/2$. Then, the eigenstates of the coupled spin system are [32]:

$$
\begin{aligned}
|1\rangle &= |\uparrow\rangle \otimes \left(\cos\left(\frac{\theta_\uparrow}{2}\right)|\uparrow\rangle - \sin\left(\frac{\theta_\uparrow}{2}\right)|\downarrow\rangle\right), \\
|2\rangle &= |\uparrow\rangle \otimes \left(\sin\left(\frac{\theta_\uparrow}{2}\right)|\uparrow\rangle + \cos\left(\frac{\theta_\uparrow}{2}\right)|\downarrow\rangle\right), \\
|3\rangle &= |\downarrow\rangle \otimes \left(\cos\left(\frac{\theta_\downarrow}{2}\right)|\uparrow\rangle - \sin\left(\frac{\theta_\downarrow}{2}\right)|\downarrow\rangle\right), \\
|4\rangle &= |\downarrow\rangle \otimes \left(\sin\left(\frac{\theta_\downarrow}{2}\right)|\uparrow\rangle + \cos\left(\frac{\theta_\downarrow}{2}\right)|\downarrow\rangle\right).
\end{aligned}
\tag{23}
$$

In the eigenbasis of the spin Hamiltonian shown in Eq. (21), the rotating-frame electron control Hamiltonian $H_c = \omega_1\hat{S}_x$ becomes

$$\tilde{H}_c = \frac{\omega_1}{2} \begin{bmatrix} 0 & 0 & \cos(\Theta) & -\sin(\Theta) \\ 0 & 0 & \sin(\Theta) & \cos(\Theta) \\ \cos(\Theta) & \sin(\Theta) & 0 & 0 \\ -\sin(\Theta) & \cos(\Theta) & 0 & 0 \end{bmatrix}. \tag{24}$$

From Eq. (24), one can see that the control Hamiltonian is able to induce all transitions between any eigenstates of the electron spin up manifold and the electron spin down manifold provided $\Theta \neq n\pi/2$, where n is an integer and eigenstates are nondegenerate. The energy level connectivity can be represented as a graph, and the complete connectivity of the graph generated by the control Hamiltonian and nondegenerate energy levels guarantee universal control of the system [34, 36, 37]. Since the spin Hamiltonian does not consider nuclear–nuclear dipolar interactions, the idea presented for 1 electron, 1 nuclear spin system can be easily extended to larger number of nuclear spins, provided that suitable and distinct hyperfine couplings exist. The loss of nuclear spin polarization due to electron T_1 in the presence of anisotropic hyperfine interaction can be intuitively understood from Eq. (24). When $\sin(\Theta)$ is non-zero, there is a finite probability for the nuclear spin to flip to its low energy state through electron-nuclear double spin relaxation.

5.3 HBAC Simulations in Electron-Nuclear Coupled Systems

The ancilla qubits for the 3-qubit dephasing QEC code must be polarized to at least 41 % in order to correct errors at all. In theory, X-band ESR algorithmic cooling at 4.2 K can yield greater than 40 % polarization on one nuclear spin using 1 electron and 4 hyperfine-coupled nuclei. This is a significant reduction in the number of necessary qubits compared to NMR case at room temperature, which required 17 protons (both examples here assume error-free controls).

In this section, we explain how to experimentally implement the control, and present proof-of-principle simulation results that reflect more realistic control and decoherence parameters to examine the feasibility of HBAC in the electron-nuclear coupled systems. Simulations were carried out for both ENDOR and AHC control schemes. We consider gamma-irradiated malonic acid in which one carbon is isotopically labelled as ^{13}C (Fig. 13) as an example. The idea can, in principle, be extended to larger electron-nuclear spin ensemble systems. More details about the feasibility test with malonic acid and its extension to 5-qubit version can be found in [31].

In the simulation, electron T_1 and T_2 processes are modelled as a Markovian dynamical map, and simulated by solving a master equation of the Lindblad form [38, 39]. Inhomogeneous line broadening of the electron spin resonances is taken into account by averaging the simulation over a set of spin Hamiltonians in which

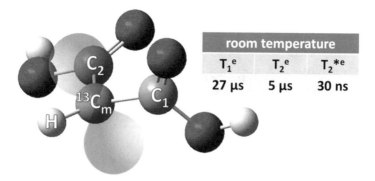

room temperature		
$T_1{}^e$	$T_2{}^e$	$T_2{}^{*e}$
27 µs	5 µs	30 ns

Fig. 13 Schematic of the gamma-irradiated malonic acid with three qubits (electron, α-^{1}H and methylene ^{13}C). The electron density distribution is represented by the *blue shaded* region. Relaxation parameters of the electron $T_1{}^e$, $T_2{}^e$, and $T_2{}^{*e}$ are measured in an X-band pulsed ESR spectrometer at room temperature

the magnitude of electron Zeeman energy is a Lorentzian-distributed random variable. We use experimentally measured electron T_1 and T_2 values to determine the Lindblad operators, and the measured ESR line width to determine the T_2^* Hamiltonian distribution.

5.3.1 HBAC Using ENDOR Control

In ENDOR, nuclear spin flip transitions are directly excited by RF pulses oscillating at the nuclear frequencies. As shown in Fig. 14, all the gates used in the PPA can be decomposed into controlled-not (CNOT) gates that are realized by transition selective π-pulses. For example, a CNOT gate with the electron as the control qubit and a nuclear spin as the target is implemented by irradiating the sample with RF pulse at the frequency that corresponds to the energy difference between $|\uparrow_e\uparrow_n\rangle$ and $|\uparrow_e\downarrow_n\rangle$, at pulse amplitude ω for duration τ such that $\omega\tau = \pi$. A Toffoli gate that flips the electron if two nuclei are both in the spin up state can be realized by exciting the transition between $|\uparrow_e\uparrow_n\uparrow_n\rangle$ and $|\downarrow_e\uparrow_n\uparrow_n\rangle$ with a MW pulse of amplitude ω for duration τ such that $\omega\tau = \pi$.

Since the spin Hamiltonian depends on the dc magnetic field orientation with respect to the crystallographic axes, we aim to select an orientation that maximizes the polarization improvement on the target spin qubit. In the ENDOR experiment, the orientation selection requirements are as follows: (1) the electron-nuclear double spin flip rate is as slow as possible by minimizing $\sin(\Theta)$ in Eq. (24); (2) all allowed transitions (as opposed to forbidden transitions) should be separated by more than the relevant ESR or NMR line width; and (3) the bandwidth of microwave control is narrow enough to obtain control faster than T_2^e, but wide enough to irradiate all relevant ESR transitions.

Using g, A^H, and A^C that are determined from continuous-wave ESR (CW ESR) measurement at X-band, we determined a crystalline orientation in which all

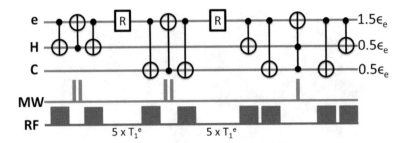

Fig. 14 Quantum circuit and corresponding pulse sequence for the 3-qubit PPA using pulsed ENDOR to control the electron, α-proton and methylene ^{13}C of gamma irradiated malonic acid. *Blue* and *red* rectangles indicate MW and RF pulses that selectively excite particular transitions for a single electron spin flip and a single nuclear spin flip, respectively. The reset (indicated by R) is accomplished by waiting for 5 times the T_1 of the electron. This single round of HBAC boosts the polarization of the electron spin approximately 1.5 times compared to its thermal equilibrium polarization

conditions above are reasonably well satisfied. We performed a simulation of 3-qubit ENDOR algorithmic cooling designed to increase the polarization of the electron (see Fig. 14).

In principle, a single round of 3-qubit HBAC increases the target spin polarization to 1.5 times the heat bath polarization. The simulation takes finite pulse width, T_1^e, T_2^e, and T_2^{*e} into account. The reset is done by waiting for 5 times the T_1 of the electron. The simulation uses 50 ns Gaussian-shaped pulses for MW, and 15 μs and 60 μs square pulses for RF. Gaussian-shaped pulses are used in the MW channel in order to maintain selectivity of a particular transition while exciting over the full ESR line width. The amplitudes of the RF pulses are chosen to reflect typical RF amplifier output power levels. Since the RF pulses are similar in duration to T_1^e at room temperature, the algorithm does not yield polarization increase at room temperature. A solution is to increase T_1^e by performing the experiment at low temperature. We use the experimentally determined value of $T_1^e = 2.6$ ms at 43 K. Taking into account all the relaxation parameters and simulating the experiment at $T = 43$ K yield a final polarization (after one round of the PPA) of 1.36 times the bath polarization.

5.3.2 HBAC Using Anisotropic Hyperfine Control

When the universal control is achieved through anisotropic hyperfine coupling and electron spin excitation [34, 35], the orientation selection criteria are modified as following: (1) the electron-nuclear double spin flip rate (i.e., forbidden rate) is strong enough that nuclear gates can be implemented quickly compared to the electron T_2; (2) however, this forbidden transition rate must also be weak enough that it does not significantly speed up the nuclear T_1 process; and (3) the frequencies

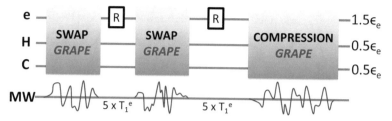

Fig. 15 Quantum circuit and corresponding pulse sequence for the 3-qubit PPA using electron, ^{1}H and ^{13}C spins and microwave-only control. Swap and compression gates are realized by shaped pulses found using the GRAPE algorithm [30]. The reset steps are done by waiting for 5 times the T_1 of the electron. One round of HBAC boosts the electron spin polarization to 1.5 times its thermal equilibrium polarization

of all transitions (allowed and forbidden) should be separated from each other by at least the ESR line width to achieve high fidelity control.

Using the same electron g-tensor and hyperfine interaction tensors, a crystal orientation can be found that satisfies new conditions above. The GRAPE algorithm [30] is then used to design the swap and compression gates via microwave control of the electron spin. The corresponding quantum circuit is illustrated in the figure below (Fig. 15). All three pulses are designed to have 99 % unitary fidelity, and the pulse lengths are 840 ns, 840 ns, and 900 ns for electron-^{1}H swap, electron-^{13}C swap, and compression, respectively.

The simulated final polarization of the electron after one round of the PPA is 1.21 times the bath polarization. The polarization improvement here is worse compared to the previous ENDOR simulation results due to the fact that T_2^e is only about 5 times longer than the duration of each GRAPE pulse, and that nuclear polarizations decay faster due to anisotropic coupling during the reset steps. On the other hand, one immediate advantage of this control scheme compared to ENDOR experiment is that the experiment can be done at room temperature since pulse durations are much shorter than room temperature T_1^e. Moreover, the ability to implement nuclear gates solely through MW pulses greatly simplifies the experimental hardware.

5.4 Prospects: Exploiting Larger Hilbert Spaces and the High Field Regime

Achieving high control fidelity and realization of electron-nuclear spin HBAC in the proof-of-principle level remains to be experimentally demonstrated. Nevertheless, given sufficient control, HBAC can potentially be explored using molecules with a greater number of nuclear spin qubits coupled to an electron. One example is the diphenyl nitroxide radical (see Fig. 16) [41, 42]. Diphenyl nitroxide as an open-shell molecular sample is an extremely stable nitroxide radical with

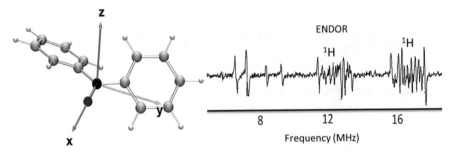

Fig. 16 *Left*: Molecular structure of the diphenyl nitroxide radical. Crystal axes are labelled as x, y, and z. *Right*: ENDOR spectrum of diphenyl nitroxide in a crystalline benzophenone matrix. 20 ENDOR peaks in the neighborhood of 12 and 16 MHz correspond to the nuclear frequencies of 10 proton spins. This spectrum indicates that all 10 nuclear spins are spectrally distinct and may be selectively controlled using ENDOR. These figures are reproduced from [40]

electron spin-1/2. Mixed single crystals of diphenyl nitroxide in benzophenone are grown with a sufficiently dilute concentration of the radical to suppress electron-electron dipolar interactions. Diphenyl nitroxide isostructurally replaces the benzophenone molecules. This provides 10 protons that are hyperfine coupled to the electron and are spectrally distinguishable through ENDOR. Nitrogen can be isotopically labelled as ^{15}N to provide an additional strongly coupled nuclear spin-1/2. This spin system therefore affords the possibility of implementing HBAC with up to 12 qubits [40].

The maximum polarization that can be reached by one nuclear spin in 12-qubit HBAC at X-band is 0.67 at room temperature. It can be improved to more than 0.99 at liquid nitrogen temperature 77 K, and a polarization arbitrarily close to 1 is possible at liquid helium temperature 4.2 K. Figure 17 shows the theoretical polarization of a target spin as a function of the number of HBAC iterations at various temperatures. One iteration of HBAC consists of a reset and a compression. Note that in order to achieve high polarization, a very large number of iterations are required unless the experiment is performed at a temperature below 77 K (see Fig. 17).

HBAC in high field ESR, such as W-band in which the Larmor frequency of the free electron is about 94 GHz, is also a possible solution to reach necessary polarization for QEC. Although high fidelity unitary quantum control in the high frequency regime has not been demonstrated, in theory only four rounds of 3-qubit HBAC at 8 K can supply a qubit with 50 % polarization, and above 80 % and 97 % polarizations at 4 K and 2 K, respectively.

6   Conclusions and Prospects

NMR experiments on spin ensembles have provided an excellent ground for developing and testing ideas of QIP in the few-qubit regime, owing to the ability to implement quantum control. However, it has lacked the ability to prepare high

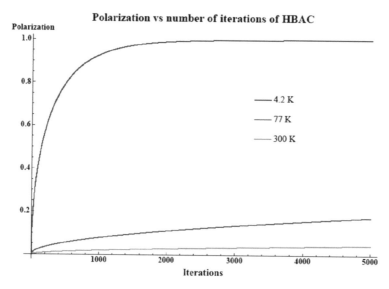

Fig. 17 Polarization of a target nuclear spin in the diphenyl nitroxide radical plotted as a function of the number of HBAC iterations at three different temperatures. Each iteration consists of one refresh and one compression step

purity ancilla qubits that are essential for QEC. The challenge for systems like NMR in which projective measurement is not available is that qubit initialization is normally only attainable via thermal equilibration, which results in very low polarizations (i.e., highly mixed qubit states). Dynamic nuclear polarization [43, 44] and algorithmic cooling are two means by which nonequilibrium polarizations can be achieved, with this review having discussed the latter. In this chapter, we reviewed HBAC, an efficient method for extracting entropy from spin qubits, allowing cooling below the cold bath temperature. The theory of HBAC has been extensively studied, and sufficient quantum control to operate several rounds of HBAC in a 3-qubit system was demonstrated using SSNMR. In standard NMR QIP, achieving qubit polarizations necessary for QEC is a practical impossibility, given the small values of thermal equilibrium nuclear polarizations even at cryogenic temperatures. Electron-nuclear hyperfine-coupled systems are more promising for HBAC than conventional NMR processors since the electron spin has about 3 orders of magnitude larger Zeeman energy, and thus its polarization and spin-lattice relaxation rates are correspondingly higher. The fast T_1 process is exploited for the reset step in HBAC. Experiments to demonstrate HBAC in electron-nuclear systems are in progress, but in this review we have presented realistic simulation results indicating that polarization enhancements on the order of the theoretical values are possible.

HBAC is an implementation independent approach, and it can also be applied in other spin systems and other QIP implementations. For example, nitrogen-vacancy centers in diamond or a photo-excited triplet state can provide highly polarized spins at room temperature by optical pumping and dynamic nuclear polarization [45–47], and HBAC can be utilized to further purify spin qubits in these systems.

Acknowledgements This work is supported by CIFAR, Industry Canada, and NSERC. We thank Dr. Tal Mor and Dr. Yossi Weinstein for helpful discussions, and Dr. Rolf Horn for proofreading the manuscript. NRB acknowledges CONACYT-COZCyT and SEP for support.

References

1. C. Negrevergne, T.S. Mahesh, C.A. Ryan, M. Ditty, F. Cyt-Racine, W. Power, N. Boulant, T. Havel, D.G. Cory, R. Laflamme, Phys. Rev. Lett. **96**, 170501 (2006)
2. B. Criger, D. Park, J. Baugh, in *Quantum Information and Computation for Chemistry*, ed. by S.A. Rice, A.R. Dinner (Wiley, New York, 2014), pp. 193–228
3. B. Criger, G. Passante, D. Park, R. Laflamme, Philos. Trans. A. Math. Phys. Eng. Sci. **370**, 4620 (2012)
4. B. Criger, O. Moussa, R. Laflamme, Phys. Rev. A **85**, 044302 (2012)
5. N.A. Gershenfeld, Science **275**, 350 (1997)
6. D.G. Cory, A.F. Fahmy, T.F. Havel, Proc. Natl. Acad. Sci. U. S. A. **94**, 1634 (1997)
7. T.D. Ladd, F. Jelezko, R. Laflamme, Y. Nakamura, C. Monroe, J.L. O'Brien, Nature **464**, 45 (2010)
8. O.W. Sørensen, J. Magn. Reson. **440**, 435 (1990)
9. O.W. Sørensen, J. Magn. Reson. **93**, 648 (1991)
10. L.J. Schulman, U.V. Vazirani, in Proceedings of Thirty-First Annual ACM Symposium on Theory of Computing—STOC '99 (ACM, New York, 1999), pp. 322–329
11. P.O. Boykin, T. Mor, V. Roychowdhury, F. Vatan, R. Vrijen, Proc. Natl. Acad. Sci. U. S. A. **99**, 3388 (2002)
12. J.M. Fernandez, S. Lloyd, T. Mor, V. Roychowdhury, Int. J. Quantum Inf. **2**, 461 (2004)
13. L.J. Schulman, T. Mor, Y. Weinstein, Phys. Rev. Lett. **94**, 120501 (2005)
14. Y. Elias, G.M. Fernandez, T. Mor, Y. Weinstein, Isr. J. Chem. **46**, 371 (2006)
15. L.J. Schulman, T. Mor, Y. Weinstein, SIAM J. Comput. **36**, 1729 (2007)
16. Y. Elias, T. Mor, Y. Weinstein, Phys. Rev. A **83**, 042340 (2011)
17. O. Moussa, *On Heat-Bath Algorithmic Cooling and Its Implementation in Solid-State NMR*, Master thesis, University of Waterloo, 2005
18. N.A. Rodríguez-Briones, R. Laflamme, Achievable polarization for heat-bath algorithmic cooling. Phys. Rev. Lett. **116**, 170501 (2016)
19. S. Raeisi, M. Michele, Asymptotic bound for heat-bath algorithmic cooling. Phys. Rev. Lett. **114**, 100404 (2015)
20. Y. Elias, H. Gilboa, T. Mor, Y. Weinstein, Chem. Phys. Lett. **517**, 126 (2011)
21. G. Brassard, Y. Elias, J.M. Fernandez, H. Gilboa, J.A. Jones, T. Mor, Y. Weinstein, L. Xiao, Experimental heat-bath cooling of spins. EPJ Plus **129**(12), 266 (2014)
22. D.E. Chang, L.M.K. Vandersypen, M. Steffen, Chem. Phys. Lett. **338**, 337–344 (2001)
23. Y. Atia, Y. Elias, T. Mor, Y. Weinstein, Algorithmic cooling in liquid-state nuclear magnetic resonance. Phys. Rev. A **93**, 012325 (2016)
24. D.G. Cory, R. Laflamme, E. Knill, L. Viola, T.F. Havel, N. Boulant, G. Boutis, E. Fortunato, S. Lloyd, R. Martinez, C. Negrevergne, M. Pravia, Y. Sharf, G. Teklemariam, Y.S. Weinstein, W.H. Zurek, Fortschritte Der Phys. **48**, 875 (2000)
25. J. Baugh, O. Moussa, C.A. Ryan, A. Nayak, R. Laflamme, Nature **438**, 470 (2005)
26. D.G. Cory, J.B. Miller, A.N. Garroway, J. Magn. Reson. **90**, 205 (1990)

27. E.M. Fortunato, M.A. Pravia, N. Boulant, G. Teklemariam, T.F. Havel, D.G. Cory, J. Chem. Phys. **116**, 7599 (2002)
28. C.A. Ryan, O. Moussa, J. Baugh, R. Laflamme, Phys. Rev. Lett. **100** (2008)
29. L. Müller, A. Kumar, T. Baumann, R.R. Ernst, Phys. Rev. Lett. **32**, 1402 (1974)
30. N. Khaneja, T. Reiss, C. Kehlet, T. Schulte-Herbrüggen, S.J. Glaser, J. Magn. Reson. **172**, 296 (2005)
31. D.K. Park, G. Feng, R. Rahimi, S. Labruyere, T. Shibata, S. Nakazawa, K. Sato, T. Takui, R. Laflamme, J. Baugh, Quant. Inform. Process. **14(7)**, 2435–2461 (2015)
32. A. Schweiger, G. Jeschke, *Principles of Pulse Electron Paramagnetic Resonance* (Oxford University Press, Oxford, 2001), p. 608
33. N. Khaneja, Phys. Rev. A **76**, 32326 (2007)
34. J. Hodges, J. Yang, C. Ramanathan, D. Cory, Phys. Rev. A **78**, 010303 (2008)
35. Y. Zhang, C.A. Ryan, R. Laflamme, J. Baugh, Phys. Rev. Lett. **107**, 170503 (2011)
36. G. Turinici, H. Rabitz, Chem. Phys. **267**, 1 (2001)
37. C. Altafini, J. Math. Phys. **43**, 2051 (2002)
38. G. Lindblad, Commun. Math. Phys. **48**, 119 (1976)
39. T.F. Havel, J. Math. Phys. **44**, 534 (2003)
40. R.R. Darabad, *Studies on Entanglement in Nuclear and Electron Spin Systems for Quantum Computing*, Doctoral thesis, Osaka University, 2006
41. Y. Deguchi, Bull. Chem. Soc. Jpn. **35**, 260 (1961)
42. Y. Deguchi, Bull. Chem. Soc. Jpn. **34**, 910 (1960)
43. A. Abragam, M. Goldman, Rep. Prog. Phys. **41**, 395 (1978)
44. A. Abragam, *Principles of Nuclear Magnetism* (Clarendon, Oxford, 1961)
45. J. Harrison, M.J. Sellars, N.B. Manson, Diam. Relat. Mater. **15**, 586 (2006)
46. K. Tateishi, M. Negoro, A. Kagawa, M. Kitagawa, Angew. Chem. Int. Ed. Engl. **52**, 13307 (2013)
47. K. Tateishi, M. Negoro, S. Nishida, A. Kagawa, Y. Morita, M. Kitagawa, Proc. Natl. Acad. Sci. U. S. A. **111**, 7527 (2014)

Printed in the United States
By Bookmasters